CHEMOMETRICS
APPLICATIONS AND RESEARCH

QSAR in Medicinal Chemistry

CHEMOMETRICS APPLICATIONS AND RESEARCH

QSAR in Medicinal Chemistry

Edited by

Andrew G. Mercader, PhD,

Pablo R. Duchowicz, PhD, and

P. M. Sivakumar, PhD

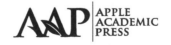

AAP | APPLE ACADEMIC PRESS

Apple Academic Press Inc. | Apple Academic Press Inc.
3333 Mistwell Crescent | 9 Spinnaker Way
Oakville, ON L6L 0A2 | Waretown, NJ 08758
Canada | USA

© 2016 by Apple Academic Press, Inc.

First issued in paperback 2021

Exclusive worldwide distribution by CRC Press, a member of Taylor & Francis Group

No claim to original U.S. Government works

ISBN-13: 978-1-77463-387-8 (pbk)
ISBN-13: 978-1-77188-113-5 (hbk)

Library and Archives Canada Cataloguing in Publication

Chemometrics applications and research : QSAR in medicinal chemistry/edited by Andrew G. Mercader, PhD, Pablo R. Duchowicz, PhD, P.M. Sivakumar, PhD.

Includes bibliographical references and index.
Issued in print and electronic formats.
ISBN 978-1-77188-113-5 (hardcover).--ISBN 978-1-4987-2259-9 (pdf)
1. QSAR (Biochemistry). 2. Pharmaceutical chemistry. 3. Chemometrics. I. Mercader, Andrew G., editor II. Duchowicz, Pablo R., author, editor III. Sivakumar, P. M., author, editor

RM301.42.C54 2015   615'.19   C2015-906689-1   C2015-906690-5

Library of Congress Cataloging-in-Publication Data

Names: Mercader, Andrew G. | Duchowicz, Pablo R. | Sivakumar, P. M.
Title: Chemometrics applications and research : QSAR in medicinal chemistry / [edited by] Andrew G. Mercader, PhD, Pablo R. Duchowicz, PhD, P.M. Sivakumar, PhD.
Description: Toronto : Apple Academic Press, 2015. | Includes index.
Identifiers: LCCN 2015036712 | ISBN 9781771881135 (alk. paper)
Subjects: LCSH: Chemometrics. | Pharmaceutical chemistry. | QSAR (Biochemistry)
Classification: LCC QD75.4.C45 C4844 2015 | DDC 615.101/543--dc23
LC record available at http://lccn.loc.gov/2015036712

Apple Academic Press also publishes its books in a variety of electronic formats. Some content that appears in print may not be available in electronic format. For information about Apple Academic Press products, visit our website at **www.appleacademicpress.com** and the CRC Press website at **www.crcpress.com**

ABOUT THE EDITORS

Andrew G. Mercader, PhD
Dr. Andrew G. Mercader studied physical chemistry at the Faculty of Chemistry of La Plata National University (UNLP), Buenos Aires, Argentina, from 1995-2001. Afterwards he joined Shell Argentina to work as Luboil, Asphalts and Distillation Process Technologist and as Safeguarding and Project Technologist, from 2001-2006. His PhD work on the development and applications of QSAR/QSPR theory was performed at the Theoretical and Applied Research Institute located at La Plata National University (INIFTA), from 2006-2009. He obtained a postdoctoral scholarship to work on theoretical-experimental studies of biflavonoids at IBIMOL (ex PRALIB), Faculty of Pharmacy and Biochemistry, University of Buenos Aires (UBA), from 2009-2012. He is currently a member of the Scientific Researcher Career in the Argentina National Research Council at INIFTA.

Pablo R. Duchowicz, PhD
Dr. Pablo R. Duchowicz studied physical chemistry from 1996-2003 at the Faculty of Exact Sciences, Chemistry Department of La Plata National University (UNLP), Buenos Aires, Argentina. His PhD work on "Physicochemical and Biological Applications of the QSPR-QSAR Theory" was performed at the Research Institute of Theoretical and Applied Physical-Chemistry (INIFTA) located at La Plata, under the supervision of Profs. Eduardo A. Castro and Francisco M. Fernández, from 2003-2005. In 2006 he obtained a postdoctoral scholarship to work on "ab initio Direct Kinetics and Molecular Dynamics Studies for Halogenated Germanes and Related Species" at INIFTA, under the supervision of Dr. Carlos J. Cobos and Prof. Adela Croce. Since 2007, he has been a member of the Scientific Researcher Career of the National Research Council of Argentina, performing research work at INIFTA.

P. M. Sivakumar, PhD
P. M. Sivakumar, PhD, is a foreign postdoctoral researcher (FPR) at RIKEN, Wako Campus, in Japan. RIKEN is Japan's largest comprehensive research institution renowned for high-quality research in a diverse range of scientific disciplines. He received his PhD from the Department of Biotechnology, Indian Institute of Technology Madras, India. He is a member of the editorial boards of

several journals and has published papers in international peer-reviewed journals and professional conferences. His research interests include drug discovery,
QSAR, and biomaterials.

CONTENTS

LIST OF CONTRIBUTORS

Stella M. Battista
Instituto de Bioquímica y Medicina Molecular (IBIMOL) (UBA-CONICET), Facultad de Farmacia y Bioquímica, Universidad de Buenos Aires, Junín 956, C1113AAD Buenos Aires, Argentina

Eduardo A. Castro
Instituto de Investigaciones Fisicoquímicas Teóricas y Aplicadas (INIFTA, CCT La Plata-CONICET), Casilla de Correo 16, Sucursal 4, 1900 La Plata, Argentina

Pratim K. Chattaraj
Department of Chemistry and Center for Theoretical Studies, Indian Institute of Technology Kharagpur, 721302, India

Kelly Chibale
Department of Chemistry, South African Medical Research Council Drug Discovery and Development Research Unit, University of Cape Town, Rondebosch 7701, South Africa
Institute of Infectious Disease and Molecular Medicine, University of Cape Town, Rondebosch 7701, South Africa

Mangesh V. Damre
Department of Pharmacoinformatics, National Institute of Pharmaceutical Education and Research (NIPER), Sect-67, S.A.S. Nagar, Punjab-160 062, India

Mukesh Doble
Department of Biotechnology, Indian Institute of Technology Madras, Adyar, Chennai 600036, India

Pablo R. Duchowicz
Instituto de Investigaciones Fisicoquímicas Teóricas y Aplicadas (INIFTA, CCT La Plata-CONICET), Casilla de Correo 16, Sucursal 4, 1900 La Plata, Argentina

Rahul P. Gangwal
Department of Pharmacoinformatics, National Institute of Pharmaceutical Education and Research (NIPER), Sect-67, S.A.S. Nagar, Punjab-160 062, India

Javier Garcia
Instituto de Investigaciones Fisicoquímicas Teóricas y Aplicadas (INIFTA, CCT La Plata-CONICET), Casilla de Correo 16, Sucursal 4, 1900 La Plata, Argentina

Ashutosh Gupta
Department of Chemistry, Udai Pratap Autonomous College, Varanasi, Uttar Pradesh, 221002 India

Nazmul Islam
Theoretical and Computational Chemistry Research Laboratory, Techno Global-Balurghat, Balurghat, Dakshin Dinajpur district, West Bengal 733103, India

Euh D. Jeong
Division of High Technology Materials Research, Busan Center, Korea Basic Science Institute (KBSI), Busan 618-230, Republic of Korea

Supratik Kar
Drug Theoretics and Cheminformatics Laboratory, Department of Pharmaceutical Technology, Jadavpur University, Kolkata 700032, India

Surendra Kumar
Computer-Aided Drug Design Lab, Department of Pharmacy, Shri Govindram Seksaria Institute of Technology and Science, Indore-452003, India

George Lambrinidis
Department of Pharmaceutical Chemistry, Faculty of Pharmacy, University of Athens, Panepistimiopolis, Zografou 15 771, Athens, Greece

P. Manivel
Organic & Medicinal Chemistry Research Laboratory, School of Advanced Sciences, VIT University, Vellore

Garima Mathur
Department of Pharmacy, Banasthali University, Banasthali 304022, Rajasthan, India

Analava Mitra
School of Medical Science and Technology, Indian Institute of Technology Kharagpur, 721302, India

Sumitra Nain
Department of Pharmacy, Banasthali University, Banasthali 304022, Rajasthan, India

F. Nawaz Khan
Organic & Medicinal Chemistry Research Laboratory, School of Advanced Sciences, VIT University, Vellore
Division of High Technology Materials Research, Busan Center, Korea Basic Science Institute (KBSI), Busan 618-230, Republic of Korea

Sarvesh Paliwal
Department of Pharmacy, Banasthali University, Banasthali 304022, Rajasthan, India

Sudip Pan
Department of Chemistry and Center for Theoretical Studies, Indian Institute of Technology Kharagpur, 721302, India

Elumalai Pavadai
Department of Chemistry, South African Medical Research Council Drug Discovery and Development Research Unit, University of Cape Town, Rondebosch 7701, South Africa

Reinaldo Pis Diez
CEQUINOR, Centro de Química Inorgánica (CONICET, UNLP), Departamento de Química, Facultad de Ciencias Exactas, UNLP, C.C. 962, 1900 La Plata, Argentina

Alicia B. Pomilio
Instituto de Bioquímica y Medicina Molecular (IBIMOL) (UBA-CONICET), Facultad de Farmacia y Bioquímica, Universidad de Buenos Aires, Junín 956, C1113AAD Buenos Aires, Argentina

Ramendra Pratap
Department of Chemistry, University of Delhi, North campus, Delhi-110007

Reeta Rai
Department of Biochemistry, All India Institute of Medical sciences, New Delhi-110029

Rajesh Rengarajan
Chemistry Department, Faculty of Science, North Jeddah, King Abdulaziz University P. O. Box 80205, Jeddah 21589, Saudi Arabia

List of Contributors

Cristian Rojas
Decanato General de Investigaciones. Universidad del Azuay, Av. 24 de Mayo 7-77 y Hernán Malo. Apartado Postal 01.01.981, Cuenca, Ecuador

Debesh R. Roy
Department of Applied Physics, S.V. National Institute of Technology, Surat 395007, India

Kunal Roy
Drug Theoretics and Cheminformatics Laboratory, Department of Pharmaceutical Technology, Jadavpur University, Kolkata 700032, India

Abhay T. Sangamwar
Department of Pharmacoinformatics, National Institute of Pharmaceutical Education and Research (NIPER), Sect-67, S.A.S. Nagar, Punjab-160 062, India

Anu Sharma
Department of Pharmacy, Banasthali University, Banasthali 304022, Rajasthan, India

Rajesh K. Sharma
Department of Chemistry, Udai Pratap Autonomous College, Varanasi, Uttar Pradesh, 221002 India

Harpreet Singh
Department of Bioinformatics, Indian Council of Medical Research, New Delhi-110029

Ponnurengam M. Sivakumar
FPR, Nanomedical Engineering Lab, RIKEN, Wako, Japan
Department of Biotechnology, Indian Institute of Technology Madras, Adyar, Chennai 600036, India

Venkatesan Subramanian
Chemical Laboratory, Central Leather Research Institute, Council of Scientific and Industrial Research, Chennai 600 020, India

Meena Tiwari
Computer-Aided Drug Design Lab, Department of Pharmacy, Shri Govindram Seksaria Institute of Technology and Science, Indore-452003, India

Piercosimo Tripaldi
Laboratorio de Química-Física de Alimentos, Facultad de Ciencia y Tecnología, Universidad del Azuay, Av. 24 de Mayo 7-77 y Hernán Malo., Apartado Postal 01.01.981, Cuenca, Ecuador

Anna Tsantili-Kakoulidou
Department of Pharmaceutical Chemistry, Faculty of Pharmacy, University of Athens, Panepistimiopolis, Zografou 157 71, Athens, Greece

Theodosia Vallianatou
Department of Pharmaceutical Chemistry, Faculty of Pharmacy, University of Athens, Panepistimiopolis, Zografou 157 71, Athens, Greece

Arturo A. Vitale
Instituto de Bioquímica y Medicina Molecular (IBIMOL) (UBA-CONICET), Facultad de Farmacia y Bioquímica, Universidad de Buenos Aires, Junín 956, C1113AAD Buenos Aires, Argentina

Dharmendra K. Yadav
Department of Chemistry, University of Delhi, North campus, Delhi-110007

LIST OF ABBREVIATIONS

2D	Two-dimensional
3D	Three-dimensional
3D-QSAR	Three-dimensional quantitative structure–activity relationship
AANT	Amino acid–nucleotide interaction database
ABC	ATP-binding cassette
AC	Accuracy
ACAT	Acyl-CoA: cholesterol O-acyltransferase
ACAT	Advanced Compartmental Absorption and Transit
ACD	Available Chemicals Directory
ACE	Angiotensin-converting enzyme
ACO	Ant colony optimization
AD	Applicability domain
ADME	Absorption, distribution, metabolism, and excretion
ADME/Tox	Absorption, distribution, metabolism, excretion, and toxicity
ADMEAP	ADME-associated proteins
ADRs	Adverse drug reactions
AffinDB	Affinity database for protein–ligand
AHS	Alternating heuristic SBS
AI	Amphypathicity index
AIC	Akaike information criterion
AIDS	Acquired immunodeficiency syndrome
Ala	alanine
ALS	Adaptive least squares
AMSP	Autocorrelation of molecular surfaces properties
ANN	Artificial neural networks
APD	Antimicrobial peptide database
API	Active pharmaceutical ingredients
AR	Adenosinereceptor
Asn	Asparagines
Asp	Aspartic acid
ATP	Adenosine triphosphate
ATR	Ataxia telangiectasia and Rad3 related
AUC	Area under the curve
aug-MIA-QSPR	Augmented Multivariate Image Analysis applied to Quantitative Structure-Activity Relationship

BDE	Bond dissociation energy
CA	Cluster analysis
CADB	Conformational angles in proteins database
CADD	Computer-aided drug design
CAMM	Computer-assisted molecular modeling
CAP	Chemicals available for purchase
CART	Classification and Regression tree analysis
CCA	Canonical correlation analysis
CCG	Chemical Computing Group
CCK	Cholecystokinin
CCKA	Cholecystokinin A-type
CCK-B	Cholecystokinin-B
CDFT	Conceptual density functional theory
CFA	Correspondence factor analysis
CFS	Conformational FS
CGO	Chemical Gaussian Overlay
ChEBI	Chemical entities of biological interest
CI	Configuration interaction
CMC	Comprehensive Medicinal Chemistry
CNPD	Chinese Natural Product Database
CNS	Central nervous system
COIN	Combined outlier index criterion
CoMFA	Comparative molecular field analysis
CoMMA	Comparative molecular moment analysis
CoMSIA	Comparative molecular similarity indices analysis
COSMO	Conductor-like screening model
CP	Combinatorial protocol
CPs	Chlorophenols
CR	Continuum regression
CRC	Cyclic redundancy check
CRM	Conformational replacement method
CS	Conformational stepwise
CSD	Cambridge structural database
CSIR	Council of Scientific and Industrial Research
CVFF	Consistent valence force field
CYP3A4	Cytochrome P450 3A4
Cys	Cysteine
DA	Discriminant analysis
DACs	Dynamic active conformations
DAIM	Decomposition And Identification of Molecules

DART	Developmental and reproductive toxicology
DART	Drug adverse reaction target
DB	Didemnin B
DCS	Desirability-credibility-similarity
DDB	Dehydrodidemnin B
DFT	Density functional theory
DHF	7,8-Dihydrofolate
DHFR	Dihydrofolate reductase
DITOP	Drug-Induced Toxicity Related Proteins
DLRP	Database of protein ligand and protein receptor pairs
DMax	Maximum residual
DOE	Design of experiments
DOPIN	Docked Proteome Interaction Network
DTC	Drug Theoretics Laboratory
DUD-E	Directory of Useful Decoys-Enhanced
EA	Electron affinity
EA	Evolutionary algorithm
ED50	50% Effective dose
EF	Enrichment factor
ELISA	Enzyme-linked immunosorbent assay
E-MSD	EBI's macromolecular structure database
EPA	Environmental Protection Agency
EPR	Electron paramagnetic resonance
E_R	Relative edulcoration
ERM	Enhanced replacement method
ES	Electrostatic energy
ESI-MS	Electrospray ionization mass spectrometry
ETGD	European Technical Guidance Documents
ET–PT	Electron transfer–proton transfer
EVA	Eigenvalue analysis
F	Fisher function
FA	Factor analysis
FA	Fraction of oral dose absorbed
FDA	Food and Drug Administration
FN	False negatives
FP	False positives
FPSA	Fractional polar surface area
FS	Full search
FS-QSAR	Fragment-similarity based QSAR
GA	Genetic algorithm

GA   Glycyrrhetinic acid
GAFEAT   GA-based feature selection procedure
GAPLS   GA-based PLS
GARGS   GA-based region selection
GEMDOCK   Generic Evolutionary Method for molecular DOCKing
GenDiS   Genomic distribution of protein structural superfamilies
GFA   Genetic function approximation
GFA   Genetic functional algorithm
GFA–MLR   Genetic function approximation and multiple linear regression
GH   Goodness of hit
GH   Guner-Henry
Glu   Glutamic acid
Gly   Glycine
GP   Genetic programming
GPCR   G-protein-coupled receptor
GPLS   Genetic partial least squares
GPQSAR   Genetic QSAR
GRIND   Grid-independent descriptors
GTD   Genomic threading database
HAART   Highly active antiretroviral therapy
HAT   Hydrogen transfer
HB   Hydrogen-bonding energy
HBA   Hydrogen bond acceptor
HBD   Hydrogen bond donor
HCV   Hepatitis C virus
HEPT   1-(2-Hydroxyethoxy)methyl-6-(phenylthio)thymine
hERG   Human ether-a-go-go-related gene
Het-PDB Navi Heteroatoms in protein structures
HF   Hartree–Fock
HHS   Hybrid heuristic SBS
HIC-Up   Hetero-compound Information Centre Uppsala
HIV   Human immunodeficiency virus
HLE   Human leukocytes elastase
HLs   Hidden layers
HMDB   The Human Metabolome Database
HOIle δ-Hydroxyl isoleucine
HOMO   Highest occupied molecular orbital
HOMSTRAD   Homologous structure alignment database
HP   Hydrophobic
HPA   Hirschfield population analysis

HQSAR	Hologram quantitative structure–toxicity relationships
HTS	High-throughput screening
IC50	50% Inhibitory concentration
IL-2	Interleukin 2
Ile	Isoleucine
IMOTdb	Spatially interacting motif database
IN	Input neuron
IP	Ionization potential
IPLF	ISIDA property-labeled fragment
IR	Infrared
IRRM	Incremental regularized risk minimization
ISE	Iterative stochastic elimination
ISSD	Integrated sequence-structure database
K	Kendall rank correlation
KBS	K-level best SBS
K_{cv}	Kendall cross-validated rank correlation
kNN	k-nearest neighbors
KohNN	Kohone's self-organizing neural network
KOWWIN	EPI
KS	Kolmogorov–Smirnov
LA	Lipid A
LBD	Ligand binding domain
LD50	Lethal Dose, 50%
LDA	Linear discriminant analysis
Leu	Leucine
LIBSVM	
LJ	Lennard-Jones potential energy
LMO	Leave-many-out
log-(RS)	Logarithm of relative sweetness
LOO	Leave-one-out
LPFC	Library of protein family core structures
LPS	Lipopolysaccharide
LRA	Linear regression analysis
LS-SVM	Least squares support vector machine
LUMO	Lowest unoccupied molecular orbital
LV	Latent variables
MAE	Mean absolute error
MCDPM	Multiconformation dynamic pharmacophore modeling
MCMM	Monte Carlo multiple minimum
MD	Molecular dynamics

MDDR	MDL Drug Data Report
MDPI	Molecular Diversity Preservation International
MDR	Multidrug resistance
MHC	Minimal hemolytic concentration
MHP	Maximum hardness principle
MIC	Minimum inhibitory concentration
MIF	Molecular interaction field
MLR	Multivariable linear regression
MLSMR	Molecular Libraries Small Molecule Repository
MLVP	Minor latent variable perturbation
MM	Molecular mechanics
MMP	Minimum magnetizability principle
MODEL	Molecular Descriptor Lab
MOE	Molecular Operating Environment
MOPAC	Molecular Orbital PACkage
MoQSAR	Multiobjective genetic QSAR
MPA	Mulliken population analysis
MPA	Multipoint attachment
MPI	Message Passing Interface
MPP	Minimum electrophilicity principle
mQSAR	Multidimensional QSAR
MR	Molar refractivity
MS	Mass spectrometry
MS/MS	Tandem mass spectrometry
MSA	Molecular shape analysis
MSECV	Mean squared error of cross validation
MSF	Most similar fragment
MS-WHIM	Molecular surface WHIM
MTC	Medullary thyroid carcinoma
MTD	Minimum topological difference
MUSEUM	Mutation and selection uncover models
MW	Molecular weight
NADPH	Nicotinamide adenine dinucleotide phosphate
NCEs	New chemical entities
nD-QSAR	n-Dimensional QSAR
NIH	National Institutes of Health
NIMAG	Number of imaginary frequencies
NIPALS	nonlinear iterative partial least squared regression
NLM	nonlinear mapping
NMR	Nuclear magnetic resonance

NNRTIs	Non-nucleoside reverse transcriptase inhibitors
NP	Natural product
NPA	Natural population analysis
NQR	Nuclear quadrupole resonance
NRTIs	Nucleoside reverse transcriptase inhibitors
NSAIDs	Nonsteroidal anti-inflammatory drugs
OECD	Organization for Economic Cooperation and Development
OLS	Ordinary least squares
OMet	S-oxomethionine
OPS	Ordered predictor selection
ORs	Olfactory receptors
OSFs	Oral slope factors
PA	Peptide association
PALI	Phylogeny and alignment of homologous protein structures
PAMPA	Parallel artificial membrane assay
PARC	Pattern recognition
PASS	Prediction of Activity Spectra for Substances
PASS2	Structural motifs of protein superfamilies
PBPK	Physiologically based pharmacokinetic modeling
PC	Phosphatidylcholine
PCA	Principal component analysis
PCDF	Polychlorinated dibenzofurans
PCET	Proton-coupled electron transfer
PCR	Principal component regression
PDB	Protein data bank
PDB_TM	Transmembrane proteins with known 3D structure
PDB-REPRDB	Representative protein chains, based on PDB entries
PDBSum	Summaries and analyses of PDB structures
PE	Phosphatidylethanolamine
PepConfDB	A database of peptide conformations
PfTMPK	Plasmodium falciparum thymidylate kinase
PG-1	Protegrin-1
P-gp	P-glycoprotein
PHDD	Polyhalogenated dibenzo-p-dioxins
Phe	Phenylalanine
PhE/SVM	Pharmacophore ensemble/support vector machine
PHYSPROP	The Physical Properties database
PLCγ1	Phospholipase Cgamma1
PLS	Partial least square

PLS-DA	Partial least squares with discriminant analysis
PLSR	Partial Least Squares Regression
PPAR	Peroxisome proliferator-activated receptor
PPIase	Peptidyl-propyl cis–trans isomerase
PPREs	Peroxisome proliferators responsive elements
PR 3	Proteinase 3
PreADMET	Prediction of ADMET
PRECLAV	Property evaluation by class variables
PRESS	Prediction sum error of square
Pro	Poline
PSO	Particle swarm optimization
QC	Quantum chemistry
QDA	Quadratic discriminant analysis
QM/MM	Quantum mechanical/molecular mechanics
QSAR	Quantitative structure–activity relationship
QSARINS	QSAR-INSUBRIA
QSFR	Quantitative structure–fate relationship
QSPkR	Quantitative structure–pharmacokinetic relationship
QSPR	Quantitative structure–property relationship
QSRR	Quantitative structure–retention relationship
QSRSR	Quantitative structure–relative sweetness relationship
QSTR	Quantitative structure–toxicity relationship
QTMS	quantum topological molecular similarity
R	Arginine
R^2	Coefficient of determination
R^2_{cv}	Coefficient of determination of cross-validation
R^{2r}_{and}	Coefficient of determination of Y-randomization
RA	Ring aromatic
RBA	Relative binding affinity
RBFNNs	Radial basis function neural networks
RDF	Radial distribution function
REACH	Registration, Evaluation and Authorization of Chemicals
RHF	Restricted Hartree–Fock
RM	Replacement method
RMSD	Root-mean-square deviation
RMSEC	Root-mean-square error of calibration
RMSEE	Root mean square error of estimate
RMSEP	Root-mean-square error of prediction
$RMSE_{cv}$	Root mean square error of cross-validation
RMSq	Residual mean squares

ROC	Receiver operating characteristic
RP-HPLC	Reversed-phase high-performance liquid chromatography
RS	Relative sweetness
RT	Regression trees
RT	Reverse transcriptase
SA-MLR	Simulated annealing based multiple linear
SAR	Specific absorption rate
SAR	Structure–activity relationship
SASA	Solvent accessible surface area
SBS	Sequential backward selection
SCC-DFTB	Self-consistent charge density functional tight binding
SCF	Self-consistent field
SCOP	Structural classification of proteins
SCOPPI	Structural classification of protein–protein interfaces
SD	Standard deviation
SDEP	Standard deviation of error of prediction
SE	Steric energies
SEE	Standard error of the estimate
SEP	Standard error of prediction
Ser	Serine
SI	Sweet index
SLR	Simple linear regression
SMF	Substructural molecular fragments
SMILES	Simplified molecular-input line-entry system
Sn	Sensitivity
SOM	Self-organizing maps
SOMFA	Self-organizing molecular field analysis
SPA	Scintillation proximity assay
SPE	Stochastic proximity embedding
SPELT	Sequential proton loss electron transfer
SPR	Structure–property relationships
SRC	Syracuse Research Corporation
S-SAR	Spectral-SAR
sst	Sum of squared error total
SURFACE	Surface residues and functions annotated, compared, and evaluated
SVM	Support vector machine
T.E.S.T	Toxicity Estimation Software Tool
T2DM	Type 2 diabetes mellitus

TCM	Traditional Chinese medicine
TDP	Thymidine diphosphate
THF	5,6,7,8-Tetrahydrofolate
Thr	Threonine
TID	Therapeutic target database
TMP	Thymidine monophosphate
TN	True negative
TNCG	Truncated-Newton conjugated gradient
TNF-α	Tumor necrosis factor-α
TOPS	Topology of protein structures database
TP	True positives
TPSA	Topological polar surface area
TQSI	Topological quantum similarity index
Trp	Tryptophan
Tyr	Tyrosine
TZDs	Thiazolidinediones
U	Relative utility.
UFS	Unsupervised forward selection
UNAIDS	United Nations Program on HIV/AIDS
UV	Ultraviolet
UVB	Ultraviolet B
Val	Valine
VEGF-R2	Vascular endothelial growth factor receptor 2
VRS	Virtual receptor site
VS	Virtual screening
VSA	van der Waals surface area
VSMP	Variable selection and modeling method based on prediction
W	Tryptophan
WHIM	weighted holistic invariant molecular
WT	Wild type

PREFACE

The quantitative structure-activity relationship can be shortly described as a theory that links the molecular structure, through molecular descriptors, to relevant biological activities in order to create regression or classification models. Hence, its importance is incalculable since being able to know or predict this link from the structure to a given biological activity has an enormous value in numerous scientific research fields. A clear example is the search for new drugs, where the ability to predict the activity of a new substance, merely by using a computer, extremely reduces the research costs, decreasing, in addition, the necessity to use animal testing.

The importance of QSAR is reflected in the growth of the number of publications on the topic, having risen by almost a factor of one hundred in the last decades. Since the first QSAR works, the theory has evolved in all of its branches, reaching a point where its usefulness is undeniable, having proved in many applications to be a successful method for the design of new compounds with enhanced biological activity. However, there is still much room for further developments, and since the available computing power is continuously increasing, QSAR's potential is enormous; limited merely by the quantity and quality of the available experimental input, which are also continuously improving.

In this book, academics, researchers, and engineering professionals present their research and development work that is relevant in QSAR and in medicinal chemistry. Contributions cover new methodologies and novel applications of existing ones, showing successful applications of the theory in different fields of high interest.

Chapter 1 presents an overview and recent developments in QSAR methodologies, showing a brief history of QSAR; an outline of fragment-based tri- and multidimensional QSAR. Descriptor selection, model generation and validation methods are presented with details, displaying some algorithms which may be useful to understand the statistical basis involved in QSAR model development and validation.

Chapter 2 covers the available web resource tools and *in silico* techniques used in virtual screening and drug discovery processes. It includes an extensive review of web resources in the following categories: databases related to chemical compounds, drug targets and ADME/Toxicity prediction; molecular modeling and drug designing; virtual screening; pharmacophore generation; molecular descriptor calculation software; software for quantum mechanics; ligand binding affinities (docking); and software related to ADME/Toxicity prediction. In addition, an overview of the drug discovery process and the importance of the previously presented resources are presented.

Chapter 3 reviews the r_m^2, a more stringent measure for the assessment of model predictivity compared to the traditional validation metrics, being specifically important since validation is a crucial step in any QSAR study. Its evolution, use and calculation are presented, along with many successful application examples.

Chapter 4 presents linear model improvement techniques that take into account the conformation flexibility of the modeled molecules. Linear models are popular in QSAR studies since they are fairly easy to obtain and have a lower tendency to overfit the training set data. Two simple alternative algorithms are presented, detailing their structure and usage. Their beneficial effects are shown by their application to several databases.

Chapter 5 summarizes the building processes of four different pharmacophore models: common-feature; 3D-QSAR; protein- and protein-ligand complexes. Pharmacophores are abstract descriptions of essential chemical features of molecules that facilitate biological activity; hence they are extremely important in hit identification and lead optimization phases of the drug discovery and development process. In addition, limitations and issues associated with pharmacophore models are presented along with some practical applications and frequently used model validation methods.

Chapter 6 shows the role of different Conceptual Density Functional Theory based chemical reactivity descriptors such as hardness, electrophilicity, net electrophilicity, and philicity in the design of different QSAR/QSPR/QSTR models. Conceptual Density Functional Theory has proven to be an important tool in the prediction of molecular properties. In addition, the synergistic effect of a mixture of antioxidant was explained using conceptual DFT.

Chapter 7 reviews the use of chemometrics in PPAR research highlighting its substantial contribution in identifying essential structural characteristics and understanding the mechanism of action. Peroxisome-Proliferator Activated Receptors (PPAR) family draws significant research interest, since they offer drug targets primarily for dyslipidemia and hyperglycaemia. In this chapter it is shown that historically PPAR structure and ligand based modelling advanced in parallel with both the resolution of X-ray crystal structures and the progress in biochemical investigation; and that currently subtle details in molecular structures are investigated through QSAR modeling, using structure and ligand based approaches or a combination of both.

Chapter 8 presents the structures and QSARs of antimicrobial and immunosuppressive cyclopeptides; discussing the balance of antimicrobial and haemolytic activities for designing new antimicrobial cyclic peptides. Cyclopeptides are natural products that display a range of structures from cyclic dipeptides to circular proteins and cyclotides with thirty amino acids.

Chapter 9 shows the relationship between DFT global descriptors and experimental toxicity of a selected group of polychlorinated biphenyls; exploring the efficacy of three DFT descriptors (global hardness, electronegativity and electrophilicity index).

Chapter 10 reviews the applications of Quantitative Structure-Relative Sweetness Relationships (QSRSR); showing that the last decade was marked by an increase in the number of studies regarding QSAR applications for both understanding the sweetness mechanism and synthesizing novel sweetener compounds for the food additive industry. Developing new sweeteners has considerable importance since they may help reducing the worldwide rise in obesity.

Chapter 11 reviews QSAR studies of 1, 4-benzodiazepine as cholecystokinin receptor CCK_A antagonists. Cholecystokinin (CCK) is a peptide hormone of the gastrointestinal system responsible for stimulating the digestion of fat and protein.

Chapter 12 presents a novel approach for docking-based scoring parameter QSAR modeling; showing its application on a dataset of bisphenylbenzimidazoles (BPBIs) as non-nucleoside reverse transcriptase inhibitors.

Chapter 13 presents a QSAR analysis of the cytotoxic effect on H460 cancer cells by a series of 1H-isochromen-1-ones and their thio analogues (1H-isochromen-1-thione).

Chapter 14 reviews QSAR studies of dihydrofolatereductase (DHFR) inhibition by different compounds. DHFR is an enzyme that reduces dihydrofolic acid to tetrahydrofolic acid; DHFR has been linked various pathologic conditions like cancer and tuberculosis.

— **Dr. Andrew G. Mercader**
Dr. Pablo R. Duchowicz
INIFTA (CONICET-UNLP), Argentina

ACKNOWLEDGMENT

The editors, AGM and PRD, thank the National Research Council of Argentina (CONICET) for financial support.

CHAPTER 1

OVERVIEW AND RECENT ADVANCES IN QSAR STUDIES

RAHUL P. GANGWAL, MANGESH V. DAMRE, and
ABHAY T. SANGAMWAR*

Department of Pharmacoinformatics, National Institute of Pharmaceutical Education
and Research (NIPER), Sect-67, S.A.S. Nagar, Punjab-160 062, India

*Corresponding author: Tel: 0172-2214682-87 Ext-2211
E-mail: abhays@niper.ac.in

CONTENTS

ABSTRACT

Quantitative structure–activity relationship (QSAR) techniques are the most prominent computational means applied for decades in the discovery and development of new drugs. The primary aim of these techniques is to develop mathematical models for the estimation of relevant properties and activities of chemicals of biological interest, especially, when they cannot be determined experimentally. The general steps involved in the QSAR studies are the generation and selection of molecular structure descriptors, construction of the models, and their validation. In the past few decades, many linear and nonlinear QSAR techniques have been developed to construct statistically reliable models based on different descriptors. This chapter seeks to provide a bird's eye view on different QSAR approaches with their merits, demerits, and brief summary on recent trends in the QSAR studies.

1.1   INTRODUCTION

The pharmaceutical companies need continuously to discover and develop new drugs, especially for new diseases and disorders, to fight the increased resistance to older drugs and newly discovered mutated infections. Traditional approaches in drug discovery involve a random screening of many compounds in search of biological properties and structural modifications of lead compounds, through substitutions, additions, or eliminations of chemical groups. This approach was not necessarily compatible; therefore, most companies tried new methods to speed up the discovery of new compounds. Quantitative structure–activity relationship (QSAR) is one of the computational approaches used by pharmaceutical companies to speed up drug discovery process in a cost-effective manner. It is a chemometrics technique that represents an attempt to correlate properties or descriptors of compounds with biological activities. In other words, it is a regression or a classification method that allows one to produce and test hypotheses to facilitate an understanding of interactions between molecules. **Figure 1** shows the general scheme of a QSAR model development.

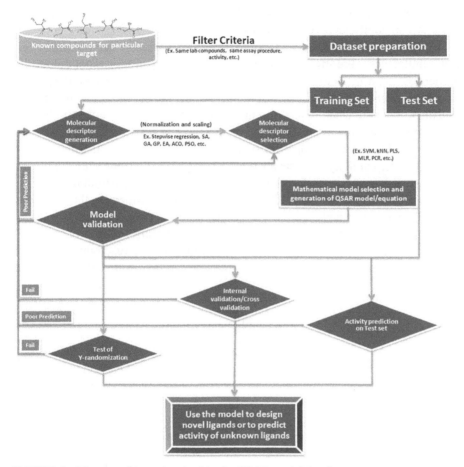

FIGURE 1　Thegeneral steps involved in the QSAR model development.

1.2　HISTORY OF QSAR DEVELOPMENT

In the eighteenth century, Crum-Brown and Fraser stated that the physiological action of a molecule is a function of its chemical composition and constitution.[1,2] In 1863, Cros noted that alcohol's toxicity increased as the solubility property of alcohol in water decreased,[3] while in 1890, Hans Horst Meyer and Charles Ernerst, working independently, observed that the toxicity of organic compound relied on their lipophilicity.[4,5] Based on biological experiments, they correlated partition coefficients with anesthetic potencies. Overton has studied the effect of functional groups in the increase or decrease of partition coefficients.[6] Afterward, Lazarev in St. Petersburg developed the an industrial hygiene standards based on partition coefficients. Lazarev has also developed a system for estimating partition coefficients from chemical structures.[7,8]

In 1893, Richet showed that cytotoxicities of a diverse set of simple organic molecules were inversely related to their corresponding water solubility property,[9,10] and in 1939 the mathematical formula was derived by Ferguson, who consequently provided a principle for toxicity. He observed the increase in anesthetic potency when moving up in a homologous series of either n-alkanes or alkanols to a point where a loss of potency, or at least no further increase occurred, using physical properties such as solubility in water, distribution between phases, capillary, and steam pressure.[11] Little additional developments in QSAR occurred until the work of Louis Hammet (1937), within the field of organic chemistry, who observed the addition of a substituent to the aromatic ring of benzoic acid had an orderly and quantitative effect on the dissociation constant. He also developed a model correlating the electronic properties of organic acid and bases with their equilibrium constants and reactivity. Based on the empirical observation, he developed the linear relationship called Hammet equation:

$$\text{Log}\frac{K}{K_0} = \rho\sigma \qquad (1)$$

where the slope ρ is a proportionality reaction constant for a given equilibrium that relates to the effect of substituent on the equilibrium to the effect on the benzoic acid equilibrium. σ describes the electronic properties of aromatic substitutions, that is, donating power.[12] Based on Hammett's relationship, electronic properties were used as descriptors for chemical structure.[13] Taft presented the first steric parameter, Es, and invented a way of separating polar, steric, and resonance effects.[14] Furthermore, Swain studied the effects of field and resonance. He studied the variation in reactivity of a given electrophilic substrate toward a series of nucleophilic reagents.[15] Free and Wilson postulated that the biological activity of a molecular set can be related to the addition of substitutions, considering the number, type, and position in the parent skeleton.[16]

In 1962, Hansch and Muir reported a structure–activity relationship between plant growth regulators and hydrophobicity. The parameter π, which is a relative hydrophobicity of substitutions, is defined in a manner analogous to the definition of sigma:

$$\pi_x = \log p_x - \log p_H \qquad (2)$$

where p_x and p_H represent the partition coefficient of derivative and the parent molecule, respectively.[17,18]

In 1964, Hansch and Fujita utilized not only these hydrophobic constants but also Hammett's electronic constants and hence developed a linear Hansch equation.[19]Hansch analysis was a powerful technique for optimizing the activity of lead molecules. An interaction between the molecule and receptor was broken down into hydrophobic, electronic, and steric components, and correlation of these components with biological activity was summarized as follows:

$$\text{Log}\frac{1}{c} = a\pi + b\sigma + cEs + d \tag{3}$$

where c is a molar concentration of compounds; π, σ, and Es are hydrophobic, electronic, and steric components, respectively. a, b, c, and d are regression coefficients.

Combination of Hansch and Free Wilson analysis has broadened the applicability of QSAR methods.[20] Currently, the QSAR technique has developed well and continues to expand as indicated by the strong upward trend in the rate of QSAR publications (**Figure 2**).

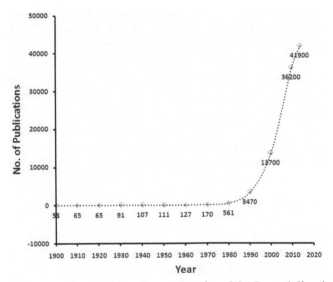

FIGURE 2   The growth of publications related to QSAR modeling based on the Google Scholar Search ("QSAR" as keyword+ excluding citations and patents) carried on December 1, 2013.

1.3 QSAR METHODOLOGIES

The goal of structure–activity relationship is to analyze and detect the deciding factor for measured activity of a particular system, so as to have an insight on the mechanism and behavior of the system. For this purpose, mathematical models are generated, which correlate experimental measurements with a set of chemical descriptors calculated from the molecular structure of the compounds. Many research groups around the world are working on the proposal of new molecular descriptors and data analysis approaches. **Table 1** provides the classificationof descriptors used in the QSAR studies based on dimensionality of their molecular representations. Based on the descriptor, different methods can be distinguished, depending on the dimension of structures employed to generate descriptors, namely: two-dimensional (2D), 3D, 4D, and nD-QSAR methods.

In traditional 2D-QSAR method (Free Wilson models), 2D molecular substitutions or fragments and their physico-chemical properties were used for quantitative predictions. Since then, the first novel 3D-QSAR method called comparative molecular field analysis (CoMFA) was presented by Cramer *et al.*, in 1988.[21] Furthermore, the CoMFA method leads to the development of other 3D-QSAR methods like comparative molecular similarity indices analysis (CoMSIA), comparative molecular moment analysis (CoMMA), and self-organizing molecular field analysis (SOMFA). As 3D-QSAR method progresses, multidimensional (nD-QSAR) methods like 4D-QSAR and 5D-QSAR were established to tackle the known 3D-QSAR problems like subjective molecular alignment and bioactive conformations. Recently, fragment-based QSAR methods have gained attention because they are simple to perform, fast, and robust.

1.4 FRAGMENT-BASED 2D-QSAR

The 2D-QSAR methods allow building of models for a wide range of ligands or compounds including cases where 3D crystal target or receptor structures are not available. In the last few decades, improved fragment-based QSAR methods were introduced. Hologram-QSAR (H-QSAR) was the first 2D molecular fragment based QSAR method introduced by Tripos. This method does not involve molecular alignment and therefore allows for automated analyses of large and diverse data sets without manual intervention. **Figure 3** show the steps involved in H-QSAR study.

TABLE 1 Classification of descriptor by the dimensionality of their molecular representation

Molecular Representation	Descriptor	Example(s)
0D	Atom count, bond count, molecular weight, sum of atomic properties	Molecular weight, average molecular weight, number of atoms, hydrogen atoms, carbon atoms, heteroatoms, nonhydrogen atoms, bonds, multiple bonds, double bond, triple bonds, aromatic bonds, rotatable bonds, rings, 3-membered ring, 4-membered ring, sum of atomic van der Waals volumes
1D	Fragment counts	Number of: primary C, secondary C, tertiary C, quaternary C, secondary C in ring, amines, ammonium groups, N in diazo groups, carbamates, nitriles, hydrazines, imides, imines, hydroxyl groups, alcohols, H-bond donor atoms, H-bond acceptor atoms, hydrophilic factor, isocyanides, thiocyanates, isothiocyanates, amides, phenols, thioesters, sulfoxides, sulfones, sulfates, disulfides, sulfonic acids
2D	Topological descriptor	Zagreb index, Wiener index, Balaban J index, connectivity chi indices, kappa shape indices, molecular walk counts, BCUT descriptors, 2D autocorrelation vector
3D	Geometrical descriptor	Molecular eccentricity, radius of gyration, E-state topological parameter, 3D Wiener index, 3D Balaban index, 3D MoRSE descriptors, radial distribution function (RDF code), WHIM descriptor, 3D autocorrelation vector, GETAWAY descriptors,
3D-surface properties		Mean molecular electrostatic potential, hydrophobicity potential, hydrogen-bonding potential
3D-grid properties		CoMFA
4D		3D coordinates + sampling of conformations

The first step to generate molecular holograms is taking counts of molecular fragments. In detail, the input dataset contains 2D structure of compounds split up into all possible fragments. Then a cyclic redundancy check (CRC) algorithm is used to assign a specific large positive integer to each unique fragment. Furthermore, all generated fragments are hashed into array bins in the range from 1 to L (total length of hologram). The term bin occupancies signify the counts of fragments in each bin. In the second step, generated hologram bins are correlated to corresponding dependent variables in the form of a mathematical equation. Leave one-out cross-validation method is used to identify the optimal number of explanatory variables for a good model. Then, the final mathematical model correlating the hologram bin values or components with the corresponding dependent variable, developed using standard partial least square (PLS) analysis method is:

$$BA_i = const + \sum_{j=1}^{L} x_{ij} C_j$$

where BA_i is the dependent variable value of the ith compound; x_{ij} is the occupancy value of the molecular hologram of the ith compound at bin j; C_j is the coefficient for the bin j derived from the PLS analysis; and L is the length of the hologram.

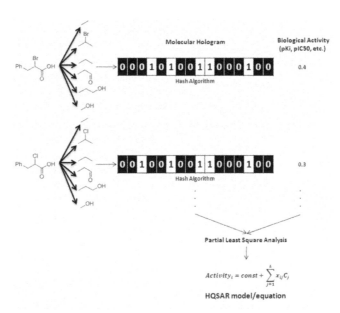

FIGURE 3 Steps involved in H-QSAR model generation.

H-QSAR suffers from the drawback of fragment collision which happens during the hashing process of fragments. Hashing process reduces the length of the hologram by placing different fragments in the same bin. The hologram length is defined by the user to control the number of bins in a hologram, which changes the pattern of bin occupancies. The 12 default hologram lengths (unique set of fragment collisions) are provided in the software program. These hologram lengths were obtained by analyzing different datasets and found to produce good predictive model.[22]

In 2009, a new molecular fragment based 2D-QSAR method was introduced by Du et al.,[23] This method uses a combination of Hansch–Fujita linear free energy equation and Free Wilson equation to develop a model. Initially, molecular fragments are generated from ligands in the dataset; then, the total binding free energy between ligand i and the receptor is calculated using the following formula:

$$\Delta G_i^0 = \sum_{\alpha=1}^{M} b_\alpha \Delta g_{i,\alpha} \tag{5}$$

where $\Delta g_{i,\alpha}$ is the free energy contribution of fragment $F_{i,\alpha}$ and b_α is the weight coefficient for each fragment. $\Delta g_{i,\alpha}$ is calculated by using following formulae:

$$\Delta g_{i,\alpha} = \sum_l \alpha_l \, p_{i,\alpha,l} \tag{6}$$

where $P_{i,\alpha,l}$ is the lth property of fragment $F_{i,\alpha}$ in molecule m_i; and α_l is the coefficient of lth property of the fragment.

In 2010 Myint et al. overcame the limitation of Free Wilson method and developed a new method called fragment-similarity based QSAR (FS-QSAR).[24] They have introduced the fragment-similarity concept in the linear regression equation to improve the traditional Free Wilson equation instead of using physico-chemical properties, which often produced nonunique solutions. In this approach, the fragment similarity was calculated using the lowest or highest eigenvalues, calculated from BCUT-matrices. The BCUT-matrices are made up of partial charges of individual atoms and their atomic connection information in each individual fragments. The modified equation for the development of FS-QSAR model is as follows:

$$-logK_i = const + \sum_{j=1}^{N} Max(Sim_{k=1}^{P_j}(F_{jk}, F_{gj})) \times A_j^{MSF} \tag{7}$$

where N is the total number of substituent positions; P_j is the total number of possible substituents at the jth substituent position; Max is the function that picks the maximum score among similarity scores; F_{jk} is the kth fragment (a known fragment in the training set) at the jth substituent position; F_{gj} is a given fragment at the jth substituent position; A_j^{MSF} is the coefficient of the most similar fragment (MSF) at the jth substituent position; $Sim[F_{jk}, F_{jg}]$ is the fragment similarity function that compares F_{jg} to F_{jk} ($e^{-|EV(F_{jk})-EV(F_{jg})|}$); and $EV(F_{jk})$ is the lowest or highest eigenvalue of the BCUT matrix of a fragment (F_{jk}).

1.5   3D-QSAR

The 3D-QSAR methods are computationally more complex. There are two types of 3D-QSAR methods, namely alignment-dependent and alignment-inde-pendent.[25] Both methods need bioactive conformations of ligands as templates for development of QSAR models. CoMFA is one of the well-known 3D-QSAR method developed by Cramer *et al.*,[21] In this method the 3D structure of ligands are superimposed, then steric and electrostatic fields are generated around each ligand. Then correlation between generated molecular field interaction energy terms and biological activities are calculated using multivariate statistical analy-ses. **Figure 4** shows the steps involved in the CoMFA model generation. Initial-ly, active molecules are placed in a 3D grid, and then the steric and electrostatic energies are measured at each grid point. PLS analysis is then performed to correlate the steric and electrostatic energies to the dependent variable making predictions.

Klebe *et al.*, introduced another 3D-QSAR method called CoMSIA. It is similar to CoMFA method in terms of using a probe atom along grid points. In CoMSIA, electrostatic, steric, hydrophobic, hydrogen bond acceptor (HBA), and hydrogen bond donor (HBD) properties are generated using a Gaussian distance function.[26] The use of Guassian-type potential function provides ac-curate information at grid points for calculating molecular fields in comparison to Lennard-Jones and Coulombic functions, which were used in CoMFA model generation.[27] However, both CoMFA and CoMSIA suffer from a major draw-back that all molecules are aligned and such alignment can affect the model generation and predictions. Also, sometimes CoMFA/CoMSIA models are non-reproducible.[27]

In 2003 Cramer *et al.*, introduced a rapid fragment based 3D-QSAR meth-od called topomer CoMFA.[28] It is useful to predict important R-groups, which can be optimized to improve the biological activities. The compound library is utilized as a source of molecular fragments to recognize such R-groups or substituents.[29] This method uses automated alignment rules. Topomers are gen-erated based on the 2D structure without any relation to a receptor site.[30] It describes both conformation and orientation of a molecular fragment. After the topomer generation, electrostatic and steric fields are calculated using a probe atom around the 3D grid. Subsequently, predictive models are generated using the PLS method.

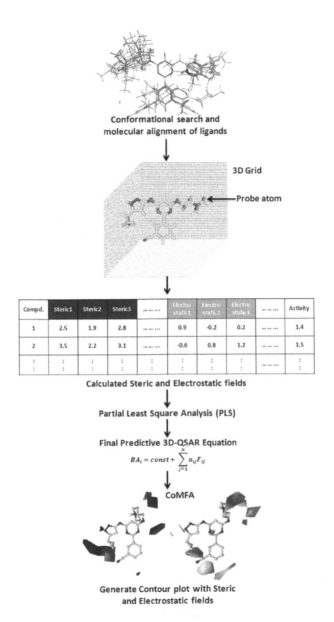

The following table appears within the figure:

Compd.	Steric1	Steric2	Steric3	... ...	Electro static1	Electro static2	Electro static3	... ...	Activity
1	2.5	1.9	2.8	... ...	0.9	-0.2	0.2	... ...	1.4
2	3.5	2.2	3.1	... ...	-0.6	0.8	1.2	... ...	1.5
:	:	:	:	:	:	:	:	... ...	:

$$BA_i = const + \sum_{j=1}^{N} a_{ij} F_{ij}$$

FIGURE 4 Steps involved in CoMFA/CoMSIA model generation.

In 1999 Robinson *et al.,* introduced another alignment-dependent method called SOMFA.[31] This method is based on molecular shape and electrostatic potentials. In detail, molecular shape and electrostatic potential values are calculated for each grid point. Shape values are binary in nature, that is, 1 for being inside and 0 for being outside the van der Waals envelope. The electrostatic potential values at each grid points are multiplied by the mean-centered activity for that molecule, which causes the most active molecules to have higher values in comparison to other molecules. Finally, the correlation between calculated property and biological response is derived via multiple linear regression (MLR) method for predictive model generation.

In 1995 Wagener et al., introduced an alignment independent 3D-QSAR method called autocorrelation of molecular surface properties (AMSP).[32] This method maps the physical properties of ligands to a van der Waals surface and individual atoms. Spatial autocorrelation of molecular properties at distinct points on the molecular surface are used as molecular descriptors to generate the model. The summation of the products of property values at various pairs of points at particular distances provide the autocorrelation coefficient. For a vector of autocorrelation, coefficient is calculated by using the following formula:

$$A\left(d_l d_u\right) = \frac{1}{L} \sum_{ij} P_i P_j \tag{8}$$

where P_i is the molecular property value at point i; P_j is the molecular property value at point j; and L is the total number of distances in the interval.

Then, a predictive multilayer neural network model is generated based on the calculated autocorrelation vectors.

In 1996, Silverman et al., introduced another alignment-independent method known as CoMMA.[33] This method uses the spatial moments of the charge and the mass distribution as descriptors for the model development. These descriptors are divided into three different classes namely descriptors relating solely to the molecular shape, descriptors relating only to the molecular charge, and descriptors relating to both shape and charge.

In 1998 Todeschini et al., developed an alignment-dependent method based on weighted holistic invariant molecular (WHIM) descriptors.[34] Molecular surface (MS)-WHIM descriptors are derived from molecular surface properties, which provide information about molecular size, shape, symmetry, and distribution of molecular surface point coordinates.[35] Initially, matrix containing Cartesian coordinates of the n atoms and diagonal matrices containing the weights are defined for the generation of QSAR model based on WHIM descriptors. Diagonal matrixes are analyzed to obtain the scoring matrix, to compute the PCA eigenvalues, and the eigenvalue proportion. Then, calculated values are correlated with the molecular size and shape.

In 2000, Pastor *et al.*, developed a new method called grid-independent descriptors (GRIND).[36] This method uses O probe and N1 probe to calculate molecular interaction fields (MIFs), calculated as follows:

$$E = \sum ES + \sum HB + \sum LJ \qquad (9)$$

where ES is the electrostatic energy; HB is the hydrogen-bonding energy; and LJ is the Lennard-Jones potential energy.

The ES, HB, and LJ are used to define a "virtual receptor site" (VRS). Then, VRS regions are programmed into GRIND so that those regions are no longer dependent upon their positions. In other words, the highest products of molecular interaction energies are stored from the generated autocorrelation descriptors of the field. This alteration is accountable for the "reversibility" of GRIND. ALMOND program is used to back the project in calculating descriptors in 3D space.

1.6   MULTIDIMENSIONAL (4D–6D) QSAR METHODS

Multidimensional QSAR methods are developed to tackle the drawbacks of 3D-QSAR methods by incorporating additional descriptors (dimension). Hopfinger *et al.*, developed a one 4D-QSAR model by using conformational Boltzmann sampling. The geometry of the receptor is essential to develop a 4D-QSAR model; which is developed using XMAP program.[24,37] In recent studies 5D- and 6D-QSAR are reported, which utilized multiple representations of the receptor and its solvation states as descriptors, respectively.[38,39] In the 5D-QSAR method, multiple representations of induced-fit hypotheses are used as the fifth dimension for the development of model. In the case of 6D-QSAR method, the different solvation models were used to develop a predictive model. The 6D-QSAR outperforms the other QSAR models in productivity; however, 5D- and 6D-QSARs are performed using Quasar and VirtualToxLab software.[40]

1.7   FEATURE OR DESCRIPTOR SELECTION

A common issue in any QSAR study is to describe molecular properties. The nature of the descriptors used and the degree to which they encrypt the structural features related to the dependent variable is a vital part of a QSAR study. Limited number of descriptors, obtained with ease and simplicity, were used in early development of QSARs. As computational power was increased over the decades, a large number of descriptors were developed maximizing the amount of information to develop a statistically reliable QSAR model. Today more than

3,000 molecular descriptors are available and mostly calculated by commercial software tool such as ADAPT, CODESSA, OASIS, and DRAGON.

Most of the time QSAR model generated using all available descriptors does not produce the most predictive model. Nonuniform or redundancy in descriptors may lead to the development of model with statistical problems, such as overfitting or chance correlation. Variable or feature selection is necessary to avoid such problems and build a reliable QSAR model. A highly predictive model developed with relatively small number of descriptors is simple and easy to interpret. In general, feature selection is based on trial and error procedure. Initially, a set of descriptors is selected according to a specific rule. Then prediction power of a model with the selected descriptors is determined by using a predefined fitness function. The trial and error is continued until a satisfactory model is developed. Some of the algorithms developed for variable selections are stepwise regression, simulated annealing, genetic algorithm (GA), genetic programming (GP), neural network pruning, evolutionary algorithm (EA), ant colony optimization (ACO) algorithm, and particle swarm optimization (PSO) technique. Among them, GA, EA, PSO, and ACO are optimization techniques simulating biological systems. Residual mean squares (RMSq), the Cp-criterion, prediction sum error of square criterion (PRESS), Akaike information criterion (AIC), and Kolmogorov–Smirnov (KS) statistics are used as fitness function or criteria during the variable selection.

1.7.1 STEPWISE REGRESSION

Stepwise regression method is the simplest among all feature selection techniques. There are two stepwise regression feature selection techniques namely, forward stepwise and backward stepwise. In forward stepwise selection procedure, new descriptors are added to the model one at a time until no more significant variables are found, whereas in backward stepwise regression the model begins with all descriptors and less informative descriptors are trimmed systematically. Commonly, F-statistics is used as fitness function or criteria to select statistically significant variables. The major drawback of stepwise regression analysis is that the algorithm fails to take into account the information of parallel effect among multiple descriptors and often finds a nonoptimal solution.

1.7.2 SIMULATED ANNEALING

Simulated annealing method is introduced by Kirkpatrik et al., and Cerny for combinatorial optimization processes.[41–43] It performs optimization by applying Metropolis criterion to a series of configurations for the system being optimized.

In simulated annealing algorithm, initially random solution is generated, and then a neighborhood sampling is repeated. The generated new solution is tested on the basis of fitness criteria. At the beginning of optimization, fitness criteria is set at high value and new solution that has worse fitness value than current solution is accepted with relatively high probability. Then the fitness criterion is gradually decreased in order to reduce probability of acceptance of such solution. As a consequence, probability of being trapped in a local minimum solution is reduced. Simulated annealing is very robust, easy to understand, and implement. In comparison to stepwise regression feature selection technique, this algorithm requires considerably higher computing power.

1.7.3 GENETIC ALGORITHM

In 1993, John Hollandhas reported the mathematical form of GA to elucidate the adaptive processes of natural systems.[44,45] Three basic steps are involved in the GA: (1) generation of chromosomes, which are represented by a binary bit string. Bit "1" denotes a selection of the corresponding variable, and bit "0" denotes no selection; (2) fitness score calculation for each chromosome in the population, which is done on the basis of predictivity of the derived model; and (3) the population of chromosomes is generated again. This step can be further divided into three processes namely selection, crossover, and mutation.

In 2001 Ozdemir *et al.,* proposed a GA based feature selection procedure (GAFEAT) for QSAR model generation in reducing the curse of dimensionality problem.[46] Hasegawa *et al.,* developed a GA-based PLS (GAPLS) program for variable selection in QSAR studies.[44] In similar fashion GA was combined with several QSAR model generation studies such as neural networks for selecting a subset of relevant descriptors, 3D H-suppressed BCUT metrics (BCUTs), counterpropagation neural network, and GA based region selection (GARGS).

1.7.4 GENETIC PROGRAMMING

Both GP and GA became popular for variable selection. The three-step procedure for GP is very similar to that of GA. However, GA and GP fundamentally differ in coding and decoding of chromosomes. Chromosomes used in GA consist of binary bit string, whereas chromosomes of GP characterize by tree structure (**Figure 5**). In GP, terminal nodes are allocated to a variable or a constant value such as X1 or 2.8, and operators such as plus or multiplication are allocated to other nodes. Due to these flexible coding and decoding of chromosome in GP, it represents more complex solutions than GA. Hence, GP can be more effective than GA for selecting variables in QSAR modeling.

1.7.5 NEURAL NETWORK PRUNING

Neural network pruning, a method for feature selection, is mainly grouped into two methods, that is, sensitivity methods[47] and penalty term methods.[48] The first method presents some measures of the importance of weights named as "sensitivities". In this method sensitivities of all weights are calculated and then the elements with the smallest sensitivities are removed. The second method modifies the error function by introducing penalty terms.[49] Kovalishyn proposed another neural network pruning method based on cascade correlation learning algorithm.

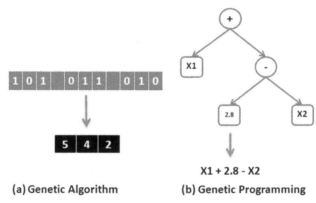

(a) Genetic Algorithm   (b) Genetic Programming

FIGURE 5   Coding of chromosomes in (a) GA (b) GP.

1.7.6 EVOLUTIONARY ALGORITHM

An EA is based on the principal of survival of the fittest. In this method, an initial population of a candidate solution is built and then each solution is evaluated by a fitness function and assigned with a value indicating its relative correctness. Kubinyi suggested an EA termed mutation and selection uncover models (MUSEUM). The major difference between MUSEUM and genetic function approximation (GFA) is the absence of a crossover operator and its reliance solely on point mutation to generate new solutions.[50]

1.7.7 ACO ALGORITHM

ACO has developed as a stochastic optimization approach. It is invented as a simulation of ant colony systems. Bonabeau *et al.*,[51] were inspired by the behavior of real ants and developed the ACO algorithms for variable selection. Ants are able to find the shortest path between a food source and their nest using deposits of pheromone as a communication agent. This basic self-organizing principle is exploited in the construction of better QSAR models. However, ACO suffers from the drawback such as long searching time and the tendency to be trapped into local optima.

1.7.8 PSO TECHNIQUE

In 1995, Eberhart and Kennedy developed the PSO algorithm based on the social behavior of bird flocking. It searches for optima by updating generations in a similar fashion to the GA and EA. However, each individual in PSO flies in the search space with a velocity that directs the flying of the particle instead of crossover and mutation operators.[52] Shen et al., developed an improved, discrete PSO algorithm to select variables in MLR and PLS based QSAR modeling.[53]

1.7.9 OTHER VARIABLE SELECTION METHODS

Many other approaches for variable selection were developed in the last few decades. In 1998, four sequential backward selection (SBS) algorithms for feature selection were assessed by Deogun et al., These four algorithms are namely, (1) best fit SBS (BFS), (2) hybrid heuristic SBS (HHS), (3) alternating heuristic SBS (AHS), and (4) K-level best SBS (KBS).[54] Xie and co-workers proposed a different method called minor latent variable perturbation (MLVP-PLS), which obviates the encountered pleonastic variables in QSAR studies.[55] A new approach for variable selection, that is, combinatorial protocol (CP) in MLR was introduced by Prabhakar,[56] where limited entry of correlated variables to the model development stage enables an efficient CP-MLR.[57] In order to obtain accurate and interpretable QSAR models, Nicolotti et al., proposed two methods based on GP.[58] The first method, genetic QSAR (or GPQSAR), derives a single linear model which represents an appropriate balance between the variance and the number of descriptors selected for the model. The other method is multiobjective genetic QSAR (MoQSAR), grounded on multiobjective GP. Livingstone and co-workers recently developed unsupervised forward selection (UFS) method for eliminating redundant variables.[59,60] Frohlich and co-workers introduced the incremental regularized risk minimization (IRRM) algorithm, a novel method for choosing subsets of descriptor by support vector machine (SVM), in classifications and regressions.[61] Byvatov et al., in 2004 proposed an SVM-based algorithm for an understanding of ligand–receptor interactions of relevant molecular features from a trained classifier.[62] Variable selection and modeling method based on prediction (VSMP) was developed by Liu et al., in which a subset selection is based on the statistic q^2 predicted in the cross alidation process.[63] Random forest technique,[64] boosting, and bagging[65] are the examples of ensemble learning techniques. Random forest technique is an extension of the recursive partitioning algorithm developed by Breiman,[66] and a new two-stage backward elimination algorithm in the random forest method for descriptor selection was proposed by Li and co-workers.[67] Mercader and co-workers recently reported enhanced replacement method (ERM) and replacement method (RM) for variable selection. ERM and RM are simple in operation and required less computational power in comparison to GA.[68] Due to unavailability of accepted rules in QSAR studies it becomes a difficult task for variable selection even in accessing various statistical methods. Models with various descriptive feature combinations were identified by numerous artificial intelligence based approaches[69,70] in which desired levels of accuracy, robustness, and interpretability were achieved.

1.8 STATISTICAL METHODS FOR GENERATION OF QSAR/QSPR MODEL

Modeling techniques are divided into two different categories. Quantitative regression techniques aim to develop correlation models by using statistical adjustments. Complementary to this, qualitative pattern recognition (PARC) techniques are devoted to the descriptive data analysis and classification. Besides, methods for the quantitative analysis of continuous properties or methods for the semiquantitative analysis of categorical properties or continuous properties partitioned into discrete classes can be applied depending on the variables being studied.

Amongst the pool of different modeling methods, the selection of the proper method for the statistical analysis is crucial. Many regression analysis methods are available in the literature. MLR, also known as ordinary least squares (OLS), is an easy interpretable regression-based method commonly used for QSAR analysis. Recently, such methods have been substituted by multivariate projection methods, namely projection to latent variables, such as principal component regression (PCR) and PLS, which in turn reduce the information content of data matrices. Thus, these techniques project multivariate data into a space of lower dimensions, obviously reducing the number of dimensions, and indeed providing insights to visualize, classify, and model a large data set. The position of the observations on the new space is given by the scores and to orientate the plane in relation to the original variables is indicated by the loadings.[71]

Also, more sophisticated methods, like adaptive least squares (ALS), canonical correlation analysis (CCA), continuum regression (CR), nonlinear GFA, and genetic partial least squares (GPLS) are also currently available. Besides, other methods are extensively developed to perform classification studies in QSAR. The so-called PARC analysis methods, that is, discriminate analysis and decision trees, can be applied to classify compounds in a model. PARC methods are based on a set of classes that contain a number of observations mapped by variables, guidelines, and rules, so that new compounds can be classified as similar or dissimilar to the members of the existing classes. The main assumptions to compare the similarity of observations within each class are the application of the principle of analogy. Thus, PARC techniques such as linear discriminant analysis (LDA), k-nearest neighbors (kNN), PCA, correspondence factor analysis (CFA), factor analysis (FA), nonlinear mapping (NLM), CCA, cluster analysis (CA), and artificial neural networks (ANN) provide qualitative information on the property–structure relationships, by means of representation techniques.[72]

1.8.1 MLR ANALYSIS

Multivariate regression procedure estimates the value of a dependent variable (biological activity) from independent variables, represented by different molecular descriptors. The first part of data analysis consists of using the data to find out values of the parameters in the models so that the models fit into the data well. Stepwise regression was commonly used to dimensionality of variable during QSAR model building. In general, the model with fewer variables is acceptable, which increases predictive power. Cross validation, a method used to estimate the true predictive power of the model, provides a rigorous internal check on the models derived using regression or PLS analysis.[73,74]

1.8.1.1 ALGORITHM FOR CALCULATING MLR

The mathematical estimation of the regression coefficients for more than single independent variables involves matrix computations. Let X be the data matrix of the predictor (independent) variables, Y represents the data vector for the dependent variable, and b is the data vector representing the regression coefficients including the constants. Then, the vector of regression coefficients is computed as

$$b = (X'X)^{-1}X'Y \qquad (10)$$

Different statistical parameters are used in the analysis of MLR. In statistical data analysis the total sum of squares (TSS or SST) is a quantity that appears as part of a standard way of presenting results of such analyses. It is defined as being the sum, over all observations, of the squared differences of each observation from the overall mean.[75]

$$sst = \sum_{i=1}^{n}(y_i - \bar{y})^2 \tag{11}$$

The sum of squared error (sse) can be calculated as follows

$$sse = \sum_{i=1}^{n}e_i^{\,2} \tag{12}$$

The mean squared error of cross validation (MSECV) can be calculated as follows

$$MSECV = sse/n \tag{13}$$

The standard error of estimate (see) can be calculated as follows

$$see = \sqrt{\frac{sse}{(n-k-1)}} \tag{14}$$

where n is the number of observations and k is the number of independent variables.

The correlation coefficient (r^2) can be calculated as follows[76]

$$\text{Correlation coefficient}\left(r^2\right) = 1 - \left(\frac{sse}{sst}\right) \tag{15}$$

The relationship between r^2 and the number of subjects (n) and predictors (k) can be readily understood. If the number of subjects equals $k + 1$, then r^2 will always be 1.0 (assuming some variance in the variables). Because of that, all subjects must fall on the regression line, plane, or hyperplane. However, there is no "freedom" to vary about the plane. As the ratio of the number of subjects to the number of variables studied increases, this "overfitting" of the data to the plane decreases. The larger the number of subjects to the number of variables, the closer will be the regression statistics estimates of the population values. Notice, however, that r^2 is biased toward overestimation. This bias becomes smaller and smaller as the ratio of subjects to variables increases.[77] This relation can be explained in term of r^2_{adjusted} which can be calculated as follows

$$r^2 \text{ adjusted} = r^2 - \frac{(1-r^2)}{(n-1)/(n-k-1)} \tag{16}$$

The Fisher (F) value for statistical analysis can be calculated by using the following formula

$$F = \frac{r^2(n-k-1)}{k*(1-r^2)} \tag{17}$$

The coefficient of cross validation (q^2) can be calculated as follows

$$q^2 = \frac{(S_y^{\,2} - MSECV)}{S_y^{\,2}} \tag{18}$$

where $S_y^{\,2}$ is the sum of squared deviation between the biological activities of the test set molecule and the mean activity of the training set molecules and MSECV is the sum of squared deviations between the observed and the predicted activities of the test molecules. The $S_y^{\,2}$ can be calculated by using the following formula

$$S_y^{\,2} = \frac{sst}{(n-1)} \tag{19}$$

1.8.2 PRINCIPAL COMPONENT ANALYSIS

The principal component analysis (PCA) method is used to extract the systematic variance in the data matrix. It helps to obtain an overview over dominant patterns and major trends in the data. The purpose behind the PCA is to generate a set of latent variables, which is smaller than the set of original variables but still explains all the variance in the matrix of the original variables.

In mathematical terms, PCA is a method to convert large number of correlated variables into a smaller number of uncorrelated variables, the so-called principal components. Prior to PCA the data is often preprocessed to convert into a form most suitable for the application of PCA. Commonly used preprocessing methods for PCA are scaling and mean centering of the data.[78]

From a geometric point of view PCA is described as: Given a data set or matrix with *n* objects and *m* variables each of the variables represents one coordinate axis, so each object can be plotted as a point in m-dimensional space. The entire data set is then a swarm of points in this space. In this point swarm, the first principal component is the line which gives the best approximation to the data, that is, it represents the maximum variance within the data. The second principal component is orthogonal to the first principal component and again has maximum variance. Further, principal components are generated accordingly.[79]

An advantage of PCA is its ability to cope with almost any kind of data matrix with many rows and few columns or vice versa. One widely used algorithm for performing PCA is the nonlinear iterative partial least squared regression (NIPALS) described as follows.

1.8.2.1   THE NIPALS ALGORITHM FOR PCA

The NIPALS algorithm extracts one principal component at a time. Each factor is obtained iteratively by repeated regressions of X on scores $\hat{t}$ to obtain improved $\hat{p}$ and of X on these $\hat{p}$ to obtain improved $\hat{t}$. The algorithm proceeds as follows: To ensure comparable noise levels, X-variables are initially scaled, for example, by subtracting the calibration means $\hat{t}'$, forming X_0. Then, for factors $a = 1, 2, ..., A$ compute $\hat{t}_a$ and $\hat{t}_a$ from X_{a-1}:.

Start:

Select start values. e.g. $\hat{t}_a$ = the column in X_{a-1} that has the highest remaining sum of squares.

Repeat points (i) to (v) until convergence

(i) Improve the estimate of loading vector $\hat{t}_a$ for this factor by projecting the matrix X_{a-1} on $\hat{t}_a$, i.e.

$$\hat{p}'_a = (\hat{t}'_a \hat{t}_a)^{-1} \hat{t}'_a X_{a-1} \tag{20}$$

(ii) Scale the length of $\hat{t}_a$ to 1.0 to avoid scaling ambiguity:

$$\hat{p}_a = \hat{p}_a (\hat{p}'_a \hat{p}_a)^{-0.5} \tag{21}$$

(iii) Improve the estimate of score $\hat{t}_a$ for this factor by projecting the matrix X_{a-1} on $\hat{p}'_a$:

$$\hat{t}_a - X_{a-1}\hat{p}_a (\hat{p}'_a \hat{p}'_a)^{-1} \tag{22}$$

(iv) Improve the estimate of the eigenvalue $\hat{T}_a$:

$$\hat{T}_a = (\hat{t}'_a \hat{t}_a) \tag{23}$$

(v) Check convergence: If $\hat{p}'_a$ minus $\hat{p}'_a$ in the previous iteration is smaller than a certain small pre-specified constant, e.g. 0.0001 times $\hat{p}'_a$, the method has converged for this factor. If not, go to step i).

Subtract the effect of this factor:

$$X_a = X_{a-1} - \hat{t}'_a \hat{t}_a \tag{24}$$

and go to *Start* for the next factor[78]

1.8.2.2   PCR EQUATION AND ALGORITHM

The aim of PCR is to predict the values of Y by extracting intrinsic effects in the data matrix X. PCR is the combination of PCA and MLR. First, PCA is carried out which yields a loading matrix P and score matrix T as described earlier. The PCA scores are inherently uncorrelated and are utilized for the generation of the MLR model.[80] The selection of relevant effects for MLR in PCR can be quite a difficult task. A straightforward approach is to take those PCA scores which have a variance above the certain threshold. The regression model can be optimized by varying the number of principal components. However, if the relevant effects are rather small compared with the irrelevant effect, they will not include in first few principal components. This problem can be solved by applying PLS regression method.[81]

1.8.2.2.1   PCR MODEL EQUATION

The general form of the PCR model is:

$$X = T.P^T + E \text{ and } y = T.b + f \tag{25}$$

The decomposition of the X matrix is carried out using PCA and the b-coefficients are calculated using MLR.

1.8.2.2.2   PCR ALGORITHM

PCR is performed as a two-step operation:
1.   First X is decomposed by PCA, see PCA Algorithm.
2.   Then the principal components regression is obtained by regressing y on the $\hat{t}$'s.

A PCR of J different Y-variable on K X-variables is equal to J separate PCR on the same K X-variables (one for each Y-variable). Thus we here only give attention to the case of one single Y-variable, y.

The principal component regression is obtained by regressing y on the $\hat{t}$'s obtained from the PCA of X. the regression coefficients for each y can be calculated according to equation

$$\hat{b} = \hat{p}(\text{diag}(1/\hat{T}_a) \tag{26}$$

Where X-loadings

$$\hat{p} = (\hat{p}_{ka}, k = 1,2,\ldots,K \text{ and } a = 1,2,\ldots, A) \tag{27}$$

represent the PCA loadings of the A factors employed, and Y-loadings

$$\hat{q} = (\hat{q}_1, \ldots\ldots\ldots, \hat{q}_A)' \tag{28}$$

are found the usual way by least squares regression of y on $\hat{T}$ from the model $y = Tq+f$.

Since the scores in $\hat{T}$ are uncorrelated, this solution is equal to

$$\hat{b} = (diag(1/\hat{T}a))^{-1}\hat{T}'_a y \tag{29}$$

Inserting this in (26) and replacing $\hat{T}$ by $X\hat{P}$, the PCR estimate of b can be written as

$$\hat{b} = \hat{P}(diag(1/\hat{T}a))^{-1}\hat{T}'aX'y \tag{30}$$

which is frequently used as definition of the PCR.

When the number of factors A equals K, the PCR gives the same $\hat{b}$ as the MLR. But the X-variables are often intercorrelated and somewhat noisy, then the optimal A is less than K:

In such cases MLR would imply division by eigenvalues n values $\hat{T}a$ close to zero, which makes the MLR estimate of b unstable. In contrast, PCR achieves a stabilized estimation of b by dropping such unreliable eigenvalues.

1.8.3   PARTIAL LEAST SQUARES

PLS is often used as the regression method in QSAR model development. There are some extra advantages of PLS such as it is less influenced by noise, more stable, increased the predictability, and improved the interpretation of the results compared to other methods (e.g., PCR, LDA), insensitive to colinearity among the predictor variables; however, in addition it allows to handle data sets where the number of variables is larger than the number of observations.[81] PLS is able to examine complex structure–activity problems to analyze data in a more real-istic way, and to interpret how molecular structure influences biological activity. The standard algorithm for computing PLS regression components (i.e., factors) are NIPALS. An alternative method for estimation of PLS components is the SIMPLS algorithm.[82]

1.8.3.1   PLS EQUATION AND ALGORITHMS (NIPALS)

PLS decomposes X and Y concurrently. It is divided into two types as listed hereunder:

- PLS2 is the most general and handles several Y-variables together and

- PLS1 is a simplification of the PLS algorithm made possible with only one Y-variable.

1.8.3.2   PLS MODEL EQUATION

The general form of the PLS model is:

$$X = T.P^T + E \text{ and } Y = T.B + F \tag{31}$$

1.8.3.3   PLS1 ALGORITHM

Orthogonalized PLSR algorithm for one Y-variable: PLS1
Calibration:
C 1 The scaled input variables **X** and y are first centered e.g.

$$X_0 = X - 1\bar{x} \quad \text{and} \quad Y_0 = Y - 1\bar{y} \tag{32}$$

Choose A_{max} to be higher than the number of phenomena expected in **X**. For each factor $a = 1,..., A_{max}$ perform steps **C 2.1 - C 2.5**:
C 2.1 Use the variability remaining in y to find the loading weights w_a, using LS and the local 'model'

$$X_{a-1} = y_{a-1} w_a' + E \tag{33}$$

and scale the vector to length 1. The solution is

$$\hat{w}_a = \chi\, X_{a-1}\, y_{a-1} \tag{34}$$

where c is the scaling factor that makes the length of the final $\hat{w}_a$ equal to 1

$$c = (ya\text{-}1' \, X_{a-1} \, X_{a-1}' \, y_{a-1})^{(-0.5)} \tag{35}$$

C 2.2 Estimate the scores t_a using the local 'model'

$$X_{a-1} = t_a \hat{w}_a' + E \tag{36}$$

this gives the solution

$$t_a = X_{a-1} \, \hat{w}_a \tag{37}$$

C 2.3 Estimate the loading p_a using the local 'model'

$$P_a = X_{a-1} \cdot t_a / t_a\, 't_a \tag{38}$$

C 2.4 Estimate the chemical loading q_a using the local 'model'

$$y_{a-1} = t_a q_a + f \tag{39}$$

this gives the solution

$$q_a = y'_{a-1} w_a / t_a' t_a \tag{40}$$

C 2.5 Create new **X** and **y** residuals by subtracting the estimated effect of this factor:

$$\hat{E} = X_{a-1} - t_a p_a \tag{41}$$

$$f = y_{a-1} - t_a q_a \tag{42}$$

Replace the former $Xa{-}1$ and $ya{-}1$ by the new residuals _ E and _f and increase a by 1, i.e.
Set

$$X_a = \hat{E} \tag{43}$$

$$y_a = f \tag{44}$$

$$a = a + 1 \tag{45}$$

C 3 Determine A, the number of valid PLS factors to retain in the calibration model.

C 4 Compute b_0 and b for A PLS factors, to be used in the predictor $y = 1b_0 + Xb$

$$b = \hat{W}(P\,\hat{W})^{-1} q \tag{46}$$

$$b_0 = \bar{y} - \bar{x}'b \tag{47}$$

PREDICTION:

Full prediction

For each new prediction object $i = 1,2,...$ perform steps P1 to P3, or, step P4.

P1 Scale input data x_i like for the calibration variables. Then compute

$$X_{i0}' = X_i' - \bar{X} \tag{48}$$

Where $\bar{X}$ is the center for the calibration objects.
For each factor $a = 1 \dots A$ perform steps **P 2.1 - P 2.2.**
P 2.1 Find $t_{i,\,a}$ according to the formula in **C 2.2** i.e.

$$t_{i,a} = X_{i,a-1} \ \hat{w}_a \tag{49}$$

P 2.2 Compute new residual

$$X_{i,a} = X_{i,a-1} - t_{i,a} p'_a \tag{50}$$

If $a < A$, increase a by 1 and go to **P 2.1**. If $a = A$, go to **P 3**.
P 3 Predict y_i

$$yi = \bar{y} + \sum_{a-1}^{A} t_{i,a} q_a \tag{51}$$

SHORT PREDICTION

P 4 Alternatively to steps P 1 - P 3, find $y\_$ by using b_0 and b in **C 4**, i.e.

$$y = 1b_0 + X_i \ b \tag{52}$$

Note that P and Q are not normalized. T and W are normalized to 1 and orthogonal.[84]

Cross validation is an approach for selecting which model, among several with different levels of complexity, is most likely to have high predictive value. It is particularly useful in PLS, to establish the number of components which optimally distinguish signal from noise. It substitutes computational power for the theoretical assumptions about data distributions in contrast with classical statistical techniques such as the F-test. It involves omitting one or more rows of input data, rederiving the model, and predicting the target property values of the omitted rows. The rederivation and prediction cycle continues until all target property values have been predicted exactly once. The root mean square error of all target predictions, the prediction error sum of squares (PRESS), is the basis for evaluating the current model.[85]

Cross validation is a widely used technique to explore the predictive ability of statistical models. The formulas used to calculate the aforementioned statistics are presented hereunder:

$$R^2_{LOO}(Q2) = 1 - \frac{PRESS}{SSY} \tag{53}$$

$$R^2_{LOO}(Q2) = 1 - \frac{\sum_{i=n}^{n} \left(y_i - \hat{y}_{i,LOO} \right)^2}{\sum_{i=n}^{n} \left(y_i - \hat{y}_{tr} \right)^2} \tag{54}$$

$$SEP = \sqrt{\frac{PRESS}{n}} \qquad (55)$$

where $\hat{\bar{y}}_{i,LOO}$ is the averaged value of the dependent variable for the training set; $\hat{y}_{i,LOO}$ is the measured values of the dependent variable over the available training set; $\hat{y}_{i,LOO}$ is the predicted values of the dependent variable over the available training set; R^2_{LOO}(Q2) is the cross validated correlation coefficient; SEP is the standard error of prediction; and PRESS is the prediction error sum of squares, which is the square difference between the predicated and measured activity of test set molecule.[85]

1.9 CONCLUSIONS

We have provided an overview and recent developments in QSAR methodologies, features selection technique, model generation, and validation methods. Since each QSAR method has its own benefits and drawbacks, researchers may select the suitable method for modeling their systems. However, given a wide range of choices, it is a challenging task to pick the appropriate models for one's studies. This chapter outlines many basic principles of QSAR methods as well as some algorithms which may be useful to many researchers to understand the statistical basis involved in QSAR model development and validation.

KEYWORDS

- **Fragment-based QSAR**
- **Molecular Descriptor**
- **nD-QSAR**
- **QSAR**
- **QSPR**

REFERENCES

1. Brown, C. A.; Fraser, T. R. Art. XXVIII.-on the connection between chemical constitution and physiological action. Part I. On the physiological action of the salts of the ammonium bases, derived from Strychnia, Brucia, Thebaia, Codeia, Morphia, and Nicotia. *Am. J. Med. Sci.* **1870,***58* (118), 502–505.

2. Abraham, D. J. *Burger's medicinal chemistry and drug discovery.* Wiley Online Library: 2003.
3. Vedani, A.; Dobler, M.; Lill, M. A. The challenge of predicting drug toxicity *in silico. Basic Clin. Pharm. Toxicol.* **2006,***99* (3), 195–208.
4. Lipnick, R. L. Narcosis: fundamental and baseline toxicity mechanism for nonelectrolyte organic chemicals. *Practical Applications of Quantitative Structure-Activity Relationships (QSAR) in Environmental Chemistry and Toxicology* **1990,***1*.
5. Borman, S. New QSAR techniques eyed for environmental assessments. *Chem. Eng. News* **1990,***68* (8), 20–23.
6. Connor, J. A.; Overton, C. Substituted 2, 2'-bipyridines as ligands. preparation and characterization of 4, 4'-disubstituted 2, 2'-bipyridine derivatives of the hexacarbonyls of chromium, molybdenum and tungsten. *J. Organomet. Chem.* **1983,***249* (1), 165–174.
7. Selassie, C. D. *History of quantitative structure-activity relationships.* 2003; Vol. 1.
8. Lipnick, R. L.; Filov, V. A. Nikolai Vasilyevich Lazarev, toxicologist and pharmacologist, comes in from the cold. *Trends Pharmacol. Sci.* **1992,***13*, 56–60.
9. Richet, C. On the relationship between the toxicity and the physical properties of substances. *Compt Rendus Seances Soc Biol* **1893,***9*, 775–776.
10. Deamer, D. W.; Kleinzeller, A.; Fambrough, D. M. *Membrane permeability: 100 years since Ernest Overton.* Academic Press: 1999; Vol. 48.
11. Ferguson, J. The use of chemical potentials as indices of toxicity. *Proc. Roy. Soc. London. Series B, Biol. Sci.* **1939,***127* (848), 387–404.
12. Hammett, L. P. The effect of structure upon the reactions of organic compounds. Benzene derivatives. *J. Am. Chem. Soc.* **1937,***59* (1), 96–103.
13. Matsui, T.; Ko, H. C.; Hepler, L. G. Thermodynamics of ionization of benzoic acid and substituted benzoic acids in relation to the Hammett equation. *Canadian J. Chem.* **1974,***52* (16), 2906–2911.
14. Kamlet, M. J.; Abboud, J. L.; Taft, R. The solvatochromic comparison method. 6. The. pi.* scale of solvent polarities. *J. Am. Chem. Soc.* **1977,***99* (18), 6027–6038.
15. Swain, C. G.; Lupton, E. C. Field and resonance components of substituent effects. *J. Am. Chem. Soc.* **1968,***90* (16), 4328–4337.
16. Free, S. M.; Wilson, J. W. A mathematical contribution to structure-activity studies. *J. Med. Chem.* **1964,***7* (4), 395–399.
17. Gao, H.; Lien, E. J.; Wang, F. Hydrophobicity of oligopeptides having un-ionizable side chains. *J. Drug Target.* **1993,***1* (1), 59–66.
18. Hansch, C.; Maloney, P. P.; Fujita, T.; Muir, R. M. Correlation of biological activity of phenoxyacetic acids with Hammett substituent constants and partition coefficients. **1962,***194*, 178–180.
19. Hansch, C.; Fujita, T. p-σ-π Analysis. A method for the correlation of biological activity and chemical structure. *J. Am. Chem. Soc.* **1964,***86* (8), 1616–1626.
20. Prabhakar, Y. S.; Gupta, M. K. Chemical structure indices in *in silico* molecular design. *Sci. Pharm.* **2008,***76*, 101–132.
21. Cramer, R. D.; Patterson, D. E.; Bunce, J. D. Comparative molecular field analysis (CoMFA). 1. Effect of shape on binding of steroids to carrier proteins. *J. Am. Chem. Soc.* **1988,***110* (18), 5959–5967.
22. Lowis, D. R. HQSAR: a new, highly predictive QSAR technique. *Tripos Tech. Notes* **1997,***1* (5), 1–15.
23. Du, Q. S.; Huang, R. B.; Wei, Y. T.; Pang, Z. W.; Du, L. Q.; Chou, K. C. Fragment-based quantitative structure–activity relationship (FB-QSAR) for fragment-based drug design. *J. Comput. Chem.* **2009,***30* (2), 295–304.

24. Myint, K. Z.; Xie, X.-Q. Recent advances in fragment-based QSAR and multi-dimensional QSAR methods. *Int. J. Mol. Sci.* **2010,***11* (10), 3846–3866.

25. Gangwal, R. P.; Bhadauriya, A.; Damre, M. V.; Dhoke, G. V.; Sangamwar, A. T. p38 Mitogen-activated protein kinase inhibitors: a review on pharmacophore mapping and QSAR studies. *Curr. Top. Med. Chem.* **2013,***13* (9), 1015–1035.

26. Klebe, G.; Abraham, U.; Mietzner, T. Molecular similarity indices in a comparative analysis (CoMSIA) of drug molecules to correlate and predict their biological activity. *J. Med. Chem.* **1994,***37* (24), 4130–4146.

27. Dudek, A. Z.; Arodz, T.; Galvez, J. Computational methods in developing quantitative structure-activity relationships (QSAR): a review. *Comb. Chem. High Throughput Screen.* **2006,***9* (3), 213–228.

28. Cramer, R. D.; Cruz, P.; Stahl, G.; Curtiss, W. C.; Campbell, B.; Masek, B. B.; Soltanshahi, F. Virtual screening for r-groups, including predicted pIC50 contributions, within large structural databases, using topomer CoMFA. *J. Chem. Inf. Model.* **2008,***48* (11), 2180–2195.

29. Ambure, P. S.; Gangwal, R. P.; Sangamwar, A. T. 3D-QSAR and molecular docking analysis of biphenyl amide derivatives as p38α mitogen-activated protein kinase inhibitors. *Mol. Divers.* **2012,***16* (2), 377–388.

30. Cramer, R. D. Topomer CoMFA: a design methodology for rapid lead optimization. *J. Med. Chem.* **2003,***46* (3), 374–388.

31. Robinson, D. D.; Winn, P. J.; Lyne, P. D.; Richards, W. G. Self-organizing molecular field analysis: A tool for structure-activity studies. *J. Med. Chem.* **1999,***42* (4), 573–583.

32. Wagener, M.; Sadowski, J.; Gasteiger, J. Autocorrelation of molecular surface properties for modeling corticosteroid binding globulin and cytosolic Ah receptor activity by neural networks. *J. Am. Chem. Soc.* **1995,***117* (29), 7769–7775.

33. Silverman, B.; Platt, D. E. Comparative molecular moment analysis (CoMMA): 3D-QSAR without molecular superposition. *J. Med. Chem.* **1996,***39* (11), 2129–2140.

34. Todeschini, R.; Gramatica, P. New 3D molecular descriptors: the WHIM theory and QSAR applications. In *3D QSAR in drug design*, Springer: 2002; pp 355–380.

35. Todeschini, R.; Lasagni, M.; Marengo, E. New molecular descriptors for 2D and 3D structures. Theory. *J. Chemom.* **1994,***8* (4), 263–272.

36. Pastor, M.; Cruciani, G.; McLay, I.; Pickett, S.; Clementi, S. GRid-INdependent descriptors (GRIND): a novel class of alignment-independent three-dimensional molecular descriptors. *J. Med. Chem.* **2000,***43* (17), 3233–3243.

37. Hopfinger, A.; Wang, S.; Tokarski, J. S.; Jin, B.; Albuquerque, M.; Madhav, P. J.; Duraiswami, C. Construction of 3D-QSAR models using the 4D-QSAR analysis formalism. *J. Am. Chem. Soc.* **1997,***119* (43), 10509–10524.

38. Fischer, P. M. Computational chemistry approaches to drug discovery in signal transduction. *Biotechnol. J.* **2008,***3* (4), 452–470.

39. Vedani, A.; Dobler, M.; Lill, M. A. Combining protein modeling and 6D-QSAR. Simulating the binding of structurally diverse ligands to the estrogen receptor. *J. Med. Chem.* **2005,***48* (11), 3700–3703.

40. Vedani, A.; Dobler, M.; Zbinden, P. Quasi-atomistic receptor surface models: A bridge between 3-D QSAR and receptor modeling. *J. Am. Chem. Soc.* **1998,***120* (18), 4471–4477.

41. Kirkpatrick, S.; Gelatt, C.; Vecchi, M. IBM Research Report RC 9355. **1982**.

42. Kirkpatrick, S.; Jr., D. G.; Vecchi, M. P. Optimization by simmulated annealing. *Science* **1983,***220* (4598), 671–680.

43. Černý, V. Thermodynamical approach to the traveling salesman problem: an efficient simulation algorithm. *J. Optimiz. Theory App.* **1985,***45* (1), 41–51.

44. Hasegawa, K.; Miyashita, Y.; Funatsu, K. GA Strategy for variable selection in QSAR studies: GA-based PLS analysis of calcium channel antagonists-. *J. Chem. Inf. Comput. Sci.* **1997,***37* (2), 306–310.

45. Lucasius, C. B.; Kateman, G. Understanding and using genetic algorithms Part 1. Concepts, properties and context. *Chemom. Intell. Lab. Syst.* **1993,***19* (1), 1–33.
46. Ozdemir, M.; Embrechts, M. J.; Arciniegas, F.; Breneman, C. M.; Lockwood, L.; Bennett, K. P. In *Feature selection for in-silico drug design using genetic algorithms and neural networks*, Soft Computing in Industrial Applications, 2001. SMCia/01. Proceedings of the 2001 IEEE Mountain Workshop on, IEEE: 2001; pp 53-57.
47. Qi Lin, W.; Hui Jiang, J.; Long Wu, H.; Shen, G.-L.; Qin Yu, R. Recent advances in chemometric methodologies for QSAR studies. *Curr. Comput.-Aided Drug Des.* **2006,***2* (3), 255–266.
48. Kovalishyn, V. V.; Tetko, I. V.; Luik, A. I.; Kholodovych, V. V.; Villa, A. E.; Livingstone, D. J. Neural network studies. 3. Variable selection in the cascade-correlation learning architecture. *J. Chem. Inf. Comput. Sci.* **1998,***38* (4), 651–659.
49. Tetko, I. V.; Villa, A. E.; Livingstone, D. J. Neural network studies. 2. Variable selection. *J. Chem. Inf. Comput. Sci.* **1996,***36* (4), 794–803.
50. Kubiny, H. Variable selection in QSAR studies. I. An evolutionary algorithm. *Quant. Struct.□ Act. Relat.* **1994,***13* (3), 285–294.
51. Bonabeau, E.; Dorigo, M.; Theraulaz, G. Inspiration for optimization from social insect behaviour. *Nature* **2000,***406* (6791), 39–42.
52. Eberhart, R.; Kennedy, J. In *A new optimizer using particle swarm theory*, Micro Machine and Human Science, 1995. MHS'95., Proceedings of the Sixth International Symposium on, IEEE: 1995; pp 39–43.
53. Shen, Q.; Jiang, J.-H.; Jiao, C.-X.; Shen, G.-l.; Yu, R.-Q. Modified particle swarm optimization algorithm for variable selection in MLR and PLS modeling: QSAR studies of antagonism of angiotensin II antagonists. *Eur. J. Pharm. Sci.* **2004,***22* (2), 145–152.
54. Deogun, J. S.; Choubey, S. K.; Raghavan, V. V.; Sever, H. Feature selection and effective classifiers. *J. Am. Soc. Inf. Sci.* **1998,***49* (5), 423–434.
55. Xie, H.-P.; Jiang, J.-H.; Cui, H.; Shen, G.-L.; Yu, R.-Q. A new redundant variable pruning approach—minor latent variable perturbation–PLS used for QSAR studies on anti-HIV drugs. *Comput. Chem.* **2002,***26* (6), 591–600.
56. Prabhakar, Y. S. A combinatorial approach to the variable selection in multiple linear regression: analysis of Selwood *et al.,* data set–a case study. *QSAR Comb. Sci.* **2003,***22* (6), 583–595.
57. Gupta, M. K.; Prabhakar, Y. S. Topological descriptors in modeling the antimalarial activity of 4-(3', 5'-disubstituted anilino) quinolines. *J. Chem. Inf. Model.* **2006,***46* (1), 93–102.
58. Nicolotti, O.; Gillet, V. J.; Fleming, P. J.; Green, D. V. Multiobjective optimization in quantitative structure-activity relationships: Deriving accurate and interpretable QSARs. *J. Med. Chem.* **2002,***45* (23), 5069–5080.
59. Whitley, D. C.; Ford, M. G.; Livingstone, D. J. Unsupervised forward selection: a method for eliminating redundant variables. *J. Chem. Inf. Comput. Sci.* **2000,***40* (5), 1160–1168.
60. Smith, P. A.; Sorich, M. J.; McKinnon, R. A.; Miners, J. O. Pharmacophore and quantitative structure-activity relationship modeling: complementary approaches for the rationalization and prediction of UDP-glucuronosyltransferase 1A4 substrate selectivity. *J. Med. Chem.* **2003,***46* (9), 1617–1626.
61. Fröhlich, H.; Wegner, J. K.; Zell, A. Towards optimal descriptor subset selection with support vector machines in classification and regression. *QSAR Comb. Sci.* **2004,***23* (5), 311–318.
62. Byvatov, E.; Schneider, G. SVM-based feature selection for characterization of focused compound collections. *J. Chem. Inf. Comput. Sci.* **2004,***44* (3), 993–999.
63. Liu, S.-S.; Liu, H.-L.; Yin, C.-S.; Wang, L.-S. VSMP: a novel variable selection and modeling method based on the prediction. *J. Chem. Inf. Comput. Sci.* **2003,***43* (3), 964–969.
64. Breiman, L. Random forests. *Mach. Learn.* **2001,***45* (1), 5–32.
65. Breiman, L. Bagging predictors. *Mach. Learn.* **1996,***24* (2), 123–140.

66. Breiman, L.; Friedman, J. H.; Olshen, R. A.; Stone, C. J. *Classification and regression trees.* Wadsworth & Brooks. *Monterey, CA* **1984**.

67. Li, S.; Fedorowicz, A.; Singh, H.; Soderholm, S. C. Application of the random forest method in studies of local lymph node assay based skin sensitization data. *J. Chem. Inf. Model.* **2005,***45* (4), 952–964.

68. Mercader, A. G.; Duchowicz, P. R.; Fernández, F. M.; Castro, E. A. Replacement method and enhanced replacement method versus the genetic algorithm approach for the selection of molecular descriptors in QSPR/QSAR theories. *J. Chem. Inf. Model.* **2010,***50* (9), 1542–1548.

69. Rogers, D.; Hopfinger, A. J. Application of genetic function approximation to quantitative structure-activity relationships and quantitative structure-property relationships. *J. Chem. Inf. Comput. Sci.* **1994,***34* (4), 854–866.

70. Hasegawa, K.; Funatsu, K. GA strategy for variable selection in QSAR studies: GAPLS and D-optimal designs for predictive QSAR model. *J. Mol. Struct.* **1998,***425* (3), 255–262.

71. Goodford, P. Multivariate characterization of molecules for QSAR analysis. *J. Chemom.* **1996,***10* (2), 107–117.

72. Stone, M.; Jonathan, P. Statistical thinking and technique for QSAR and related studies. Part I: General theory. *J. Chemom.* **1993,***7* (6), 455–475.

73. Kubinyi, H. QSAR and 3D QSAR in drug design Part 1: methodology. *Drug Discov. Today* **1997,***2* (11), 457–467.

74. Liu, S.-S.; Yin, C.-S.; Wang, L.-S. Combined MEDV-GA-MLR method for QSAR of three panels of steroids, dipeptides, and COX-2 inhibitors. *J. Chem. Inf. Comput. Sci.* **2002,***42* (3), 749–756.

75. Everitt, B. S. *The Cambridge Dictionary of Statistics.* CUP, 2002. ISBN 0-521-81099-X.

76. Luco, J. M.; Ferretti, F. H. QSAR based on multiple linear regression and PLS methods for the anti-HIV activity of a large group of HEPT derivatives. *J. Chem. Inf. Comput. Sci.* **1997,***37* (2), 392–401.

77. Eriksson, L.; Johansson, E. Multivariate design and modeling in QSAR. *Chemom. Intell. Lab. Syst.* **1996,***34* (1), 1–19.

78. Mevik, B.-H.; Wehrens, R. The pls package: principal component and partial least squares regression in R. *J. Stat. Softw.* **2007,***18* (2), 1–24.

79. Risvik, H. Principal component analysis (PCA) & NIPALS algorithm. 2007.

80. Hwang, J. G.; Nettleton, D. Principal components regression with data chosen components and related methods. *Technometrics* **2003,***45* (1), 70–79.

81. Maitra, S.; Yan, J. *Principle component analysis and partial least squares: two dimension reduction techniques for regression.* 2008; p 79–90.

82. Geladi, P.; Kowalski, B. R. Partial least-squares regression: a tutorial. *Anal. Chim. Acta* **1986,***185*, 1–17.

83. Wold, S.; Johansson, E.; Cocchi, M. PLS—partial least squares projections to latent structures. *3D QSAR in drug design* **1993,***1*, 523–550.

84. Abdi, H. Partial least squares regression and projection on latent structure regression (PLS Regression). *WIREs. Comp. Stats.* **2010,***2* (1), 97–106.

85. Shao, J. Linear model selection by cross-validation. *J. Am. Stat. Assoc.* **1993,***88* (422), 486–494.

CHAPTER 2

SOFTWARE AND WEB RESOURCES FOR COMPUTER-AIDED MOLECULAR MODELING AND DRUG DISCOVERY

DHARMENDRA K. YADAV[1*], REETA RAI[2], RAMENDRA PRATAP[1], and HARPREET SINGH[3]

[1]Department of Chemistry, University of Delhi, North campus, Delhi-110007

[2]Department of Biochemistry, All India Institute of Medical sciences, New Delhi-110029

[3]Department of Bioinformatics, Indian Council of Medical Research, New Delhi-110029

* Corresponding Author: Department of Chemistry, North campus, University of Delhi-110007; Tel.: +91 11 27666646 Ext. (178); E-mail: dharmendra30oct@gmail.com

CONTENTS

ABSTRACT

Computer-aided molecular modeling and drug design plays a crucial role in drug discovery and has become an essential tool in the pharmaceutical industry. This chapter covers the available web resource tools and *in silico* techniques used in virtual screening (VS) and drug discovery processes to reduce the wet lab economy and time. Computational chemists can use these tools/databases and web resources in the molecular modeling and drug designing field for the purposes of discovering new leads. However, in spite of despite wet lab experiments, application of molecular docking, quantitative structure–activity relationship, and absorption, distribution, metabolism, and excretion /toxicity studies used in the prediction of VS and biological evaluation are proving beneficial in drug discovery process. This chapter covers drug design software and resources related to drug discovery approaches, with special importance on structure- and ligand-based drug design, chemoinformatics tools, and chemical databases.

2.1 INTRODUCTION

Currently, drug design and development is driven by the modernization and knowledge of a combination of experimental and computational approaches. The mechanism of action of target protein and its structural interaction with potential drugs is fundamental in this approach [1, 2]. The process starts with consideration of a hypothesis where the structural features of a series of compounds and their biological activity are correlated. Without a complete understanding of the biochemical processes responsible for activity, the hypothesis is generally refined by examining structural similarities and differences for active and inactive molecules. This is followed by selection of compounds on the basis of functional groups, which are responsible for their activity. The physico-chemical properties (total energy, dipole movement, steric energy, binding affinity, etc.) of the compounds represent their biological activity. Rational drug design and development process through *in silico* approaches aim at thoroughly studying the biological activity of a broad range of small molecules on a wide range of macromolecular targets [3]. A number of computational approaches is used worldwide in drug discovery process, that is, similarity searching, molecular modeling, pharmacophores, quantitative structure–activity relationship (QSAR) models, data mining, machine learning, drug discovery databases, and network and data analysis tools that use computers and intellectuals. These methods have also been used in optimization of unknown compounds' target identification, clarification of absorption, distribution, metabolism, excretion, and toxicity properties as well as physico-chemical characterization. Currently, these *in silico* approaches are used for virtual ligands and target-based high throughput through virtual screening (VS) to predict biological activity of new derivatives without experimental analysis.

Because the size of the existing data and of the new compounds produced is too large for manual manipulation, information technologies here play a crucial role in planning, analyzing, and predicting these biochemical data. This focus of this chapter is on different predictive *in silico* approaches and recently used web resources in drug design and discovery process. Chemoinformatics and bioinformatics tools help in the identification of complementary leads and targets. These approaches facilitate lead discovery against individual targets using molecular docking, [2, 3] pharmacophores, [4] quantitative or qualitative "structure–activity" relationships, and machine learning methods [4, 5].

Combinatorial approaches straightforwardly conduct parallel searches against each individual target to find virtual hits that simultaneously interact with multiple targets. Bioinformatics and systems biology approaches are becoming increasingly important along with the above mentioned chemoinformatics methods to study the therapeutic potential of medicinal plants [6]. These approaches are used to select targets for docking studies, and to identify relationships between the revealed actions of phytochemical targets and the known therapeutic effects of medicinal plants. Thus, another aim of this chapter is a critical consideration of the various available databases and *in silico* tools for their utilization in new computer-aided molecular modeling and drug discovery processes based on their worldwide usage.

2.2 DRUGS DISCOVERY

Most drugs are discovered by the following methods:
1. By natural products
2. By chance
3. By structure–activity relationships
4. By rational drug design
5. By systematic screening

However, drug discovery process involves the following six steps:
1. Disease selection
2. Target hypothesis
3. Lead identification
4. Lead optimization
5. Preclinical trial
6. Clinical trial

Combinatorial chemistry systematically and repetitively yields a large collection of compounds from sets of different types of reagents called "building block" [4–6]. For this reason, varieties of structural processing technologies for a diversity of analysis were created and applied. These types of computational methods are known as cheminformatics [6]. Natural sources of secondary metabolites are found through high-throughput screening (HTS) methods as shown in **Table 1–2**. A type of web resources related to drug designing and drug discovery is the structural databases of small molecules. It has been observed that many drug-like compounds—which should be potential candidates—do not come up as hits when they are screened against biological targets. It is believed that further refinement of the filtering technologies should be made in order to recognize lead-like compounds instead of drug-like compounds. Intrinsically, lead-likeness and drug-likeness are descriptors of potency, selectivity, absorption, distribution, metabolism, toxicity, and scalability. Moreover, conventional methodology takes years to discover new compounds and is much more expensive. Therefore, efforts must be made to reduce the economic burden and time of research during wet lab experiments by using computer-aided molecular modeling. Rational drug designing methods improve the drug pipeline and weed out candidates early in the process; thus discovering bad candidates as soon as possible in order to reduce costs.

TABLE 1   Databases related to chemical compounds

S. No.	Database	Description	URL
1.	ChEBI	Chemical entities of biological interest	http://www.ebi.ac.uk/chebi/
2.	ChEMBL	Database of bioactive drug-like small molecules	https://www.ebi.ac.uk/chembl/
3.	CSD (Cambridge structural database)	World repository of 500,000 small molecule crystal structures. Crystal structure information for organic and metal-organic compounds	http://www.ccdc.cam.ac.uk/prods/csd/csd.html
4.	ChemBank	Database of small molecules and small-molecule screens	http://chembank.broadinstitute.org/
5.	HIC-Up	Hetero-compound Information Centre – Uppsala. Freely accessible resource for structural biologists who are dealing dealing with hetero-compounds.	http://xray.bmc.uu.se/hicup

TABLE 1   (*Continued*)

6.	AANT	Amino acid–nucleotide interaction database	http://aant.icmb.utexas.edu/
7.	KEGG LI-GAND	Database consisting of COMPOUND, GLYCAN, REACTION, RPAIR, RCLASS, and ENZYME	http://www.genome.jp/ligand/
8.	Klotho	Collection and categorization of biological compounds	http://www.biocheminfo.org/klotho
9.	ChEBI	Chemical entities of biological interest	http://www.ebi.ac.uk/chebi/
10.	ChEMBL	Database of bioactive drug-like small molecules	https://www.ebi.ac.uk/chembl/
11.	CSD (Cambridge structural database)	World repository of 500,000 small molecule crystal structures. Crystal structure information for organic and metal-organic compounds	http://www.ccdc.cam.ac.uk/prods/csd/csd.html
12.	ChemBank	Database of small molecules and small-molecule screens	http://chembank.broadinstitute.org/
13.	HIC-Up	Hetero-compound Information Centre – Uppsala	http://xray.bmc.uu.se/hicup
		Freely accessible resource for structural biologists who are dealing dealing with hetero-compounds	
14.	ACD	Available Chemicals Directory: Chemical sourcing database or CAP (chemicals available for purchase)	http://www.mdli.com/products/experiment/available_chem_dir/index.jsp
			http://accelrys.com/products/
15.	ASINEX	Lead generation and lead optimization	http://www.asinex.com/
16.	Bionet Database	Screening compounds database	http://www.keyorganics.ltd.uk/scdownloads.htm
17.	ChemDB (UCI)	Chemical dataset	http://cdb.ics.uci.edu/CHEMWeb/
18.	ChemStar	Provides synthetic organic dompounds for HTS, building blocks for combinatorial chemistry, custom synthesis, preplated library, virtual database	http://www.chemstar.ru/en/

TABLE 1 (*Continued*)

19.	Peptaibol	Peptaibol (antibiotic peptide) sequences	http://www.cryst.bbk.ac.uk/peptaibol/welcome.html
20.	APD	Antimicrobial peptide database	http://aps.unmc.edu/AP/main.php
21.	DART	Drug adverse reaction target database	http://xin.cz3.nus.edu.sg/group/drt/dart.asp
22.	MetaRouter	Compounds and pathways related to bioremediation	http://pdg.cnb.uam.es/MetaRouter
23.	LIGAND	Chemical compounds and reactions in biological pathways	http://www.genome.ad.jp/ligand/
24.	PDB-Ligand	3D structures of small molecules bound to proteins and nucleic acids	http://www.idrtech.com/PDB-Ligand/
25.	PubChem	Structures and biological activities of small organic molecules	http://pubchem.ncbi.nlm.nih.gov/
26.	ZINC	Database of commercially available compounds for VS	http://zinc.docking.org/
27.	IBS	Inter Biosceen Database: Chemical library for screening	http://www.ibscreen.com/
28.	Maybridge Database	Designs and produces innovative chemical building blocks and screening compounds, and provides medicinal chemistry for the drug discovery industry	http://www.maybridge.com/
29.	ChemSpider	Providing access to millions of chemical structures. It is the richest single source of structure-based chemistry information and an invaluable source of spectral information	http://www.chemspider.com/
30.	BindingDB	Database of measured binding affinities, focusing chiefly on the interactions of protein considered to be drug targets with small, drug-like molecules. BindingDB contains 648,915 binding data, for 5,662 protein targets and 284,206 small molecules	http://www.bindingdb.org/bind/index.jsp

TABLE 1   (*Continued*)

31.	CoCoCo	Suite of molecular databases for high throughput VS purposes. It collects molecular structural information of commercial compounds.	http://cococo.unimore.it/tiki-index.php
32.	ChemBioFinder	Suite of databases provided by Cambridgesoft, there being about 500,000 compounds indexed from a variety of databases	http://chembiofinder.cambridgesoft.com/chembiofinder/SimpleSearch.aspx
33.	MDPI	Molecular Diversity Preservation International: compounds database	http://www.mdpi.org/cumbase.htm
34.	MSDchem	Consistent and enriched library of ligands, small molecules, and monomers that are referred to as residues and hetgroups in any protein data bank entry	http://www.ebi.ac.uk/msd-srv/chempdb/cgi-bin/cgi.pl
35.	Relibase (CCDC)	Ligand overlays and binding mode comparisons	http://relibase.ccdc.cam.ac.uk/
36.	SPRESI database	Containing over 6.1 million molecules, 3.85 million reactions, 636,000 references, and 164,000 patents	http://www.spresi.com/
37.	eMolecules	Search over 8.0 million unique chemical structures	http://www.emolecules.com/
38.	MDDR (MDL Drug Data Report)	Database covering the patent literature, journals, meetings, and congresses	http://www.mdl.com/products/knowledge/drug_data_report/index.jsp
39.	FDA (Food and Drug Administration) Drug	List of drugs approved by the FDA	http://www.centerwatch.com/patient/drugs/druglsal.html
40.	Accelrys databases	Accelrys chemical sourcing, synthesis, and bioactivity database	http://accelrys.com/
41.	MedChem	Database contains compounds with names and CAS numbers, log P values, pKa values, activities, and Rubicon 3D coordinates	http://www.daylight.com/products/medchem.html

TABLE 1   (*Continued*)

42.	WDI (World Drug Index)	Drug database of almost 80,000 drugs and pharmacologically active compounds, including all marketed drugs	http://www.daylight.com/products/wdi.html
43.	CHEMnet-BASE	Dictionary of drug	http://www.chemnetbase.com/
44.	DrugBank	Combined information on drugs and drug targets	http://www.drugbank.ca/
45.	Drug@FDA	Information about FDA approved drug products	http://www.accessdata.fda.gov/scripts/cder/drugsatfda/
46.	NCI Drug Dictionary	Contains technical definitions and synonyms for drugs/agents used to treat patients with cancer or conditions related to cancer	http://www.cancer.gov/drug-dictionary/
47.	Rx List	The Internet drug list	http://www.rxlist.com/drugs/alpha_a.htm
48.	ANTIMIC	Database of natural antimicrobial peptides	http://research.i2r.a-star.edu.sg/Templar/DB/ANTIMIC/
49.	GLIDA	G-protein coupled receptors ligand database	http://gdds.pharm.kyoto-u.ac.jp:8081/glida/
50.	PharmGKB	Pharmacogenomics knowledge base: effect of genetic variation on drug responses. Integrated resource about how variation in human genetics leads to variation in response to drugs.	http://www.pharmgkb.org/
51.	SuperDrug	Two-dimensional (2D) and 3D chemical structures of drugs. Contains compounds with conformers	http://bioinformatics.charite.de/superdrug http://bioinf.charite.de/superdrug/
52.	SuperNatural	Natural compounds and their suppliers	http://bioinformatics.charite.de/supernatural
53.	CMC- MDL	CMC (Comprehensive Medicinal Chemistry) MDL	http://www.mdl.com/products/knowledge/medicinal_chem/index.jsp

TABLE 2   Molecular modeling and drug designing related web resource

S. No.	Resources	URL
1.	Structure-based drug design	http://www.biocryst.com/structure_baseddrugdesign.htm
2.	Structure based drug design and molecular modeling	http://www.imb-jena.de/~rake/Bio-informatics_WEB/dd_introduction.html
3.	Target based rational drug design	http://www.pharmacy.umaryland.edu/courses/PHAR531/lectures_old/compchem_1.html
4.	The drug discovery pipeline	http://www.newdrugdesign.com/Rachel_Theory_04.html
5.	The rational basis of drug design	http://www.rosalindfranklin.edu/cms/biochem/walters/walters_lect/walters_lect.html
6.	Designing a drug	http://www.louisville.edu/~mjwell04/design.html
7.	Docking and scoring	http://www.dddc.ac.cn/embo04/material/EMBO040921.ppt
8.	Drug design	http://www.chemsoc.org/exemplarchem/entries/2003/nottingham_russell/6.html
9.	Drug design	http://en.wikipedia.org/wiki/Drug_design
10.	Historical events—some events in the history of drugs	http://www.druglibrary.org/schaffer/History/histsum.htm
11.	Biocomputing and drug design	http://www.techfak.uni-bielefeld.de /bcd/ForAll/ Introd/ drugdesign.html#net
12.	Brief history of drugs	http://www.chamisamesa.net/drughist.html
13.	Computational techniques in the drug design	http://www.ccl.net/cca/documents/dyoung/topics-orig/drug.html
14.	Computers in drug design	http://www.cem.msu.edu/~parrill/design/drugdesign.html#drug
15.	QSAR and drug design	http://www.netsci.org/Science/Compchem/feature12.html
16.	Rational drug design	http://www.wellcome.ac.uk/en/genome/tacklingdisease/hg09b002.html

TABLE 1   (*Continued*)

17. Rationalizing combi-chem	http://pubs.acs.org/subscribe/journals/mdd/v05/i02/html/02lesney.html
18. Searching for new drugs in virtual molecule databases	http://www.ercim.org/publication/Ercim_News/enw43/rarey.html
19. Lead optimization solutions	http://www.chemdiv.com/test/optimization/
20. Lead optimization	http://www.metabolon.com/Metabolomic-Applications-Lead-Optimization.htm
21. Leads and target tissues	http://www.louisville.edu/~mjwell04/leads.htm
22. Molecular drug design (the robotics way)	http://www.cs.rpi.edu/~sakella/rmp03/presentations/1
23. QSAR	http://www.louisville.edu/~mjwell04/QSAR.htm

2.3   DRUG DESIGNING PROCESS

Drug designing process starts with the preparation of a library ranging from hundreds to thousands compounds from various sources, like nature, previous drug data, or from traditional remedies. These molecules are searched for drug-like properties. These steps start from virtual HTS followed by evaluating large chemical databases in order to identify potent drug candidates. A large data set of proposed potent drug candidates is used for screening, which is subjected to QSAR for decreasing the chances of selecting a wrong candidate by establishing the relationship between the structure and their activity. After screening, only a few compounds are left, which are further screened for their absorption, distribution, metabolism, and excretion (ADME) properties. Consequently, this further eliminates about one-third of the candidates, and leaves only the desired candidates [6]. **Figure 1** shows how different methods are used during drug designing process.

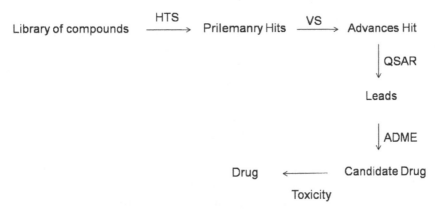

FIGURE 1   High throughput VS methods in drug design and development.

2.3.1   LEAD IDENTIFICATION

The first step in drug discovery is the search of a suitable lead compound that binds with the target protein showing good binding affinity. Most lead compounds are found by chance. However, they may come from many other sources, that is, identification of chemical compounds having certain biological activity, metabolic products, combinatorial chemistry techniques, chemical compound databases, and natural resources like bacteria, plants, species of marine biology, andBactria, and start from the natural ligand or modulator, enhancing a side effect as shown in **Table 2** [4–6]. Most of the pharmaceutical companies are using 384 and 1536-well multiple microtiter plate assay for screening of large number of compounds simultaneously. The varieties of fluorescent probes available that allow detection of substrates in the picomolar range assure that most positive hits will be observed. Some of the technologies used for the bioassay endpoints are enzyme-linked immunosorbent assay (ELISA), fluorescent-based calorimetric assays, and scintillation proximity assay (SPA). Most biological assays are based on affinity screening of small molecules to the target, using physical properties such as ultraviolet (UV) or fluorescence as the binding endpoint detection. Most tools will pass potential leads through various filters in an attempt to discard those hits that may fail based on an undesirable "druggability" profile through VS, nuclear magnetic resonance (NMR)-based screening, combinatorial chemistry, and pharmacophores mapping (cheminformatics) [7–11].

2.3.2 HIGH THROUGHPUT VS

To search the potential leads against a specific target using a computer is called "VS". VS technology uses high-throughput docking, homology searching, and pharmacophores searches of 3D databases [9–11]. Molecular docking simulations have the potential to save time and cost involved in identifying candidate drug leads that interact with potential active sites on target protein structures that are selected by their relevance in an indication and/or disease setting. VS to identify candidate drug leads using molecular docking simulations has significant limitations. Chief among them is the lack of integration of the vast amount of biological information available, which is being accumulated at a rate exceeding Moore's law and, therefore, outstripping current computer hardware capacity for storage and analysis. Such a vast amount of data provides a route to more successful homology-based prediction methodologies by learning from known biological information instead of trying to accurately model complex biological systems. Moreover, conventional docking approaches cannot predict binding interactions between all available biomolecular structures from one species against all of the available candidate small molecule drugs, in a computationally efficient manner. This significantly limits their use in identifying putative drugs in the modern genomics era of personalized medicine [12]. A key requirement for a successful VS is accession to a large and a diverse library or database as shown in **Table 3**. Databases of compounds with millions of small molecules are available commercially as well as on the Web for public use.

TABLE 3   Web resources related to VS database

S. No.	Database	Description	URL
1.	ChemID Plus	Allows users to search compound identifiers such as chemical name or CAS registry number on the NLM ChemIDplus database of over 370,000 chemicals	http://chem.sis.nlm.nih.gov/chemidplus/
2.	ChemBank	Allows users to search small compounds, assays, and proteins	http://chembank.broadinstitute.org/chemistry/search/
3.	ZINC	Contains over 8 million purchasable compounds in ready-to-dock, 3D formats	http://zinc.docking.org/
4.	IB Screen database	Chemical library for screening	http://www.ibscreen.com/

TABLE 3 (*Continued*)

5.	Maybridge Database	Designs and produces innovative chemical building blocks and screening compounds, and provides medicinal chemistry for the drug discovery industry	http://www.maybridge.com/default.aspx
6.	MDL SCD	Consolidated supplier catalogs for high-throughput screening	http://www.mdl.com/products/experiment/screening_compounds/index.jsp
7.	Bioscreening	Online searchable database of available compounds	http://www.bioscreening.com/Structure-Search.html
8.	TimTec	Synthetic organic compound library	http://www.timtec.net/screening-compound-libraries.html
9.	RPBS ADME Tox	ADME-Tox (poor absorption, distribution, metabolism, elimination [ADME] or toxicity) filtering for small compounds	http://bioserv.rpbs.jussieu.fr/RPBS/cgi-bin/Ressource.cgi?chzn_lg=an&chzn_rsrc=ADMETox
10.	PDB Chemical Search	Substructure search against 8,458 chemical compounds from PDB	http://www.ebi.ac.uk/msd-srv/msdmotif/chem/
11.	ChemDB	Chemical dataset	http://cdb.ics.uci.edu/CHEM/Web/
12.	Pharme	Free open source pharmacophore search technology that can search millions of chemical structures in seconds	http://smoothdock.ccbb.pitt.edu/pharmer/
13.	Catalyst	Pharmacophore modeling and analysis; 3D database building and searching; ligand conformer generation and analysis tools; geometric, descriptor-based querying; shape-based screening	http://accelrys.com/products/discovery-studio/pharmacophore.html
14.	ACPC	Open source tool for ligand based VS using autocorrelation of partial charges	https://github.com/UnixJunkie/ACPC/blob/master/README.md
15.	DecoyFinder	Graphical tool which helps finding sets of decoy molecules for a given group of active ligands	http://urvnutrigenomica-ctns.github.io/DecoyFinder/
16.	Corina	Generates 3D structures for small- and medium-sized, drug-like molecules. Distributed by molecular networks	http://www.molecular-networks.com/products/corina

TABLE 3   (*Continued*)

17.	PyRX	VSsoftware for computational drug discovery that can be used to screen libraries of compounds against potential drug targets	http://pyrx.sourceforge.net/
18.	MOLA	Free software for VSusing AutoDock4/Vina in a computer cluster using nondedicated multiplatform computers	http://www.esa.ipb.pt/bio-chemcore/index.php/ds/m
19.	Screen Suite	Ligand-based screening tool using fingerprints, 2D, and 3D descriptors	http://www.chemaxon.com/products/screen/
20.	MolSign	Program for pharmacophore identification and modeling. Can be used for querying databases as a pharmacophore-based search	http://www.vlifesciences.com/products/Functional_products/Molsign.php
21.	REDUCE	Tool to filter compounds from libraries using descriptors and functional groups. Part of the Molecular FORECASTER package	http://fitted.ca/
22.	QUASI	Generates pharmacophores and performs pharmacophore based VS. Distributed by De Novo Pharmaceuticals	http://www.denovopharma.com/page2.asp?PageID=485
23.	Tuplets	Pharmacophore based VS.	http://www.certara.com/products/molmod/sybyl-x/simpharm/
24.	VSDMIP	Virtual Screening Data Management on an Integrated Platform. Comes with a PyMOL graphical user interface.	http://ub.cbm.uam.es/software/vsdmip.php
25.	New Human GPCR modeling and virtual screening database	Web server to use the new human G-protein-coupled receptor (GPCR) modeling and VS database as well as a new function similarity detection algorithm to screen all human GPCRs against the ZINC8 nonredundant (TC<0.7) ligand set combined with ligands from the GLIDA database (a total of 88,949 compounds)	http://cssb.biology.gatech.edu/skolnick/webservice/gpcr/index.html

TABLE 3   (*Continued*)

26.	FINDSITE-COMB	Web service for large scale virtual ligand screening using a threading/structure-based FINDSITE-based approach.	http://cssb.biology.gatech.edu/FINDSITE-COMB

2.3.3   PHARMACOPHORE MODELING

The pharmacophore search finds molecules with overall different chemistries, which have the functional groups in the correct geometry. A reasonable qualitative prediction of binding can be made by specifying the spatial arrangement of a small number of atoms or functional groups. Such arrangement is called a pharmacophore. Pharmacophore modeling is one of the most powerful techniques to classify and identify key features from a group of molecules such as active and inactive compounds. Chemical features in the hypothesis or pharmacophore model will furnish a new insight to design novel molecules that can enhance or inhibit the function of the target and will be useful in drug discovery strategies. A pharmacophore is the ensemble of steric and electronic features that is necessary to ensure the optimal supramolecular interactions with a specific biological target structure and to trigger (or to block) its biological response. Pharmacophore mapping is one of the major elements of drug design in the absence of structural data of the target receptor. The tool initially applied to discovery of lead molecules, now extends to lead optimization. Pharmacophores can be used as queries for retrieving potential leads from structural databases (lead discovery), for designing molecules with specific desired attributes (lead optimization), and for assessing similarity and diversity of molecules using pharmacophore fingerprints. They can also be used to align molecules based on the 3D arrangement of chemical features or to develop predictive 3D QSAR models [13, 14].

2.3.4   COMBINATORIAL CHEMISTRY

The combinatorial chemistry is a concept that produces a large collection of potential chemical compounds, and then these combinatorial libraries are quickly evaluated to find a desirable property by using a technique known as virtual high throughput screening [15, 16]. As shown in **Figure 2**, a scaffold is employed that contains a portion of the molecules that remains constant. Subsite groups (shown in different shapes) are potential sites for derivatization. We can generate an enormous number of chemical compounds with this scaffold since it contains three sites of derivatization and the library contains 10 groups per site, and more than 1,000 diverse combinations are theoretically possible through this process. For these reasons, it is an important and powerful technique that chemists can use to aid in the modification of the lead compounds [14, 17–19].

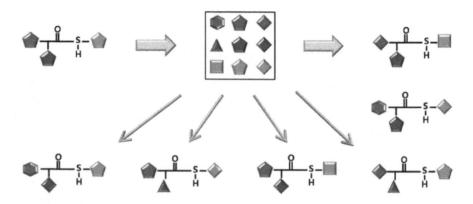

FIGURE 2   Development of compound library through combinatorial chemistry approaches.

2.3.5. LEAD IDENTIFICATION AND OPTIMIZATION

VS is a part of chemoinformatics and is used in lead identification. It involves protein structure based compound screening or docking and chemical-similarity search based on small molecules. Important features to be considered while developing a VS system are (1) knowledge about the compounds that you may screen against your receptor; (2) knowledge about the receptor structure and receptor–ligand interactions in general; and (3) standard knowledge about drugs and drug characteristics. These lead compounds undergo more extensive optimization in a subsequent step of drug discovery called lead optimization [20, 21]. The drug discovery process generally follows the following path that includes a hit to lead stage: target validation, assay development, HTS, hit to lead, lead optimization, preclinical drug development, and clinical drug development. Lead identification/optimization is one of the most important steps in drug development. The chemical structure of the lead compound is used as a starting point for chemical modifications in order to improve potency, selectivity, or pharmacokinetic parameters. Once a molecule is identified, the next step is to check its adsorption, distribution, metabolism, excretion, and toxicity (ADMET) properties. If the molecule has neither toxicity nor mutagenicity, then it has the potential for use as a lead molecule. Further optimization gives better quality of lead molecules. These may subsequently be developed as drug(s). Lead optimization is one of the major bottlenecks of the drug discovery process.

Chemical diversity integrates its wealth of organic, medicinal, and computational chemistry and its technological capabilities, to offer a platform for the most efficient lead optimization solution(s). This is possible by both wet lab and computationally predicted molecular structure to decide the side effect and activity of compounds [21, 22]. This type of technique is mostly used to improve the drug discovery process.

2.3.6 QSAR MODELING

More than 50 years have passed since the field of QSARs modeling was founded by Corwin Hansch [23]. More than 50 years of continuous improvements, interdisciplinary breakthroughs, and community-driven developments have contributed to make QSAR as one of the commonly employed approaches to model the physical and biological properties of chemicals in use. In the 1890s, Hans Horst Meyer from the University of Marburg and Charles Ernest Overton from the University of Zurich, working independently, noted that the toxicity of organic compounds depends on their lipophilicity. QSAR allows the use of statistics to lower the trial and error factor in drug designing [24, 25]. QSAR modeling is widely practiced in academy, industry, and government institutions around the world. Recent observations suggest that following years will be of strong dominance by the structure-based methods, the value of statistically based QSAR approaches in helping to guide lead optimization is starting to be appreciatively reconsidered by leaders of several larger computer-aided drug design (CADD) groups [26]. A growing trend is to use QSAR early in the drug discovery process as a screening and enrichment tool to estimate from further development those chemicals lacking drug-like properties or those chemicals predicted to elicit a toxic response. The fundamental assumption of QSAR is that variations in the biological activity of a series of chemicals that target a common mechanism of action are correlated with variations in their structural, physical, and chemical properties calculated through software as shown in **Table 4**. Structurally related properties of a chemical can be determined by experimental or computational means comparatively much more efficiently than its biological activity using in vivo or in vitro approaches. A statistically validated QSAR model is capable of predicting the biological activity of unknown chemical compounds of the same series and can be used before their synthesis and biological evaluation as shown in **Figure 3**. This involves the cooperation between different software modules within the data mining environment, such as quantum chemical calculation, molecular descriptor calculation, QSAR model development, and QSAR prediction [27]. For example, QSAR studies for the inhibition of inflammatory targets

(COX 2) by a series of aceclofenac, amodiaquine, aspirin, celecoxib, diclofenac, ibuprofen, mefenamic, naproxen, paramethasone, berberine, and indometacin were studied and statistical calculations were done by Scigress Explore. Correlation between the observed inhibition values and the calculated ones were found good enough statistically (r^2=0.857808, r^2_{CV}=0.76784). The obtained results were compared with those where the descriptors have been calculated with Scigress Explore 7.7 (CAChe). Mostly it would be better to consider the following classes of chemical structure descriptors while developing QSAR model based on the above descriptors. In this regard, as an example, development of a highly improved multiple linear regression QSAR model related to anti-inflammatory activity was successful by using activity data of known anti-inflammatory drugs as shown in Table 5.

Predicted anti-inflammatory = +0.167357 × Dipole vector × (debye)
activity log (LD_{50})   +0.00695659 × Steric energy (kcal/mole)

−0.00249368 × Heat of formation (kcal/mole)

+0.852125 × Size of smallest ring

−1.1211 × Group count (carboxyl)

−1.24227

$$[r^2CV=0.767 \text{ and } r^2=0.857]$$

where r^2 refers to regression coefficient as a parameter for showing correlation between activity and dependent variables, and r^2CV refers to cross validated regression coefficient as a parameter for prediction accuracy estimation of model. In the above example of QSAR model, dipole moment (debye), steric energy (kcal/mole), heat of formation (kcal/mole), size of smallest ring, and group count (carboxyl) are the dependent descriptors and thus are used in the regression equation as shown in **Table 5**. Cross-validation value indicates how well the equation might predict unknown molecules. Based on the calculation of descriptor values structural representations are derived. and dimensionally based methods of QSAR are categorized into the following classes:

1. 1D-QSAR correlating activity with global molecular properties like pKa, log P, and so on
2. 2D-QSAR correlating activity with structural patterns like connectivity indices, 2D-pharmacophores, without taking into account the 3D representation of these properties
3. 3D-QSAR correlating activity with noncovalent interaction fields surrounding the molecules
4. 4D-QSAR additionally including ensemble of ligand configurations in 3D-QSAR

5. 5D-QSAR explicitly representing different induced-fit models in 4D-QSAR

6. 6D-QSAR further incorporating different solvation models in 5D-QSAR

Linear regression analysis methods are the most easily interpretable among various statistical methods for QSAR. These regressions represent direct correlation of independent variables (x) with a dependent variable (y). These models can be considered for prediction of y from the data of x variables and belong to qualitative or quantitative set of system [28]. Inclusive variants can be simple linear regression (SLR), multiple linear regression (MLR), and stepwise MLR. The following are the regression analysis methods:

Linear regression analysis (LRA): SLR, MLR, and stepwise multiple linear regression.

Multivariate data analysis: Principal component analysis (PCA), principal components regression (PCR), partial least square analysis (PLS), and genetic function approximation (GFA).

Genetic partial least squares (G/PLS)

Pattern recognition: Cluster analysis, artificial neural networks (ANNs), k-Nearest neighbor (kNN)

TABLE 4   Web resources for pharmacophore generation and QSAR modeling

S. No.	Resources	Description	URL
1.	ACD/Percepta	Prediction of ADME/T and physico-chemical properties	http://www.acdlabs.com/products/percepta
2.	ADMET Predictor	Prediction of ADME/T and physico-chemical properties	http://www.simulations-plus.com
3.	Chemistry Development Kit (CDK)	The CDK is a Java library for structural chemo- and bioinformatics applications. It includes the generation of 260 types of descriptors.	http://cdk.sourceforge.net
4.	Chembench	Chemoinformatics research support by integrating robust model builders, generators of descriptors, property and activity predictors, virtual libraries of available chemicals with predicted biological and drug-like properties, and special tools for chemical library design	http://chembench.mml.unc.edu

TABLE 4   (*Continued*)

5.	Discovery Studio	QSAR modeling and pharmaco-phore generation, for data analysis and structure optimization	http://accelrys.com/prod-ucts/discovery-studio
6.	GUSAR	QSAR modeling, antitarget interactions, and LD 50 value prediction based on atom-centric quantitative	http://www.way2drug.com/GUSAR
		neighbourhoods of atoms (QNA) and multilevel neighbourhoods of atoms (MNA) descriptors	
7.	KNIME	Graphical workbench for the entire analysis process, including plug-ins for descriptor generation,	http://www.knime.org
		creation of QSAR models, and work with SD files:	
8.	Molecular Operating Environment (MOE)	Calculates over 600 molecular descriptors including topological indices, structural keys, E-state indices, physical properties, topological polar surface area (TPSA), the Chemical Computing Group's (CCG's file), and van der Waals surface area (VSA) descrip-tors. MOE includes tools for the creation of QSAR/QSPR models using probabilistic methods and decision trees, PCR, and PLS methods	http://www.chemcomp.com/software-chem.htm
9.	Molinspiration	Cheminformatics software with tools supporting molecule manipu-lation and processing, including SMILES and SD conversion, normalization of molecules, generation of tautomers, molecule fragmentation, and calculation of various molecular properties needed in QSAR, molecular mod-eling, and drug design	http://www.molinspiration.com
10.	OpenTox	Interoperable, standards-based framework for the support of pre-dictive toxicology including APIs and services for compounds, data sets, features, algorithms, models,	http://www.opentox.org

TABLE 4　(*Continued*)

		ontologies, tasks, validation, and	

		reporting which may be combined into multiple applications satisfying a variety of different user needs	
11.	Prediction of Activity Spectra for Substances (PASS)	PASS is software for the creation of SAR models based on MNA descriptors and modified Bayesian algorithm. It predicts several thousand types of biological activity, including pharmacological effects, mechanisms of action, toxic and adverse effects, interaction with metabolic enzymes and transporters, and influence on gene expression.	http://www.way2drug.com
12.	PreADMET	Calculates more than 2,000 2D and 3D descriptors, with prediction of ADME/T and drug-likeness properties	http://preadmet.bmdrc.org
13.	PredictFX	QSAR modeling and simulation suite that provides prediction of off-target pharmacology, associated side effect profile, and aunity profiles on 4,790 targets for drug lead compounds	http://ww.certara.com/products/molmod/predictfx
14.	MedChem Studio	Cheminformatics platform supporting lead identification and prioritization, de novo design, scaffold hopping, and lead optimization	http://www.simulationsplus.com/Products.aspx?grpID=1&cID=13&pID=12
15.	Scigress Explorer, SCIGRESS	Molecular and QSAR modeling including generation of physicochemical descriptors for small organic molecules, inorganics, polymers, materials systems, and whole proteins	http://www.fqs.pl/ chemistry_materials_life_science/products/scigress_explorer

TABLE 4   (*Continued*)

16.	Selnergy	Combination of docking software to predict interaction energies of a ligand with a protein, database of	http://www.greenpharma. com/services/selnergy-tm
		7,000 protein structures with annotated biological properties and Greenpharma Core Database	
17.	Small-molecule drug discovery suite	2D/3D QSAR with a large selection of fingerprint options, shape-based screening, with or without atom	http://www.schrodinger. com/productsuite/1
		properties, ligand-based pharmacophore modeling, docking, and R-group analysis	
18.	StarDrop	QSAR modeling, data analysis and structures optimization, R-group analysis, and ADME/T prediction	http://www.optibrium.com
19.	SYBYL-X Suite	QSAR modeling, pharmacophore hypothesis generation, molecular alignment, conformational	http://www.tripos.com
		searching, ADME prediction, docking, and VS	
20.	Toxicity Estimation Software Tool (T.E.S.T.)	Estimation of toxicity values and physical properties of organic chemicals based on the molecular structure of the organic chemical entered by the user	http://www.epa.gov/nrmrl/ std/qsar/q sar.html
21.	cQSAR	A regression program that has dual databases of over 21,000 QSAR models	http://www.biobyte.com/bb/ prod/cqsar.html
22.	GALAHAD	GA-based program to develop pharmacophore hypotheses and structural alignments from a set of molecules that bind at a common site	http://www.certara.com/ products/molmod/sybyl-x/ simpharm/
23.	clogP	Program for calculating log Poct/ water from structure	http://www.biobyte.com/bb/ prod/clogp40.html

TABLE 4 (*Continued*)

24.	Almond	3D-QSAR approach using GRIND. Starting with a set of 3D structures, Almond employs GRID3 force field to generate molecular interaction fields (MIFs). The information in the MIFs is transformed to generate information-rich descriptors independent of the location of the molecules within the grid.	http://www.certara.com/products/molmod/sybyl-x/qsar/
25.	ClogP/CMR	Estimates Molar Refractivity and log P	http://www.certara.com/products/molmod/sybyl-x/
26.	QSAR with CoMFA	Builds statistical and graphical models that relate the properties of molecules (including biological activity) to their structures. Several structural descriptors can be calculated, including EVA and the molecular fields of CoMSIA	http://www.certara.com/products/molmod/sybyl-x/qsar/
27.	Topomer CoMFA	3D QSAR tool that automates the creation of models for predicting the biological activity or properties of compounds. Distributed by Tripos.	http://www.certara.com/products/molmod/sybyl-x/qsar/
28.	Surflex-Sim	Performs the alignment of molecules by maximizing their 3Dsimilarity. Surflex-Sim uses a surface based morphological similarity function while minimizing the overall molecular volume of the aligned structures.	http://www.certara.com/products/molmod/sybyl-x/simpharm/
29.	QSARPro	QSAR software for evaluation of several molecular descriptors along with facility to build the QSAR equation (linear or nonlinear regression) and use it for predicting the activities of test/new set of molecules. Performs 2D and 3D QSAR, and provides GQSAR, a group based QSAR approach establishing a correlation of chemical group variation at different molecular sites of interest with the biological activity.	http://www.vlifesciences.com/products/QSARPro/Product_QSARpro.php

TABLE 4   (*Continued*)

30.	Hologram QSAR (HQSAR)	Program using molecular holograms and PLS to generate fragment-based structure–activity relationships. Unlike other 3D-QSAR methods, HQSAR does not require alignment of molecules.	http://www.certara.com/products/molmod/sybyl-x/qsar/
31.	Open3DQSAR	Program aimed at high-throughput generation and chemometric analysis of MIFs. Free open source software for Windows, Linux, and Mac.	http://open3dqsar.source-forge.net/
32.	Codessa	Derives descriptors using quantum mechanical results from AMPAC. These descriptors are then used to develop QSAR/QSPR models.	http://www.semichem.com/codessa/default.php
33.	smirep	System for predicting the structural activity of chemical compounds	http://www.karwath.org/systems/smirep.html
34.	BlueDesc	Free and open source molecular descriptor calculator. Converts an MDL SD file into ARFF and LIBSVM format for machine learning and data mining purposes using CDK and JOELib2.	http://www.ra.cs.uni-tuebingen.de/software/bluedesc/welcome_e.html
35.	Molegro Data Modeller	A program for building regression or classification models, performing feature selection and cross-validation, PCA, high-dimensional visualization, clustering, and outlier detection	http://www.clcbio.com/products/clc-drug-discovery-workbench/
36.	KeyRecep	Estimates the characteristics of the binding site of the target protein by superposing multiple active compounds in 3D space so that the physico-chemical properties of the compounds match maximally with each other. Can be used to estimate activities and vHTS	http://www.immd.co.jp/en/product_2.html
37.	PaDEL-Descriptor	Free software to calculate molecular (797) descriptors and (10) fingerprints. Can be used from command lines or GUI	http://padel.nus.edu.sg/software/padeldescriptor/

TABLE 4   (*Continued*)

38.	CODESSA Pro	Program for developing QSAR/ QSPR. Distributed by Compu-Drug.	http://www.compudrug.com/
39.	OpenMol-GRID	Uses a grid approach to deal with large-scale molecular design and engineering problems. The methodology used relies on QSPR/ QSAR.	http://www.openmolgrid. org/?m=1&s=11
40.	McQSAR	Free program to generate QSAR equations using the genetic function approximation paradigm	http://users.abo.fi/mivainio/ mcqsar/
41.	Molconn-Z	Standard program for generation of molecular connectivity, shape, and information indices for QSAR analyses	http://www.edusoft-lc.com/ molconn/
42.	OCHEM Database	Online Chemical Modeling Environment project. Online database of experimental measurements integrated with a modeling environment. User can submit experimental data or use the data uploaded by other users to build predictive QSAR models for physico-chemical or biological properties.	https://www.ochem.eu/ home/show.do
43.	MOLE db	Molecular Descriptors Data Base is a free online database comprised of 1,124 molecular descriptors calculated for hundreds of thousands of molecules.	http://michem.disat.unimib. it/mole_db/

TABLE 4   (*Continued*)

44.	E-Dragon	Online version of DRAGON, which is an application for the calculation of molecular descriptors developed by the Milano Chemometrics and QSAR Research Group. These descriptors can be used to evaluate molecular	http://www.vcclab.org/lab/edragon/
		structure–activity or structure–property relationships, as well as for similarity analysis and HTS of molecule databases.	

(*Continued*)

45.	3-D QSAR	3D QSAR MODELS DATABASE for VS. Users can process their own molecules by drawing or uploading them to the server and selecting the target for the VS and biological activity prediction.	http://www.3d-qsar.com/
46.	MOLFEAT	Web service to compute molecular fingerprints and molecular descriptors of molecules from their 3D structures, and for computing activity of compounds of specific chemical types against selected targets based on published QSAR models. Currently covers 1,114 fingerprints, 3,977 molecular descriptors, and 23 QSAR models for 16 chemical types against 14 targets.	http://jing.cz3.nus.edu.sg/cgi-bin/molfeat/molfeat.cgi
47.	Partial Least Squares Regression (PLSR)	Generates model construction and prediction of activity/property using the PLS regression technique	http://www.vcclab.org/lab/pls/
48.	OSIRIS Property Explorer	Integral part of Actelion's inhouse substance registration system. Calculates on-the-fly various drug-relevant properties for drawn chemical structures, including cLog P and water solubility.	http://www.organic-chemistry.org/prog/peo/

TABLE 5 Development of anti-inflammatory model, predicted chemical descriptors (shadow), and their biological activity correlated through derived QSAR model equation

Compound Name	Compound ID No.	Exp. LD_{50} (mg/kg)	Exp. log. LD_{50} (mg/kg)	Dipole Vector X (debye)	Dipole Vector Y (debye)	Dielectric Energy (kcal/mole)	Steric Energy (kcal/mole)	Heat of Formation (kcal/mole)	HOMO Energy (eV)	Log P	Size of Smallest Ring	Group Count (sec-amine)	Group Count (car-boxyl)	Pred. log LD_{50} (mg/kg)
Aceclofenac	CID_71771	130	2.114	-0.848	1.6	-0.579	-6.66	-130.614	-8.801	3.539	6	1	1	2.402
Amodiaquine	CID_2165	550	2.74	-1.639	2.005	-0.411	4.302	9.686	-8.32	4.193	6	1	0	2.875
Aspirin	CID_2244	200	2.301	-0.493	-0.039	-0.56	-15.821	-145.255	-9.937	1.244	6	0	1	2.677
Celecoxib	CID_2662	2000	3.301	3.548	-3.459	-1.125	-1.645	-126.329	-9.988	4.252	5	0	0	3.189
Clindamycin	CID_29029	1832	3.263	-1.355	-2.655	-0.672	23.46	-242.376	-9.328	1.209	5	1	0	3.075
Diclofenac	CID_3033	250	2.398	-1.44	1.517	-0.382	-4.888	-54.158	-8.769	3.965	6	1	1	2.125
Ibuprofen	CID_3672	636	2.803	1.644	-0.24	-0.326	-18.725	-101.384	-9.551	3.83	6	0	1	2.905
Indometha-cin	CID_3715	12	1.079	-0.708	-0.687	-0.583	-23.13	-112.576	-8.698	3.969	5	0	1	1.172
Ketoprofen	CID_3825	360	2.556	0.856	3.877	-0.551	-15.842	-82.13	-9.97	3.461	6	0	1	2.503
Lornoxicam	CID_5282204	573	2.758	0.911	0.381	-0.799	42.917	-57.228	-8.963	0.976	5	1	0	2.886
Meclof-enamate	CID_4037	100	2	-2.152	1.915	-0.412	-1.87	-56.707	-8.69	4.5	6	1	1	2.033
Mefenamic acid	CID_4044	525	2.72	0.449	-0.878	-0.321	-10.165	-53.929	-8.238	3.931	6	1	1	2.404
Meloxicam	CID_5281106	470	2.672	0.646	0.442	-0.94	30.848	-56.717	-9.198	0.902	5	1	0	2.756
Nabumetone	CID_4409	3880	3.589	1.603	0.906	-0.405	-17.441	-49.887	-8.66	3.37	6	0	0	3.657
Naproxen	CID_156391	360	2.556	-0.173	-1.929	-0.412	-29.356	-97.745	-8.767	2.989	6	0	1	2.276

TABLE 5 (*Continued*)

Nimesulide	CID_4495	200	2.301	-5.98	-1.732	-1.361	-9.18	-56.062	-9.691	2.195	6	1	0	2.461
Aristolochic Acid	CID_2236	81	1.908	3.028	2.374	-0.885	-2.455	-124.659	-9.07	2.785	5	0	1	1.729
Azimexon	CID_47294	170	2.23	-0.92	-1.113	-0.767	280.397	51.497	-10.154	-0.271	3	0	0	2.498
Berberine	CID_2353	23	1.362	-2.129	2.183	-2.101	18.846	81.035	-11.74	2.681	5	0	0	1.38
Ciamexon	CID_71759	130	2.114	-1.652	-4.507	-0.691	139.832	50.144	-9.362	1.613	3	0	0	1.401
Imemixon	CID_68791	150	2.176	4.865	-3.143	-1.443	113.293	23.614	-9.992	-0.805	3	0	0	2.373
Indometacin	CID_3715	12	1.079	-0.771	-0.741	-0.571	-23.111	-112.584	-8.696	3.969	5	0	1	1.162
Isopteropodin	CID_122813	162	2.21	1.68	1.735	-0.582	2.761	-120.992	-8.936	0.959	5	1	0	2.409

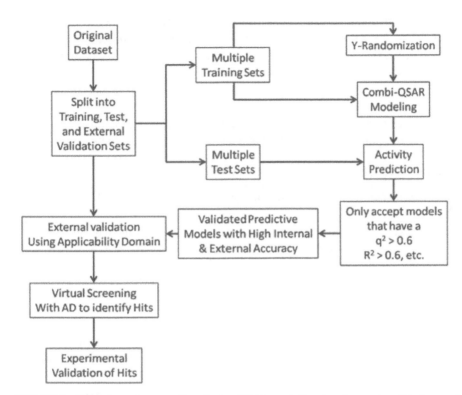

FIGURE 3   Workflow diagram of predictive SQAR modeling development, validation, and interpretation.

2.3.6   MOLECULAR CHEMICAL DESCRIPTORS

Chemical descriptors are at the core of QSAR modeling, and so many different types of chemical descriptors reflecting various levels of chemical structure representation have been proposed so far. These levels range from molecular formula (1D) to the most popular among chemists 2D structural formula to 3D, conformation-dependent (3D), and even higher levels taking into account mutual orientation and time-dependent dynamics of molecules (4D and higher; for discussion see study of Polanski [29]). A comprehensive collection of molecular descriptors, along with their description and compilation of calculation software are shown in **Tables 6 and 7**. Some of the most important descriptors used in QSAR modeling are listed hereunder:

1. Constitutional descriptors (molecular weight, halogenated atom counts, and functional group counts (amine, carbonyl, carboxylic acid, hydroxyl, nitrile, nitro group, etc.)

2. Electrostatic descriptors (partial charges, charged surface areas, etc.)
3. Topological descriptors Kier & Hall connectivity indices, that is, zero order, first order, and second order and valence connectivity indices, that is, zero order, first order, second order, etc.)
4. Geometrical descriptors (solvent accessible surface, isosurface volume, molar volume, etc.)
5. Quantum-chemical descriptors, that is, dipole moment, quadrupole moment, polarizibility, HOMO and LUMO energies, dielectric energy, etc.

TABLE 6   Molecular descriptor calculation software

S. No.	Software	Description	URL
1.	ADAPT	A computational model platform developed for pharmacokinetic and pharmacodynamic applications	http://bmsr.usc.edu/Software/ADAPT/ADAPT.html
2.	AFGen	A fragment based descriptor generator with three diff erent types of topologies: paths, acyclic subgraphs, and arbitrary topology subgraphs	http://glaros.dtc.umn.edu/gkhome/afgen/overview
.3.	Dragon	An application for the calculation of molecular descriptors	http://www.talete.mi.it/products/dragon_all_about.htm
4.	CODESSA	Calculation of over 500 types of constitutional, topological, geometrical, electrostatic, thermodynamic, and quantum-chemical descriptors	http://www.codessa-pro.com
5.	DRAGON	Calculation of almost all types of descriptors (4,885 types of descriptors in total)	http://www.talete.mi.it
6.	E-DRAGON	A remote version of DRAGON	http://www.vcclab.org
7.	MolconZ	Standard program for generation of molecular connectivity, shape, and information indices for QSAR analyses	http://www.edusoft-lc.com/molconn/
8.	MOE	Integrates tools for computer-assisted drug discovery	http://www.chemcomp.com/
9.	ISIDA	Calculation of substructural molecular fragments (SMFs) and ISIDA property-labeled fragment (IPLF) descriptors	http://infochim.u-strasbg.fr/spip.php?rubrique49
10.	OpenMolGrid	Drug-design using Grid technology	http://www.openmolgrid.org/?m=2&s=242

TABLE 6 *(Continued)*

11.	Molecular Descriptor Lab (MODEL)	Web service for calculating approximately 4,000 molecular descriptors based on the 3D structure of a molecule	http://jing.cz3.nus.edu.sg/cgi-bin/model/model.cgi
12.	VLife MDS	Workbench for computer-aided drug design (CADD) and molecule discovery	http://www.vlifesciences.com/vlife_tech/mds.htm
13.	Codessa	Advanced, fully featured QSAR program that ties information from AMPAC™ and other quantum mechanics programs with experimental data	http://www.semichem.com/codessa/default.php
14.	Mold2	Calculation of over 700 descriptors	http://www.fda.gov/ScienceResearch/BioinformaticsTools/Mold2
15.	JoeLib	Cheminformatics algorithm library, which was designed for prototyping, data mining, graph mining, and of course algorithm development	http://joelib.sourceforge.net/wiki/
16.	CDK	Open source Java computational chemistry package which supports chemical structure drawing and the graphical layout of 2D chemical structures	http://crdd.osdd.net/cdk.sourceforge.net/
17.	MOLGEN	Web service for calculating 708 arithmetical, topological, and geometrical descriptors	http://molgen.de
18	PreADMET	Descriptor calculation, drug likeness prediction: rule-based drug-like screening, ADME prediction: examination of various ADME properties of drug candidates, chemical library design: powerful workspace, molecular set, and molecular table	http://preadme.bmdrc.org/sales/main.htm
19.	Open Babel	Molecular fingerprint generation and similarity searching	http://openbabel.org
20.	ADMET-Works ModelBuilder	A tool for building mathematical models that can later be used for predicting various chemical and biological properties of compounds	http://www.fqs.pl/life_science/admeworks_modelbuilder
21.	CAChe	Computer-aided chemistry modeling package designed for experimental chemists conducting research in life science, materials, and chemistry	http://www.fqs.pl/chemistry/cache

TABLE 6 (*Continued*)

22.	VolSurf	A computational procedure aimed to produce and to explore the physico-chemical property space of a molecule (or library of molecules) starting from 3D maps of interaction energies between the molecule and chemical probes	http://www.moldiscovery.com/accounts/login/?next=/product/manual/volsurf/descriptors.html
23.	PaDEL	Calculates 729 1D, 2D, and 134 3D descriptors, and 10 types of finger-prints	http://padel.nus.edu.sg/software/padeldescriptor
24.	TSAR	A fully integrated QSAR package for library design and lead optimization	http://accelrys.com/products/informatics/
25.	Almond	Program specifically developed for generating and handling alignment in-dependent descriptors called GRIND (GRid INdependent Descriptors)	http://www.moldiscovery.com/software/pentacle
26.	JKlustor	A Java software for diversity calcula-tions and clustering	http://www.jchem.com/doc/admin/JKlustor.html

TABLE 7   Software for quantum mechanics

S. No.	Software	Description	URL
1.	AMPAC 4.0 with GUI	Set of tools to study molecular structure and chemical reactions	http://www.netsci.org/Resources/Software/Modeling/QM/ampac.html
2.	GAMESS	A general ab initio quantum chem-istry package	http://www.netsci.org/Resources/Software/Modeling/QM/gamess.html
3.	Gaussian	Predicts the energies, molecu-lar structures, and vibrational frequencies of molecular systems, along with numerous molecular properties derived from these basic computation types	http://www.gaussian.com/
4.	Huckel	Calculates electronic properties of molecules	http://www.oraxcel.com/projects/huckel/
5.	hmo10	Huckel molecular orbital calculator	http://www.simtel.net/pub/pd/42108.html
6.	Jaguar	Rapid ab initio electronic structure package	http://www.schrodinger.com/
7.	MOPAC	A semiempirical quantum chemis-try program based on Dewar and Thiel's NDDO approximation	http://openmopac.net/

2.3.8 MOLECULAR DOCKING

Docking is finding a binding geometry between two interactive molecules of similar structure. Molecular docking is a key tool in structural molecular biology and computer-assisted drug design. The goal of ligand–protein docking is to predict the predominant binding mode of a ligand with a protein of known 3D structure as shown in **Figures 4 & 5**. Successful docking methods search high-dimensional spaces effectively using a scoring function that correctly ranks candidates. Docking can be used to perform VS on large libraries of compounds, rank the results, and propose structural hypotheses of how the ligands inhibit the target, which is invaluable in lead optimization. The setting up of the input structures for the docking is just as important as the docking itself, and analyzing the results of stochastic search methods can sometimes be unclear. The best possible starting point is an X-ray crystal structure of the target site. If the molecular model of the binding site is precise enough, one can apply docking algorithms that simulate the binding of drugs to the respective receptor site [30]. This analysis reveals important, primitive information on how the compound actually binds to the target and the nature and extent of changes induced in the target by the binding. These data, in turn, suggest ways to refine the lead compound to improve its binding to the target protein [31–34]. The experimental drug is then ready for conventional drug development (e.g., studies in safety assessment, formulation, clinical trials, etc.). This reiterative analysis and compound modifications are possible because of the structural data obtained by X-ray crystallography at each stage. This capability renders structure-based drug design a powerful tool for rapid and efficient development of drugs that are highly specific for particular protein target sites as shown in Table 8. Most commonly used docking softwares worldwide for binding affinity studies are listed hereunder:

1. AutoDOCK [35]
2. GLIDE [36]
3. DOCK [37]
4. Accelry's DS-LigandFit [38]
5. GOLD [39]
6. Fujitsu's Scigress Explorer (previously CaChe) [40]
7. FlexX [41]

Algorithms used while docking are (i) genetic algorithms (e.g., GOLD, Auto Dock, and Gambler), (ii) fast shape matching (e.g., DOCK and Eudock), (iii) Monte Carlo simulations (e.g., MCDock and QXP), (iv) Tabu search (e.g., PRO_LEADS and SFDock), and (v) incremental construction (e.g., FlexX, Hammerhead, and SLIDE). Some software are also available online to calculate the ligands binding as shown in Table 9.

Structure-based drug design is an improvement over traditional drug screening techniques. By identifying the target protein in advance and by discovering the chemical and molecular structure of the protein, it is possible to design optimal drugs to interact with the protein. Some important docking applications are (1) determine the lowest free energy structures for the receptor–ligand complexes; (2) search databases and rank hits for lead generation; (3) calculate the differential binding of a ligand to two different macromolecular receptors; (4) study the geometry of a particular complex; (5) propose modification of lead molecules to optimize its potency or other properties; (6) de novo design for lead generation; and (7) library design. The principal techniques currently available are (1) molecular dynamics; (2) Monte Carlo methods; (3) genetic algorithms; (4) fragment-based methods; (5) point complementarity methods; (6) distance geometry methods; (7) tabu searches; and (8) systematic searches [42]. In addition, molecular docking is often used as VS approach [43], whereby large virtual libraries of compounds are reduced in size to a manageable subset, which, if successful, includes molecules with high binding affinities to a target receptor [44].

TABLE 8 Databases related to of drug targets

S. No.	Database	Description	URL
1.	ArchDB	Automated classification of protein loop structures	http://gurion.imim.es/archdb
2.	ASTRAL	Sequences of domains of known structure, selected subsets, and sequence-structure correspondences	http://astral.stanford.edu/
3.	BAliBASE	A database for comparison of multiple sequence alignments	http://www-igbmc.u-strasbg.fr/BioInfo/BAliBASE2/index.html
4.	BioMagRes-Bank	NMR spectroscopic data for proteins and nucleic acids	http://www.bmrb.wisc.edu/
5.	CADB	Conformational angles in proteins database	http://cluster.physics.iisc.ernet.in/cadb/
6.	CATH	Protein domain structures database	http://www.biochem.ucl.ac.uk/bsm/cath_new
7.	CE	3D protein structure alignments	http://cl.sdsc.edu/ce.html
8.	CKAAPs DB	Structurally similar proteins with dissimilar sequences	http://ckaap.sdsc.edu/

TABLE 8 (*Continued*)

9.	CoC	Conservation of conservation: universally conserved residues in selected protein folds	http://kulibin.mit.edu/coc/
10.	Columba	Annotation of protein structures from the PDB	http://www.columba-db.de
11.	Dali	Protein fold classification using the Dali search engine	http://www.bioinfo.biocenter.helsinki.fi:8080/dali/
12.	Decoys 'R' Us	Computer-generated protein conformations	http://dd.stanford.edu/
13.	DisProt	Database of protein disorder: proteins that lack fixed 3D structure in their native states	http://divac.ist.temple.edu/disprot
14.	DMAPS	A database of multiple alignments for protein structures	http://bioinformatics.albany.edu/~dmaps
15.	DomIns	Domain insertions in known protein structures	http://www.domins.org/
16.	DSDBASE	Native and modeled disulfide bonds in proteins	http://www.ncbs.res.in/~faculty/mini/dsdbase/dsdbase.html
17.	DSMM	Database of simulated molecular motions	http://projects.villa-bosch.de/dbase/dsmm/
18.	eF-site	Electrostatic surface of functional site: electrostatic potentials and hydrophobic properties of the active sites	http://ef-site.protein.osaka-u.ac.jp/eF-site
19.	FSN	Flexible structural neighborhood, structural neighbors of proteins identified by FATCAT tool	http://fatcat.ljcrf.edu/fatcat-cgi/cgi/struct_neibor/fatcatStructNeibor.pl
20.	GenDiS	Genomic distribution of protein structural superfamilies	http://caps.ncbs.res.in/gendis/home.html
21.	Gene3D	Precalculated structural assignments for whole genomes	http://cathwww.biochem.ucl.ac.uk:8080/Gene3D/
22.	GTD	Genomic threading database: structural annotations of complete proteomes	http://bioinf.cs.ucl.ac.uk/GTD
23.	GTOP	Protein fold predictions from genome sequences	http://spock.genes.nig.ac.jp/~genome/
24.	Het-PDB Navi	Heteroatoms in protein structures	http://daisy.nagahama-i-bio.ac.jp/golab/hetpdb-navi.html

TABLE 8   (*Continued*)

25.	HOMSTRAD	Homologous structure alignment database: curated structure-based alignments for protein families	http://www-cryst.bioc.cam.ac.uk/homstrad
26.	IMB Jena Image Library	Visualization and analysis of 3D biopolymer structures	http://www.imb-jena.de/IMAGE.html
27.	IMGT/3 Dstructure-DB	Sequences and 3D structures of vertebrate immunoglobulins, T cell receptors, and MHC proteins	http://imgt3d.igh.cnrs.fr/
28.	IMOTdb	Spatially interacting motif database	http://caps.ncbs.res.in/imotdb/
29.	ISSD	Integrated sequence-structure database	http://www.protein.bio.msu.su/issd
30.	LPFC	Library of protein family core structures	http://www-smi.stanford.edu/projects/helix/LPFC
31.	MMDB	NCBI's database of 3D structures, part of NCBI Entrez	http://www.ncbi.nlm.nih.gov/Structure
32.	E-MSD	EBI's macromolecular structure database	http://www.ebi.ac.uk/msd
33.	ModBase	Annotated comparative protein structure models	http://salilab.org/modbase
34.	MolMovDB	Database of macromolecular movements: descriptions of protein and macromolecular motions, including movies	http://bioinfo.mbb.yale.edu/MolMovDB/
35.	PALI	Phylogeny and alignment of homologous protein structures	http://pauling.mbu.iisc.ernet.in/~pali
36.	PASS2	Structural motifs of protein superfamilies	http://ncbs.res.in/~faculty/mini/campass/pass.html
37.	PepConfDB	A database of peptide conformations	http://www.peptidome.org/products/list.htm
38.	PDB	Protein structure databank: all publicly available 3D structures of proteins and nucleic acids	http://www.rcsb.org/pdb
39.	PDB-REPRDB	Representative protein chains, based on PDB entries	http://mbs.cbrc.jp/pdbreprdb-cgi/reprdb_menu.pl

TABLE 8 (*Continued*)

40.	PDBsum	Summaries and analyses of PDB structures	http://www.ebi.ac.uk/thornton-srv/databases/pdbsum/
41.	PDB_TM	Transmembrane proteins with known 3D structure	http://pdbtm.enzim.hu/
42.	PMDB	3D protein models obtained from structure predictions	http://a.caspur.it/PMDB/
43.	Protein Folding Database	Experimental data on protein folding	http://pfd.med.monash.edu.au
44.	SCOP	Structural classification of proteins	http://scop.mrc-lmb.cam.ac.uk/scop
45.	SCOPPI	Structural classification of protein–protein interfaces	http://www.scoppi.org
46.	Sloop	Classification of protein loops	http://www-cryst.bioc.cam.ac.uk/~sloop/
47.	STING report	Amino acid properties in proteins of known structure	http://sms.cbi.cnptia.embrapa.br/SMS/STINGm/SMSReport/
48.	Structure Superposition Database	Pairwise superposition of TIM-barrel structures	http://ssd.rbvi.ucsf.edu/
49.	SUPERFAMILY	Assignments of proteins to structural superfamilies	http://supfam.org/
50.	SURFACE	Surface residues and functions annotated, compared, and evaluated: a database of protein surface patches	http://cbm.bio.uniroma2.it/surface
51.	SWISS-MODEL Repository	Database of annotated 3D protein structure models	http://swissmodel.expasy.org/repository
52.	TargetDB	Target data from worldwide structural genomics projects	http://targetdb.pdb.org/
53.	3D-GENOMICS	Structural annotations for complete proteomes	http://www.sbg.bio.ic.ac.uk/3dgenomics
54.	TOPS	Topology of protein structures database	http://www.tops.leeds.ac.uk
55.	TTD	Therapeutic target database	http://xin.cz3.nus.edu.sg/group/cjttd/ttd.asp

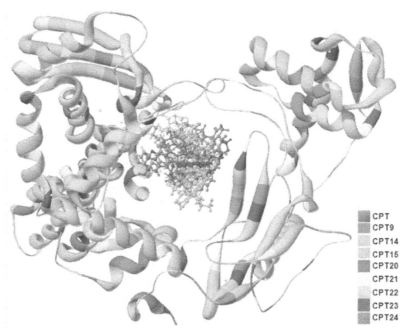

FIGURE 4 Superimposition of most favorable confirmation of predicted active camptothecin and its derivative docked on the same binding site residues of anticancer target Topoisomerase I.

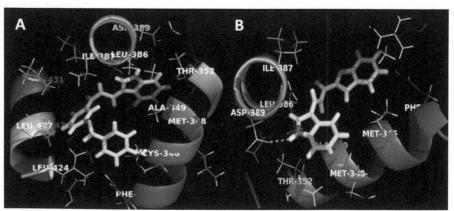

FIGURE 5 *In silico* molecular docking studies elucidating the possible mechanisms of chalcone derivatives induced modulation of liver cancer protein (LRH-1) receptor (PDB:3PLZ). The docking studies were carried out using SYBYL-X 2.0, Tripos International. These compounds docked on LRH-1 form a H-bond of length 2.4 Å to the binding pocket residue Asp-389 and total scores of 7.9867 (A) and 5.2861 (B) were observed.

TABLE 9 Web resources related to Ligand Binding Affinities (docking)

S. No	Resources	Description	URL
1.	AutoDock	Molecular modeling simulation software including protein–ligand docking	http://autodock.scripps.edu/
2.	FlexX	Prediction of protein–ligand inter-actions (docking)	http://www.biosolveit.de/ FlexX
3.	Glide	Schr"odinger's ligand–protein docking software	http://www.schrodinger. com/productpage/14/5/21
4.	GOLD	Prediction of protein–ligand inter-actions (docking), VS, lead optimi-zation, and identifying the correct binding mode of active molecules	http://www.ccdc.cam.ac.uk/ Solutions/GoldSuite/Pages/ GOLD.aspx
5.	LigandScout	VS based on 3D chemical feature pharmacophore models	http://www.inteligand.com/
6.	Molegro Vir-tual Docker	Prediction of protein–ligand inter-actions	http://www.molegro.com/ mvd-product.php
7.	OEDocking	Molecular docking tools and their associated workflows	http://www.eyesopen.com/ oedocking
8.	AffinDB	Affinity database for protein–ligand	http://pc1664.pharmazie. uni-marburg.de/
9.	SCIGRESS	Desktop/server molecular model-ing software suite employing linear scaling semiempirical quantum methods for protein optimization and ligand docking	http://www.fqs.pl/Chem-istry_Materials_Life_Sci-ence/products/scigress
10.	BindingDB	Web-accessible database of experi-mentally determined protein–ligand binding affinities	http://www.bindingdb.org/ bind/index.jsp
11.	DLRP	Database of protein ligand and pro-tein receptor pairs that are known to interact with each other	http://dip.doe-mbi.ucla.edu/ dip/DLRP.cgi
12.	GlamDock	Docking program based on a Monte Carlo with minimization (basin hopping) search in a hybrid interac-tion matching/internal coordinate search space	http://www.chil2.de/Glam-dock.html
13.	eHiTS	Exhaustive search based docking program	http://www.simbiosys.ca/ ehits/index.html
14.	GEMDOCK	Generic Evolutionary Method for molecular DOCKing	http://gemdock.life.nctu. edu.tw/dock/

TABLE 9   (*Continued*)

15.	ParaDockS	Parallel Docking Suite, for docking small, drug-like molecules to a rigid receptor employing either the knowledge-based potential PMF04 or the empirical energy function p-Score	http://www.paradocks.org/
16.	iGEMDOCK	Graphic environment for the docking, VS, and postscreening analysis	http://gemdock.life.nctu. edu.tw/dock/igemdock.php
17.	VLifeDock	Multiple approaches for protein–ligand docking	http://www.vlifesciences. com/products/VLifeMDS/ VLifeDock.php
18.	HomDock	Progam for similarity-based docking, based on a combination of the ligand based GMA molecular alignment tool and the docking tool GlamDock	http://www.chil2.de/Hom-Dock.html
19.	DAIM-SEED-FFLD	DAIM (Decomposition And Identification of Molecules) decomposes the molecules into molecular fragments that are docked using SEED (Program for docking libraries of fragments with solvation energy evaluation)	http://www.biochem-caflisch.uzh.ch/download/
20.	DOCK	Anchor-and-Grow based docking program. Free for academic usage. Flexible ligand. Flexible protein. Maintained by the Soichet group at the UCSF	http://dock.compbio.ucsf. edu/
21.	BDT	Graphic front end application which controls the conditions of AutoGrid and AutoDock runs. Maintained by the Universitat Rovira i Virgili	http://www.quimica.urv. cat/~pujadas/BDT/index. html
22.	Autodock Vina plugin for PyMOL	Allows defining binding sites and export to Autodock and VINA input files, doing receptor and ligand preparation automatically, starting docking runs with Autodock or VINA from within the plugin, viewing grid maps generated by autogrid in PyMOL, handling multiple ligands and setup VSs, and setup docking runs with flexible side chains	http://wwwuser.gwdg. de/~dseelig/adplugin.html

TABLE 9 (*Continued*)

23.	GriDock	VS front end for AutoDock 4. GriDock was designed to perform the molecular dockings of a large number of ligands stored in a single database (SDF or Zip format) in the lowest possible time	http://159.149.85.2/cms/ index.php?Software_ projects:GriDock
24	Computer-Aided Drug-Design Platform using PyMOL	PyMOL plugins providing a graphical user interface incorporating individual academic packages designed for protein preparation (AMBER package and Reduce), molecular mechanics applications (AMBER package), and docking and scoring	http://people.pharmacy. purdue.edu/~mlill/software/ pymol_plugins/install.shtml
25.	DockoMatiC	GUI application that is intended to ease and automate the creation and management of AutoDock jobs for high-throughput screening of ligand/receptor interactions	http://dockomatic.source-forge.net/
26.	ICM	Docking program based on pseudo-Brownian sampling and local minimization. Ligand and protein flexible	http://www.molsoft.com/ docking.html
27.	FITTED	Suite of programs to dock flexible ligands into flexible proteins	http://fitted.ca/
28.	Fleksy	Program for flexible and induced fit docking using receptor ensemble (constructed using backbone-dependent rotamer library) to describe protein flexibility	http://www.cmbi.ru.nl/software/fleksy/
29.	FlexX, Flex-Ensemble (FlexE)	Incremental build based docking program. Flexible ligand. Protein flexibility through ensemble of protein structure	http://www.biosolveit.de/ flexx/index.html?ct=1
30.	BetaDock	Molecular docking simulation software based on the theory of b-complex	http://voronoi.hanyang. ac.kr/software.htm
31.	HADDOCK	HADDOCK is an approach that makes use of biochemical and/or biophysical interaction data such as chemical shift perturbation data resulting from NMR titration experiments, mutagenesis data, or bioinformatic predictions	http://www.nmr.chem. uu.nl/haddock/

TABLE 9 (*Continued*)

32.	ADAM	Automated docking tool. Can be used for vHTS. Distributed by IMMD.	http://www.immd.co.jp/en/product_2.html
33.	ASEDock	Docking program based on a shape similarity assessment between a concave portion (i.e., concavity) on a protein and the ligand	http://www.ncbi.nlm.nih.gov/pubmed/18278891
34.	Hint!	Numerically and graphically evaluates binding of drugs or inhibitors into protein structures and scores DOCK orientations, constructs hydropathic (LOCK and KEY) complementarity maps that can be used to predict a substrate from a known receptor or protein	http://www.edusoft-lc.com/hint/
35.	ISE-Dock	Docking program which is based on the iterative stochastic elimination (ISE) algorithm	http://www.ncbi.nlm.nih.gov/pubmed/18058908
36.	DockVision	Docking package including Monte Carlo, genetic algorithm, and database screening docking algorithms	http://www.dockvision.com/
37.	Hammerhead	Automatic, fast fragment-based docking procedure for flexible ligands, with an empirically tuned scoring function and an automatic method for identifying and characterizing the binding site on a protein	http://www.ncbi.nlm.nih.gov/pubmed/8807875
38.	PLANTS	Docking algorithm based on a class of stochastic optimization algorithms called ant colony optimization (ACO)	http://www.tcd.uni-konstanz.de/research/plants.php
39.	FLOG	Rigid body docking program using databases of pregenerated conformations	http://www.ncbi.nlm.nih.gov/pubmed/8064332
40.	ADDock	Anchor dependent molecular docking method	http://www.biodelight.com.tw/English/addock_index.html
41.	EUDOC	Program for identification of drug interaction sites in macromolecules and drug leads from chemical databases	http://www.ncbi.nlm.nih.gov/pubmed/12116409

TABLE 9 (*Continued*)

42.	EADock	Hybrid evolutionary docking algorithm with two fitness functions, in combination with a sophisticated management of the diversity	http://www.ncbi.nlm.nih.gov/pubmed/17380512
43.	FINDSITE-LHM	Homology modeling approach to flexible ligand docking. It uses a collection of common molecule substructures, compounds in similarity-based ligand binding pose prediction	http://cssb.biology.gatech.edu/findsitelhm
44.	Rosetta Ligand	Monte Carlo minimization procedure in which the rigid body position and orientation of the small molecule and the protein side chain conformations are optimized simultaneously	https://www.rosettacommons.org/software
45.	MS-Dock	Free multiple conformation generator and rigid docking protocol for multistep virtual ligand screening	http://www.mti.univ-paris-diderot.fr/recherche/plate-formes/logiciels
46.	Surflex-Dock.	Docking program based on an idealized active site ligand (a protomol), used as a target to generate putative poses of molecules or molecular fragments	http://www.certara.com/products/molmod/sybyl-x/sbd/
47.	GalaxyDock	Protein–ligand docking program that allows flexibility of preselected side chains of ligand	http://galaxy.seoklab.org/softwares/galaxydock.html
48.	CDocker	CHARMm based docking program. Random ligand conformations are generated by molecular dynamics and the positions of the ligands are optimized in the binding site using rigid body rotations followed by simulated annealing	http://accelrys.com/
49.	YASARA Structure	Adds support for small-molecule docking to YASARA view/model/dynamics using Autodock and Fleksy	http://www.yasara.org/
50.	LigandFit	CHARMm based docking program. Ligand conformations generated using Monte Carlo techniques are initially docked into an active site based on shape, followed by further CHARMm minimization	http://accelrys.com/

TABLE 9 (*Continued*)

51.	Lead Finder	Program for molecular docking, VS, and quantitative evaluation of ligand binding and biological activity	http://www.moltech.ru/
52.	rDock	Fast, versatile, and open source program for docking ligands to proteins and nucleic acids. Free and open source.Developed by the University of Barcelona.	http://rdock.sourceforge.net/
53.	MOE	Suite of medicinal chemistry tools like ligand–receptor docking, Protein/ligand interaction diagrams, multifragment search, ligand and structure-based query editor, high-throughput conformation generation, pharmacophore search	http://www.chemcomp.com/
54.	POSIT	Ligand guided pose prediction. POSIT uses bound ligand information to improve pose prediction	http://www.eyesopen.com/oedocking
55.	idock	Free and open source multithreaded VS tool for flexible ligand docking for computational drug discovery	https://github.com/HongjianLi/idock
56.	VinaMPI	Massively parallel Message Passing Interface (MPI) program based on the multithreaded virtual docking program AutodockVina	http://cmb.ornl.gov/~sek/
57.	HYBRID	Docking program similar to FRED, except that it uses the Chemical Gaussian Overlay (CGO) ligand-based scoring function	http://www.eyesopen.com/oedocking
58.	FlipDock	GA based docking program using FlexTree data structures to represent a protein–ligand complex for flexible ligand and flexible protein	http://flipdock.scripps.edu/
59.	FRED	FRED performs a systematic, exhaustive, and nonstochastic examination of all possible poses within the protein active site, filters for shape complementarity and pharmacophoric features before selecting and optimizing poses using the Chemgauss4 scoring function	http://www.eyesopen.com/oedocking

TABLE 9 (*Continued*)

60.	BioDrugScreen	Computational drug design and discovery resource and server. The portal contains the DOPIN (Docked Proteome Interaction Network) database constituted by millions of predocked and prescored complexes from thousands of targets from the humans	http://www.biodrugscreen.org/
61.	LPCCSU	Analysis of interatomic contacts in ligand–protein complexes	http://bip.weizmann.ac.il/oca-bin/lpccsu
62.	PLATINUM	Calculates hydrophobic properties of molecules and their match or mismatch in receptor–ligand complexes. These properties may help to analyze results of molecular docking.	http://model.nmr.ru/platinum/
63.	GPCRauto-model	Web service that automates the homology modeling of mammalian olfactory receptors (ORs) based on the six 3D structures of G-protein-coupled receptors (GPCRs) available, performs the docking of odorants on these models	http://genome.jouy.inra.fr/GPCRautomdl/cgi-bin/welcome.pl
64.	Pose & Rank	Web server for scoring protein–ligand complexes	http://modbase.compbio.ucsf.edu/ligscore/
65.	iScreen	Web service for docking and screening the small molecular database on traditional Chinese medicine (TCM) on user's protein	http://iscreen.cmu.edu.tw/
66.	Score	Allows to calculate some different docking scores of ligand–receptor complex that can be submitted as a whole file containing both interaction partners or as two separated files	http://159.149.85.2/score.htm
67.	idTarget	Web server for identifying biomolecular targets of small chemical molecules with robust scoring functions and a divide-and-conquer docking approach	http://idtarget.rcas.sinica.edu.tw/
68.	MetaDock	Online docking solution and docking results analysis service. Docking is done with GNU/GPL-licensed AutoDock v.4 and Dock6 under academic license	http://dock.bioinfo.pl/

TABLE 9   (*Continued*)

69.	SwissDock	SwissDock, a Web service to predict the molecular interactions that may occur between a target protein and a small molecule	http://www.swissdock.ch/
70.	DockingServer	DockingServer offers a Web-based, easy to use interface that handles all aspects of molecular docking from ligand and protein setup	http://www.dockingserver.com/web
71.	BSP-SLIM	Web service for blind molecular docking method on low-resolution protein structures. The method first identifies putative ligand binding sites by structurally matching the target to the template holo-structures	http://zhanglab.ccmb.med.umich.edu/BSP-SLIM/
72.	1-Click Docking	Free online molecular docking solution. Solutions can be visualized online in 3D using the WebGL/Javascript based molecule viewer of GLmol	https://mcule.com/apps/1-click-docking/?utm_source=ccl&utm_medium=maillist&utm_campaign=1-click-docking
73.	MEDock	Maximum-Entropy based docking Web server for efficient prediction of ligand binding sites	http://medock.csbb.ntu.edu.tw/
74.	Blaster	Public access service for structure-based ligand discovery. Uses DOCK as the docking program and various ZINC database subsets as the database	http://blaster.docking.org/
75.	Docking At UTMB	Web-driven interface for performing structure-based VS with AutoDock Vina	http://docking.utmb.edu/
76.	PatchDock	Web server for structure prediction of protein–protein and protein–small molecule complexes based on shape complementarity principles	http://bioinfo3d.cs.tau.ac.il/PatchDock/
77.	Pardock	All-atom energy based Monte Carlo, rigid protein ligand docking, implemented in a fully automated, parallel processing mode which predicts the binding mode of the ligand in receptor target site	http://www.scfbio-iitd.res.in/dock/pardock.jsp

TABLE 9 (*Continued*)

78.	FlexPepDock	High-resolution peptide docking (refinement) protocol, implemented within the Rosetta framework. The input for this server is a PDB file of a complex between a protein receptor and an estimated conformation for a peptide	http://flexpepdock.furman-lab.cs.huji.ac.il/
79.	PatchDock	Web server for structure prediction of protein–protein and protein–small molecule complexes based on shape complementarity principles	http://bioinfo3d.cs.tau.ac.il/PatchDock/

The potential for a docking algorithm to be used as a VS tool is based on both speed and accuracy. Another application is the screening of the side effects that can be caused by the interactions with other proteins, like proteases, Cytochrome P450, and others. It is also possible to check the specificity of a potential drug against homologous proteins through docking. Docking is also a widely used tool in predicting protein–protein interactions. Knowledge of the molecular associations, aids in understanding a variety of pathways taking place in vivo and in revealing of the possible pharmacological targets. QSAR modeling and docking applications by *in silico* studies of phytochemicals from plants used in traditional Indian medicine have been fulfilled. Several papers have been published in which QSAR modeling was used for studying the properties of Indian herbal medicines [45–48]. Most of these studies combine QSAR modeling of the appropriate therapeutic activity with docking for revealing the possible targets or mechanisms of action of the studied phytochemicals.

2.3.8.1 MOLECULAR DOCKING APPLICATIONS

QSAR and molecular docking studies were performed to explore antimalarial novel artemisinin derivatives. The QSAR model showed a high correlation (r^2 = 0.83 and rCV^2 = 0.81) and indicated that connectivity index (order 1, standard), connectivity index (order 2, standard), dipole moment (debye), dipole vector X (debye), and LUMO energy (electron volt) correlate well with activity. High binding likeness on antimalarial target plasmepsin was detected through molecular docking. Active artemisinin derivatives showed significant activity and indicated compliance with standard parameters of oral bioavailability and ADMET. The active artemisinin derivatives namely, β-Artecyclopropylmether HMCP (A3), β-Artepipernoylether (PIP-1) (A4), and 9-(β-Dihydroartemisinoxy)methyl anthracene (A5) were semisynthesized and characterized based on its ^{1}H and

^{13}C NMR spectroscopic data and later on their activity; tested in vivo on infected mice with multidrug resistant strain of *Plasmodium yoelii nigeriensis*. Thus, successfully validating the predicted results by in vivo experiments [45].

A different QSAR model was developed on the basis of forward stepwise multiple linear regression method for the prediction of anticancer activity of 18β-glycyrrhetinic acid derivatives against the human breast cancer cell line MCF-7. The QSAR model for antiproliferative activity against MCF-7 showed high correlation (r^2=0.89 and rCV^2=0.85) and indicates that chemical descriptors namely, dipole moment (debye), steric energy (kcal/mole), heat of formation (kcal/mole), ionization potential (electron volt), LogP, LUMO energy (electron volt), and shape index (basic kappa, order 3) correlate well with activity. The QSAR predicted virtually active derivatives were first semisynthesized and characterized on the basis of their ^{1}H and ^{13}C NMR spectroscopic data and then were in vitro tested against MCF-7 cancer cell line. In particular, derivative of some glycyrrhetinic acid has marked cytotoxic activity against MCF-7 similar to that of standard anticancer drug "paclitaxel". The biological assays of active derivative selected by VS showed significant experimental activity [46].

A QSAR model and docking study was performed for the prediction of anticancer activity of glycyrrhetinic acid (GA) analogs against the human lung cancer cell line (A-549), the QSAR model was developed by forward stepwise multiple linear regression methodology. The regression coefficient (r^2) and prediction accuracy (rCV^2) of the QSAR model were 0.94 and 0.82, respectively. The QSAR study indicated that the dipole moments, size of smallest ring, amine counts, hydroxyl, and nitro functional groups are correlated well with cytotoxic activity. Docking studies showed high binding affinity of the predicted active compounds against the lung cancer target epidermal growth factor receptor. These active glycyrrhetinic acid derivatives were then semisynthesized, characterized, and in vitro tested for anticancer activity. The experimental results were in agreement with the predicted values and the ethyl oxalyl derivative of GA showed equal cytotoxic activity to that of standard anticancer drug "paclitaxel" [47].

QSAR models of camptothecin derivatives against Topoisomerase-I were developed by multiple linear regression method using leave-one-out validation approach. The r^2 and rCV^2 of the model were 0.89 and 0.86, respectively. The QSAR study indicated that chemical descriptors, viz. connectivity index (order 1, standard), electron affinity (electron volt), molecular weight, and group count (ether), correlate well with the activity. Further, screening for drug likeness, ADME, and toxicity showed that the compounds CPT9, CPT14, CPT20, CPT21, and CPT22 exhibit marked anticancer activity and possesses twice the potency of the standard drug camptothecin. The docking study showed high binding affinity of the predicted active derivatives that showed H-bond formation with GLY363, ARG364, LYS374, GLN421, ARG488, and ASP-533 thus considered as the most stable and potent anticancer compounds. The obtained results in this study will be helpful for the design of new potent and selective inhibitors of DNA Topoisomerase-I [48].

2.3.9 ADME/TOXICITY

In silico ADMET properties are now computable, and the accuracy of some of the software predictions, for physico-chemical properties in particular, is close to that of measured data. There is, however, a universal agreement that additional experimental ADME/T data are needed for the *in silico* model development, since models are only as good as the data on which they are based [49]. The traditional approach to drug discovery focused primarily on potency, and only later in the development process were ADME/T properties and toxicity considered. This inevitably led to numerous costly failures and so, in the late 1980s and early 1990s, earlier consideration began to be given to ADME/T. Initially this was mostly a measure of physico-chemical properties (e.g., aqueous solubility) and in vitro testing. Poor ADME properties and toxicities still accounted for 60% of new chemical entities (NCEs) failures [50]. At around the same time, combinatorial chemical techniques were producing huge increases in NCEs, and although HTS helped to filter out chemicals with undesirable properties, this was not sufficient, thereby creating the so-called ADME bottleneck. *In silico* ADME/T prediction techniques may be categorized into methods that model the reactions relevant for both ADME and toxicity, that is, (a) molecular modeling or pharmacophore modeling databases, where the interaction, or "best fit", of a small molecule within or with the active site of a typical protein receptor, has proven especially useful for the detection and evaluation of new leads, (b) techniques based on cumulative observations, that is, expert systems, and (c) methods that utilize predictions based on experimental data and training sets, the so-called data driven systems. These systems utilize QSAR/QSPR modeling techniques, complemented with data mining techniques such as ANNs, Bayesian modeling, decision and regression trees, and support vector machines [51].

2.3.9.1 PHYSICAL PROPERTIES OF ADME

Physical properties of a molecule can profoundly affect its oral absorption, that is, distribution, metabolism, excretion, and toxicology properties; hence, these properties play a very critical role in the bioavailability and action duration of new drugs, thereby determining their clinical success. Lipinski's "Rule of 5"

[52] provided a rallying point for the majority of scientists to even consider that a strategy for oral absorption was feasible by utilizing basic physico-chemical properties of a molecule. This set of guidelines, rather than rules, suggested that absorption and permeability issues were more likely to occur when two or more of the following criteria were true for the compounds: molecular weight exceeding 500 amu; calculated log P greater than 5; more than 5 hydrogen bond donors; and more than 10 hydrogen bond acceptors. Using a number of ADME descriptors—for example, solubility, permeability, bioavailability, volume of distribution, plasma protein binding, central nervous system (CNS) penetration (i.e., blood–brain barrier permeability), brain tissue binding, p-glycoprotein efflux, hERG inhibition, and CYP inhibition—Gleeson from GlaxoSmithKline has put together what he calls a set of simple, interpretable ADME/T rules of thumb[53].

The bioavailability of compounds from their physico-chemical properties and structures using computational approaches has recently gained considerable attention. Computational methods are currently available to estimate solubility, metabolism, toxicity, pKa, blood–brain barrier permeability, other ADME, and physico-chemical parameters as shown in **Table 10–12**. Such information is saving time and money in drug discovery projects at all levels. Therefore, ADME/T information during the early stages of the drug design process will help to determine the ultimate fate of a valuable lead. The need for high-throughput approaches in ADME prediction is driven by the impact of combinatorial chemistry and HTS to the drug discovery process. It is a highly valuable tool that can predict biological (in vitro/in vitro) activity through *in silico* approaches. For example, the recent QSAR model for predicting human oral bioavailability of many structurally diverse drugs [54] involves ADME/T in the discovery and development process as shown in Figure 6. *In silico* ADME/T predictions may be utilized, although the reliability of *in silico* predictions for such complex endpoints such as hepatotoxicity, neurotoxicity, and developmental toxicity are severely limited. The following list shows typical ADME and toxicology studies:

Typical ADME studies: Physico-chemical parameters, chemical stability; biological matrices, permeability studies-Caco-2; MDCK; LLC-PK1, metabolic stability—microsomes, hepatocytes, and S9; recombinant CYPs; UGTs, reaction phenotyping with CYPs and UGTs, CYP inhibition and induction, metabolite profiling and identiication, plasma protein binding, blood-plasma partitioning, transporter studies, for example, PgP, BCRP, bioanalytical, PK, tissue distribution*, PK/PD, PBPK, reactive metabolite screening.

Typical toxicology studies: Cytotoxicity, hERG/in vivo QTc studies, genetic toxicity studies including mutagenicity, hepatotoxicity screening, tolerability studies: increasing single dose and multiple day, multiple dose studies in rodent plus a second animal species, Safety Pharmacology inc. CNS, cardiovascular, and GI, carcinogenicity, developmental and reproductive toxicology (DART) studies, 1-month, 3-month, 6-month rat studies and 9-month dog/monkey studies, industrial toxicology studies, neurotoxicity, nuclear receptor screening.

TABLE 10   Software related to ADME/toxicity prediction

S. No.	Software	Description	URL
1.	IMPACT-F.	Expert system to estimate oral bioavailability of drug-candidates in humans. IMPACT-F is composed of several QSAR models to predict oral bioavailability in humans.	http://www.pharmainformatic.com/html/impact-f.html
2.	q-ADME.	Predicts the following properties: drug half-life (T1/2); fraction of oral dose absorbed (FA); Caco-2 permeability; volume of distribution (VD); octanol/water distribution coefficient (Log P)	http://q-pharm.com/category/uncategorized/
3.	DDDPlus	Models and simulates the in vitro dissolution of active pharmaceutical ingredients (API) and formulation excipients dosed as powders, tablets, capsules, and swellable or nonswellable polymer matrices under various experimental conditions	http://www.simulationsplus.com/Products.aspx?DDDPlus&grpID=2&cID=14&pID=14
4.	PredictFX	Program to identify and address safety issues. Predicts the profile of affinities against a panel of biological targets, the profile of side effects, and the link between side effects and target profile	http://www.certara.com/products/predictfx/
5.	ADMET Predictor	Software for advanced predictive modeling of ADMET properties. ADMET predictor estimates a number of ADMET properties from molecular structures, and is also capable of building predictive models of new properties from user's data via its integrated ADMET Modeler module. Distributed by Simulations Plus, Inc.	http://www.simulationsplus.com/Products.aspx?grpID=1&cID=11&pID=13

TABLE 10 (*Continued*)

6.	ACD/ADME Suite	Predicts of ADME properties from chemical structure, like Predict P-gp specificity, oral bioavailability, passive absorption, blood–brain barrier permeation, distribution, P450 inhibitors, substrates and inhibitors, maximum recommended daily dose, Abraham-type (Absolv) solvation parameters	http://www.acdlabs.com/products/percepta/physchem_adme_tox/
7.	q-TOX	Computes toxic effects of chemicals solely from their molecular structure (LD50, MRDD, side effects)	http://q-pharm.com/category/uncategorized/
8.	ADMET Modeler	Integrated module of ADMET predictor that automates the process of making high quality predictive structure–property models from sets of experimental data. It works seamlessly with ADMET predictor structural descriptors as its inputs, and appends the selected final model back to ADMET predictor as an additional predicted property	http://www.simulations-plus.com/Products.aspx?pID=13&mID=14
9.	Filter-it	Command-line program for filtering molecules with unwanted properties out of a set of molecules. The program comes with a number of preprogrammed molecular properties that can be used for filtering	http://silicos-it.com/software/software.html
10.	Virtual LogP	Bernard Testa's Virtual logP calculator. Provided by the Drug Design Laboratory of the University of Milano.	http://159.149.85.2/vlogp.htm
11.	MolScore-Drugs	Expert system to identify and prioritize drug candidates	http://www.pharmainformatic.com/html/molscore-drugs.html
12.	Discovery Studio TOPKAT Software	Cross-validated models for the assessments of chemical toxicity from chemical's molecular structure	http://accelrys.com/products/discovery-studio/admet.html

TABLE 10 *(Continued)*

13.	ADMEWORKS ModelBuilder	Builds QSAR/QSPR models that can later be used for predicting various chemical and biological properties of compounds. Models are based on values of physico-chemical, topological, geometrical, and electronic properties derived from the molecular structure, and can be imported into ADMEWORKS predictor.	http://www.fqs.pl/Chemistry_Materials_Life_Science/products/admeworks_modelbuilder
14.	Molcode Toolbox	Molcode toolbox allows prediction of medicinal and toxicological endpoints for a large variety of chemical structures, using proprietary QSAR models	http://www.molcode.com/?mid=18
15.	ACD/Tox Suite	Collection of software modules that predict probabilities for basic toxicity endpoints. Several modules including hERG inhibition, CYP3A4 inhibition, genotoxicity, acute toxicity, aquatic toxicity, eye/skin irritation, endocrine system disruption, and health effects	http://www.acdlabs.com/products/percepta/physchem_adme_tox/
16.	ACD/PhysChem Suite	Predicts basic physico-chemical properties, like pKa, log P, log D, aqueous solubility, and other molecular properties in seconds, uses fragment-based models	http://www.acdlabs.com/products/percepta/
17.	Derek Nexus	Predicts toxicity properties using QSAR and other expert knowledge rules	http://www.lhasalimited.org/products/derek-nexus.htm
18.	Metabolizer Preview	Enumerates all the possible metabolites of a given substrate, predicts the major metabolites and estimates metabolic stability	http://www.chemaxon.com/products/metabolizer/
19.	MedChem Studio	Cheminformatics platform for computational and medicinal chemists supporting lead identification and optimization, *in silico* ligand based design, and clustering/classifying of compound libraries. It is integrated with MedChem Designer and ADMET predictor	http://www.simulationsplus.com/Products.aspx?MedChem%20Studio&grpID=1&cID=13&pID=12

TABLE 10　(*Continued*)

20.	MedChem Designer	Tool that combines molecule drawing features with a few free ADMET property predictions from ADMET predictor	http://www.simulations-plus.com/Products.aspx?grpID=1&cID=20&pID=25
21.	MetabolExpert	Predicts the most common metabolic pathways in animals, plants, or through photodegradation	http://www.compudrug.com/?q=node/36
22.	FAF-Drugs2	Free package for *in silico* ADMET filtering	http://www.mti.univ-paris-diderot.fr/recherche/plate-formes/logiciels
23.	PrologP/PrologD	Predicts the log P/log D values using a combination of linear and neural network methods	http://www.compudrug.com/?q=node/42
24.	pKalc	Program for predicting acidic and basic pKa	http://www.compudrug.com/?q=node/38
25.	ACD/DMSO Solubility	Predicts solubility in DMSO solution	http://www.acdlabs.com/products/percepta/
26.	HazardExpert Pro	Predicts the toxicity of organic compounds based on toxic fragments	http://www.compudrug.com/?q=node/35
27.	Meteor	Predicts metabolic fate of chemicals using other expert knowledge rules in metabolism	http://www.lhasalimited.org/products/meteor-nexus.htm
28.	COMPACT	Identifies potential carcinogenicity or toxicities mediated by CYP450s	http://www.ncbi.nlm.nih.gov/pubmed/7678916
29.	PK-Sim	Predicts ADMET properties	http://www.systems-biology.com/products/pk-sim/packages.html
30.	PASS	Identification of probable targets and mechanisms of toxicity	http://pharmaexpert.ru/Passonline/index.php
31.	Cloe Predict	Pharmacokinetic prediction using physiologically based pharmacokinetic modeling (PBPK), and prediction of human intestinal absorption using solubility, pKa, and Caco-2 permeability data	http://www.cyprotex.com/insilico/
32.	ADMEWORKS Predictor	QSAR based virtual (*in silico*) screening system intended for simultaneous evaluation of the properties of compounds	http://www.fqs.pl/chemistry_materials_life_science/products/admeworks_predictor

TABLE 10   (*Continued*)

33.	Natural product likeness calculator	Calculates natural product (NP)-likeness of a molecule, that is, the similarity of the molecule to the structure space covered by known natural products. NP-likeness is a useful criterion to screen compound libraries and to design new lead compounds	http://sourceforge.net/projects/np-likeness/
34.	Leadscope	Estimates toxiticy using QSAR	http://www.leadscope.com/data_management/
35.	MEXAlert	Identifies compounds that have a high probability of being eliminated from the body in a first pass through the liver and kidney	http://www.compudrug.com/
36.	Discovery Studio ADMET Software	The ADMET collection provides components that calculate predicted ADMET properties for collections of molecules	http://accelrys.com/products/discovery-studio/admet.html
37.	SimCYP	The SimCYP population-based ADME simulator is a platform for the prediction of drug–drug interactions and pharmacokinetic outcomes in clinical populations	http://www.simcyp.com/
38.	KnowItAll - ADME | Tox Edition	Prediction of ADME toxicological properties using consensus modeling	http://www.bio-rad.com/
39.	KOWWIN - EPI Suite	Estimates the log octanol–water partition coefficient of chemicals using an atom/fragment contribution method. Distributed by the EPA's Office of Pollution Prevention Toxics and Syracuse Research Corporation (SRC) as part of the EPI Suite	http://www.epa.gov/opptintr/exposure/pubs/episuite.htm
40.	ToxTree	Full-featured and flexible user friendly open source application to estimate toxic hazard by applying a decision tree approach	http://toxtree.sourceforge.net/
41.	ADRIANA Code	Program to calculate physico-chemical properties of small molecules: number of H-bonds donor and acceptors, log P, log S, TPSA, dipole moment, polarizability, etc.	http://www.molecular-networks.com/products/adrianacode

TABLE 10 (*Continued*)

42.	OncoLogic	Evaluates the likelihood that a chemical may cause cancer, using SAR analysis, experts' decision mimicking, and knowledge of how chemicals cause cancer in animals and humans. Distributed for free by the US Environmental Protection Agency (EPA).	http://www.epa.gov/oppt/sf/pubs/oncologic.htm
43.	isoCYP	Software for the prediction of the predominant human cytochrome P450 isoform by which a given chemical compound is metabolized in phase I	http://www.molecular-networks.com/products/isocyp
44.	QikProp	Provides rapid ADME predictions of drug candidates	http://www.schrodinger.com/
45.	SMARTCyp	SMARTCyp predicts the sites in molecules that are most liable to cytochrome P450 mediated metabolism	http://www.farma.ku.dk/smartcyp/download.php
46.	MetaDrug	Predicts toxicity and metabolism of compounds using >70 QSAR models for ADME/Tox properties	http://lsresearch.thomson-reuters.com/pages/solutions
47.	SimCYP for iPhone	The SimCYP population-based ADME simulator is a platform for the prediction of drug–drug interactions and pharmacokinetic outcomes in clinical populations	https://itunes.apple.com/gb/app/simcyp-adme-prediction-toolbox/id496818712?mt=8
48.	VolSurf	Calculate ADME properties and create predictive ADME models	http://www.tripos.com/index.php?family=modules,SimplePage,,,&page=Volsurf+
49.	StarDrop	Allows the identification of the region of a molecule that is the most vulnerable to metabolism by the major drug metabolising isoforms of cytochrome P450	http://www.optibrium.com/stardrop/stardrop-p450-models.php
50.	GastroPlus	Simulates the oral absorption, pharmacokinetics, and pharmacodynamics for drugs in human and preclinical species. The underlying model is the Advanced Compartmental Absorption and Transit (ACAT) model	http://www.simulations-plus.com/Products.aspx?GastroPlus&grpID=3&cID=16&pID=11

TABLE 10 (*Continued*)

| 51. | MetaSite | Computational procedure that predicts metabolic transformations related to cytochrome-mediated reactions in phase I metabolism and predicts the structures of the most likely metabolites and warns about the potential of CYP mechanism-based inhibition | http://www.moldiscovery.com/software/metasite |

Table 11 Web resources related to ADME/toxicity prediction

S. No.	Resources	Description	URL
1.	ADME-Tox	ADME-Tox (poor ADME or toxicity) filtering for small compounds, based on a set of elementary rules	http://mobyle.rpbs.univ-paris-diderot.fr/cgi-bin/portal.py?form=admetox#welcome
2.	OSIRIS Property Explorer	Calculates on-the-fly various drug-relevant properties for drawn chemical structures, including some toxicity and drug-likeness properties	http://www.organic-chemistry.org/prog/peo/
3.	XScore-LogP	Calculates the octanol/water partition coefficient for a drug, based on a feature of the X-Score program	http://mobyle.rpbs.univ-paris-diderot.fr/cgi-bin/portal.py?form=PASS#welcome
4.	Lazar	Lazy Structure Activity Relationships. Derives predictions from toxicity databases by searching for similar compounds	http://lazar.in-silico.de/predict
5.	AquaSol	Predicts aqueous solubility of small molecules using UG-RNN ensembles	http://cdb.ics.uci.edu/cgibin/tools/AquaSolWeb.py
6.	Toxicity checker	Webserver for searching substructures commonly found in toxic and promiscuous ligands. Based on more than 100 SMARTS toxic matching rules	https://mcule.com/apps/toxicity-checker/

TABLE 10   (*Continued*)

7.	ToxCreate	Web service to create computational models to predict toxicity. Provided by OpenTox.	http://www.toxcreate.net/create
8.	DrugMint	Web server predicting the drug-likeness of compounds	http://crdd.osdd.net/oscadd/drugmint/
9.	admetSAR	admetSAR provides the manually curated data for diverse chemicals associated with known ADME and toxicity profiles	http://www.admetexp.org/
10.	Property calculator	Creates a physico-chemical property profile for a compound	https://mcule.com/apps/property-calculator/
11.	Chemicalize	Calculates or predict molecular properties, including log P, tautomers, PSA, pK, lipinskilike filters, etc.	http://www.chemicalize.org/
12.	PharmMapper	To identify potential target candidates for the given probe small molecules (drugs, natural products, or other newly discovered compounds with binding targets unidentified) using pharmacophore mapping approach	http://59.78.96.61/pharmmapper/
13.	ALOGPS	Online prediction of log P, water solubility, and pKa(s) of compounds for drug design (ADME/T and HTS) and environmental chemistry studies	http://www.vcclab.org/lab/alogps/
14.	Free ADME Tools	ADME Prediction Toolbox of the SimCYP application	http://www.simcyp.com/ProductServices/FreeADMETools/
15.	ToxPredict	Web service to estimate toxicological hazard of a chemical structure	http://apps.ideaconsult.net:8080/ToxPredict
16.	ToxiPred	A server for prediction of aqueous toxicity of small chemical molecules in *Tetrahymena pyriformis*	http://crdd.osdd.net/oscadd/toxipred/

TABLE 10 (*Continued*)

17.	MetaPred	MetaPred server predicts metabolizing CYP isoform of a drug molecule/substrate, based on support vector machine models developed using CDK descriptors	http://crdd.osdd.net/oscadd/metapred/
18.	Molinfo	Calculates or predict molecular properties other than 3D structure	http://cdb.ics.uci.edu/cgibin/tools/MolInfoWeb.py
19.	VirtualToxLab	"*In silico*" tool for predicting the toxic (endocrine-disrupting) potential of existing and hypothetical compounds (drugs, chemicals, natural products) by simulating and quantifying their interactions toward a series of proteins known to trigger adverse effects using automated, flexible docking combined with multidimensional QSAR (mQSAR).	http://www.biograf.ch/index.php?id=projects&subid=virtualtoxlab
20.	SMARTCyp Web Service	SMARTCyp predicts the sites in molecules that are most liable to cytochrome P450 mediated metabolism	http://www.farma.ku.dk/smart-cyp/

TABLE 12 Database related to ADME/toxicity prediction

S. No.	Database	Description	URL
1.	DTome	Provides a computational framework to effectively construct a drug–target networks by integrating the drug–drug interactions, drug–target interactions, drug–gene associations and target/gene–protein interactions	http://bioinfo.mc.vanderbilt.edu/DTome/
2.	Cloe Knowledge	Open access ADME/PK database for a range of marketed drugs	https://www.cloegateway.com/services/cloe_knowledge/pages/search.php

TABLE 10   (*Continued*)

3.	SuperHapten	Comprehensive database for small immunogenic compounds. Contains currently 7,257 haptens, 453 commercially available related antibodies, and 24 carriers. Provided by Charité Berlin, Institute of Molecular Biology and Bioinformatics.	http://bioinformatics.charite.de/superhapten/
4.	WOMBAT-PK	Database for clinical pharmacokinetics and drug target information. Its 2010 contains 1,260, totaling over 9,450 clinical pharmacokinetic measurements; it further includes 2,316 physico-chemical properties; 932 toxicity endpoints, and 2,186 annotated drug–target bioactivities	http://www.sunset-molecular.com/index.php?option=com_content &view=article&id=16 &Itemid=11
5.	PHYSPROP	The Physical Properties database contains chemical structures, names, and physical properties for over 41,000 chemicals. Physical properties are collected from a wide variety of sources, and include experimental, extrapolated, and estimated values for melting point, boiling point, water solubility, octanol–water partition coefficient, vapor pressure, pKa, Henry's law constant, and OH rate constant in the atmosphere	http://www.srcinc.com/?id=133
6.	PACT-F	The database contains 8,296 records, which describe in detail the results of clinical trials in humans and preclinical trials in animals	http://www.pharmainfor-matic.com/html/pact-f.html
7.	SIDER	Contains information on marketed medicines and their recorded adverse drug reactions. The available information include side effect frequency, drug and side effect classifications as well as links to further information, for example drug–target relations	http://sideeffects.embl.de/
8.	SuperTarget Database	Database of about 332,828 drug–target relations	http://bioinf-apache.charite.de/supertarget_v2/

TABLE 10 (*Continued*)

9.	ACToR	Database of all publicly available chemical toxicity data that can be used to find potential chemical risks to human health and the environment. ACToR aggregates data from over 500 public sources on over 500,000 environmental chemicals searchable by chemical name, other identifiers and by chemical structure	http://actor.epa.gov/actor/faces/ACToRHome.jsp
10.	DART	A database for facilitating the search for drug adverse reaction target. It contains information about known drug adverse rection targets, functions, and properties	http://xin.cz3.nus.edu.sg/group/drt/dart.asp
11.	ADMEAP	A database for facilitating the search for drug ADME-associated proteins	http://bidd.nus.edu.sg/group/admeap/admeap.asp
15.	ADME DB	Database containing data on interactions of substances with Drug Metabolizing Enzymes and Drug Transporters. It is designed for use in drug research and development, including drug–drug interactions and ADME studies.	http://www.fqs.pl/chemistry_materials_life_science/products/adme_db
12.	SAR Genetox Database	Genetic toxicity database to be used as a resource for developing predictive modeling training sets	http://www.leadscope.com/product_info.php?products_id=77
13.	The ADME databases	Databases for benchmarking the results of experiments, validating the accuracy of existing ADME predictive models, and building new predictive models	http://modem.ucsd.edu/adme/databases/databases.htm
14.	HMDB	The Human Metabolome Database (HMDB) is a freely available electronic database containing detailed information about small molecule metabolites found in the human body.	http://www.hmdb.ca/
15.	Leadscope	Toxicity database. Database of 160,000 chemical structures with toxicity data	http://www.leadscope.com/product_info.php?products_id=78

TABLE 10 (*Continued*)

16.	DITOP	(Drug-Induced Toxicity Related Proteins). Database of proteins that mediate toxicities through their interaction with drugs or reactive metabolites. Can be searched using keywords of chemicals, proteins, or toxicity terms	http://bioinf.xmu.edu.cn:8080/databases/DITOP/index.html
17.	SuperCyp	Comprehensive database on Cyto-chrome P450 enzymes including a tool for analysis of CYP–drug interactions.	http://bioinformatics.charite.de/supercyp/index.php?site=home
22.	t3db	Combines detailed toxin data with comprehensive toxin target information. The database currently houses over 2,900 toxins described by over 34,200 synonyms, includ-ing pollutants, pesticides, drugs, and food toxins, which are linked to over 1,300 corresponding toxin target records.	http://www.t3db.org/
18.	SAR Carci-nogenicity Database	Carcinogenicity database with validated structures to be used as a resource for preparing training sets	http://www.leadscope.com/product_info.php?products_id=65
19.	PROMISCU-OUS	Exhaustive resource of protein–pro-tein and drug–protein interactions with the aim of providing a uniform data set for drug repositioning and further analysis	http://bioinformatics.charite.de/promiscuous/
20.	TOXNET	Databases on toxicology, hazard-ous chemicals, environmental health, and toxic releases that can be accessed using a common search interface	http://toxnet.nlm.nih.gov/index.html
21.	SuperToxic	Collection of toxic compounds from literature and Web sources. The cur-rent version of this database com-piles approx. 60,000 compounds with about 100,000 synonyms. These molecules are classified according to their toxicity based on more than 2,500,000 measurements.	http://bioinformatics.charite.de/supertoxic/index.php?site=home

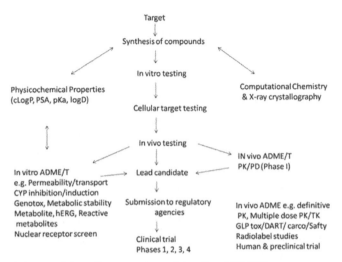

FIGURE 6   Scheme of drug discovery through *in silico* ADME/T.

Among the physico-chemical properties that the medicinal chemist will try to consider and manipulate is lipophilicity. **Table 10** shows the parameter or descriptor, important for the permeability across membranes and therefore critical for absorption, distribution, metabolism, and excretion. Initially, the log P value is an important indicator of lipophilicity and hence permeability, although it is better described by log D, usually at pH 7.4, especially for ionizable compounds. Actually, medicinal chemists are most adept at making permeable compounds and these may be assessed by comparatively high throughput methods such as Caco-2, MDCK, and LLPK-1 cell lines or PAMPA (parallel artificial membrane assay) or more laboriously with isolated in situ gut loops or everted gastrointestinal sacs from preclinical species. While the use of Caco-2 cells has proven useful for permeability and possibly absorption predictions, the same cannot be said for the prediction of efflux substrates where discrepancies between Caco-2 cells, MDCK, and LLPK-1 cell lines have occurred with some important ramifications not only for passage across the gastrointestinal tract but across the blood–brain barrier as well [52]. The properties determining permeability, that is, gaining passage across a membrane include the size of the molecule, the capacity to make H-bonds (diminishing the number of hydrogen bonds with the aqueous environment enhance permeability), the overall lipophilicity of the molecule, the shape and flexibility of the molecule, that is, number of rotatable bonds. The databases listed in **Table 12** can be used for measurement of this parameter in low solubility compounds which is a challenge although a number of computer programs are available, not only for pKa, but also for solubility, log

P, log D, polar surface area, molecular volume, for example, Pipeline Pilot, Bio-Loom, Know-It-All, ACD LogD Suite, and QikProp [55].

2.4 CONCLUSION

Nowadays, the drug design methods are of importance for prediction of biological profile, leads generation, leads identification, and to accelerate the optimization of compounds into drug candidates. Generally, the process of drug development has revolved around a screening approach, as it is highly unpredictable that which molecules or methods could serve as a drug or therapy. Drug discovery process is time consuming and takes about 10 to 15 years to develop a new medicine. For conventional screening and standardization of a new and successfull drug, average cost falls around $1.2 billion or more. Through rational drug designing, researchers can predict biological activity of designed molecules, using the above-mentioned tools before going across experimental laboratory work. The breadth of tools and Web resources along with traditional approaches described in this chapter will be highly useful for understanding of different kinds of *in silico* approaches. The aforementioned computational resources are valuable for drug design processes and to greatly reduce the wet lab expenses and time.

KEYWORDS

- **Combinatorial chemistry**
- **Computer-aided molecular modeling**
- **Molecular docking**
- **QSAR modeling**
- **Virtual screening**

REFERENCES

1. Guido, R. V., Oliva, G. & Andricopulo, A. D. (2008) Virtual screening and its integration with modern drug design technologies, *Current medicinal chemistry.* **15**, 37–46.
2. Yadav, D. K., Meena, A., Srivastava, A., Chanda, D., Khan, F. & Chattopadhyay, S. K. (2010) Development of QSAR model for immunomodulatory activity of natural coumarinolignoids, *Drug design, development and therapy.* **4**, 173–86.
3. Sakthivel, G., Dey, A., Nongalleima, K., Chavali, M., Rimal Isaac, R. S., Singh, N. S. & Deb, L. (2013) In vitro and in vivo evaluation of polyherbal formulation against Russell's viper and cobra venom and screening of bioactive components by docking studies, *Evidence-based complementary and alternative medicine : eCAM.* **2013**, 781216.

4. Rollinger, J. M., Schuster, D., Danzl, B., Schwaiger, S., Markt, P., Schmidtke, M., Gertsch, J., Raduner, S., Wolber, G., Langer, T. & Stuppner, H. (2009) *In silico* target fishing for rationalized ligand discovery exemplified on constituents of Ruta graveolens, *Planta medica.* **75**, 195–204.

5. Yadav, D. K., Khan, F. & Negi, A. S. (2012) Pharmacophore modeling, molecular docking, QSAR, and *in silico* ADMET studies of gallic acid derivatives for immunomodulatory activity, *Journal of molecular modeling.* **18**, 2513–2525.

6. Barlow, D. J., Buriani, A., Ehrman, T., Bosisio, E., Eberini, I. & Hylands, P. J. (2012) In-silico studies in Chinese herbal medicines' research: evaluation of in-silico methodologies and phytochemical data sources, and a review of research to date, *Journal of ethnopharmacology.* **140**, 526–534.

7. Xu, J. & Hagler, A. (2002) Chemoinformatics and drug discovery, *Molecules.* **7**, 566–600.

8. Friedrich Cramer, F. & Fischer's, E. (2007) Lock-and-Key Hypothesis after 100 years - Towards a Supracellular Chemistry'. Perspectives in Supramolecular Chemistry: the lock-and-key Principle, *John Wiley & Sons, Ltd,* . **1**, 1–23.

9. Chuaqui, C., Deng, Z. & Singh, J. (2005) Interaction profiles of protein kinase-inhibitor complexes and their application to virtual screening, *Journal of medicinal chemistry.* **48**, 121–133.

10. Bock, J. R. & Gough, D. A. (2005) Virtual screen for ligands of orphan G protein-coupled receptors, *Journal of chemical information and modeling.* **45**, 1402–1414.

11. Jain, S. K. & Chincholikar, A. (2004) Pharmacophore mapping and drug design, *Indian journal of Pharmaceutical sciences.* **66**, 11–17.

12. Lill, M. (2013) Virtual screening in drug design, *Methods in molecular biology.* **993**, 1–12.

13. Crossley, R. (2004) The design of screening libraries targeted at G-protein coupled receptors, *Current topics in medicinal chemistry.* **4**, 581–588.

14. Clark, M. (2005) Generalized fragment-substructure based property prediction method, *Journal of chemical information and modeling.* **45**, 30–38.

15. Wilson, S.R. & Czarnik, A. W. (1997) Combinatorial Chemistry-Synthesis and Application, *Wiley & Sons: New York.*

16. Czarnik, A. W. & DeWitt, S. H. A. (1997) A Practical Guide to Combinatorial Chemistry, *American Chemical Society: Washington, DC.*

17. Crossley, R. (2004) The design of screening libraries targeted at G-protein coupled receptors, *Current topics in medical chemistry.* **4**, 581–588.

18. Steindl, T. M., Schuster, D., Laggner, C. & Langer, T. (2006) Parallel screening: a novel concept in pharmacophore modeling and virtual screening, *Journal of chemical information and modeling.* **46**, 2146–2157.

19. Koch, M. A., Schuffenhauer, A., Scheck, M., Wetzel, S., Casaulta, M., Odermatt, A., Ertl, P. & Waldmann, H. (2005) Charting biologically relevant chemical space: a structural classification of natural products (SCONP), *Proceedings of the national academy of sciences of the United States of America.* **102**, 17272–17277.

20. Keseru, G. M. & Makara, G. M. (2006) Hit discovery and hit-to-lead approaches, *Drug discovery today.* **11**, 741–748.

21. Bleicher, K. H., Bohm, H. J., Muller, K. & Alanine, A. I. (2003) Hit and lead generation: beyond high-throughput screening, *Nature reviews drug discovery.* **2**, 369–378.

22. Gillet, V., Johnson, A. P., Mata, P., Sike, S. & Williams, P. (1993) SPROUT: a program for structure generation, *Journal of computer-aided molecular design.* **7**, 127–153.

23. Wang, J., Krudy, G., Xie, X. Q., Wu, C. & Holland, G. (2006) Genetic algorithm-optimized QSPR models for bioavailability, protein binding, and urinary excretion, *Journal of chemical information and modeling.* **46**, 2674–2683.

24. Votano, J. R., Parham, M., Hall, L. H., Kier, L. B. & Hall, L. M. (2004) Prediction of aqueous solubility based on large datasets using several QSPR models utilizing topological structure representation, *Chemistry biodiversity.* **1**, 1829–1841.

25. Singh, S., Khadikar, P. V., Scozzafava, A. & Supuran, C. T. (2009) QSAR studies for the inhibition of the transmembrane carbonic anhydrase isozyme XIV with sulfonamides using PRECLAV software, *Journal of enzyme inhibition and medicinal chemistry.* **24**, 337–349.

26. Cramer, R. D. (2012) The inevitable QSAR renaissance, *Journal of computer-aided molecular design.* **26**, 35–38.

27. Katritzky, A. R., Victor, S., Lobanov & Karelson, M. (1995) QSPR: the correlation and quantitative prediction of chemical and physical properties from structure, *Chemical society reviews.* **24**, 279–287.

28. Berk, R. A. (2003) Simple Linear Regression. Regression Analysis: a Constructive Critique, *SAGE Publications Ltd: London, pp,* 21–38.

29. Polanski, J. (2009) Receptor dependent multidimensional QSAR for modeling drug--receptor interactions, *Current medicinal chemistry.* **16**, 3243–3257.

30. Fernandez, A. (2005) Incomplete protein packing as a selectivity filter in drug design, *Structure.* **13**, 1829–1836.

31. de Beer, T. A., Wells, G. A., Burger, P. B., Joubert, F., Marechal, E., Birkholtz, L. & Louw, A. I. (2009) Antimalarial drug discovery: *in silico* structural biology and rational drug design, *Infectious disorders drug targets.* **9**, 304-18.

32. Bondensgaard, K., Ankersen, M., Thogersen, H., Hansen, B. S., Wulff, B. S. & Bywater, R. P. (2004) Recognition of privileged structures by G-protein coupled receptors, *Journal of medicinal chemistry.* **47**, 888–899.

33. Deng, Z., Chuaqui, C. & Singh, J. (2004) Structural interaction fingerprint (SIFt): a novel method for analyzing three-dimensional protein-ligand binding interactions, *Journal of medicinal chemistry.* **47**, 337–44.

34. Jambon, M., Imberty, A., Deleage, G. & Geourjon, C. (2003) A new bioinformatic approach to detect common 3D sites in protein structures, *Proteins.* **52**, 13745.

35. Morris, G. M., Goodsell, D. S., Halliday, R. S., Huey, R., Hart, W. E., Belew, R. K. & Olson, A. J. (1998) Automated docking using a Lamarckian genetic algorithm and an empirical binding free energy function, *Journal of computational chemistry.* **19**, 1639–1662.

36. Friesner, R. A., Banks, J. L., Murphy, R. B., Halgren, T. A., Klicic, J. J., Mainz, D. T., Repasky, M. P., Knoll, E. H., Shelley, M., Perry, J. K., Shaw, D. E., Francis, P. & Shenkin, P. S. (2004) Glide: a new approach for rapid, accurate docking and scoring. 1. Method and assessment of docking accuracy, *Journal of medicinal chemistry.* **47**, 1739–1749.

37. Ewing, T. J. A. & Kuntz, I. D. (1997) *Critical evaluation of search algorithms used in automated molecular docking, Journal of computational chemistry* **18**, 1175–1189.

38. Venkatachalam, C. M., Jiang, X., Oldfield, T. & Waldman, M. (2003) LigandFit: a novel method for the shape-directed rapid docking of ligands to protein active sites, *Journal of molecular graphics & modelling.* **21**, 289–307.

39. Jones, G., Willett, P., Glen, R. C., Leach, A. R. & Taylor, R. (1997) Development and validation of a genetic algorithm for flexible docking, *Journal of molecular biology.* **267**, 727–748.

40. Stewart, J. P. (2009) Mopac93, Fujitsu Ltd., Tokyo, Japan *Scigress Explorer v77047.*

41. Rarey, M., Kramer, B. & Lengauer, T. (1999) Docking of hydrophobic ligands with interaction-based matching algorithms, *Bioinformatics.* **15**, 243–250.

42. Hoppe, C., Steinbeck, C. & Wohlfahrt, G. (2006) Classification and comparison of ligand-binding sites derived from grid-mapped knowledge-based potentials, *Journal of molecular graphics & modelling.* **24**, 328–340.

43. Walters, W. P., Stahl, M. T. & Murcko, M. A. (1998) Virtual screening—an overview, *Drug discovery today.* **3**, 160–178.

44. Fukunishi, Y., Kubota, S. & Nakamura, H. (2006) Noise reduction method for molecular interaction energy: application to *in silico* drug screening and *in silico* target protein screening, *Journal of chemical information and modeling.* **46**, 2071–2084.
45. Yadav, D. K., Dhawan, S., Chauhan, A., Qidwai, T., Sharma, P., Bhakuni, R. S., Dhawan, O. P. & Khan, F. (2014) QSAR and docking based semi-synthesis and in vivo evaluation of artemisinin derivatives for antimalarial activity, *Current drug targets.* **15**, 753–761.
46. Yadav, D. K., Kalani, K., Singh, A. K., Khan, F., Srivastava, S. K. & Pant, A. B. (2014) Design, synthesis and in vitro evaluation of 18beta-glycyrrhetinic acid derivatives for anticancer activity against human breast cancer cell line MCF-7, *Current medicinal chemistry.* **21**, 1160-1170.
47. Yadav, D. K., Kalani, K., Khan, F. & Srivastava, S. K. (2013) QSAR and docking based semi-synthesis and in vitro evaluation of 18 beta-glycyrrhetinic acid derivatives against human lung cancer cell line A-549, *Medicinal Chemistry.* **9**, 1073–1084.
48. Yadav, D. K. & Khan, F. (2013) Docking and ADMET studies of Camptothecin derivatives as inhibitors of DNA Topoisomerase-I, *Journal of chemometrics* **27**, 21–33.
49. Dearden, J. C. (2007) *In silico* prediction of ADMET properties: how far have we come?, *Expert Opinion on Drug Metabolism and Toxicology.* **3**, 635–639.
50. Kennedy, T. (1997) Managing the drug discovery/development interface, *Drug discovery today.* **2**, 436–444.
51. Sato, T., Matsuo, Y., Honma, T. & Yokoyama, S. (2008) *In silico* functional profiling of small molecules and its applications, *Journal of medicinal chemistry.* **51**, 7705–7716.
52. Willmann, S., Lippert, J. & Schmitt, W. (2005) From physicochemistry to absorption and distribution: predictive mechanistic modelling and computational tools, *Expert opinion on drug metabolism & toxicology.* **1**, 159–168.
53. Gleeson, M. P. (2008) Generation of a set of simple, interpretable ADMET rules of thumb, *Journal of medicinal chemistry.* **51**, 817–834.
54. Sun, J. R., Lan, P., Sun, P. H. & Chen, W. M. (2011) 3D-QSAR and docking studies on pyrrolopyrimidine derivatives as LIM-kinase 2 inhibitors, *Letters in drug design & discovery.* **8**, 229–240.
55. Khan, F., Yadav, D. K., Maurya, A., Sonia & Srivastava, S. K. (2011) Modern methods & web resources in drug design & discovery, *Letters in drug design & discovery.* **8**, 469–490.

CHAPTER 3

THE r_m^2 METRICS FOR VALIDATION OF QSAR/QSPR MODELS

KUNAL ROY[*] and SUPRATIK KAR

Drug Theoretics and Cheminformatics Laboratory, Department of Pharmaceutical Technology, Jadavpur University, Kolkata 700032, India.

Tel.: +91-98315 94140; fax: +91-33-2837 1078; [*]E-mail: kunalroy_in@yahoo.com, kroy@pharma.jdvu.ac.in; URL: http://sites.google.com/site/kunalroyindia/

CONTENTS

ABSTRACT

Quantitative structure–activity/property relationship (QSAR/QSPR) models being used for the prediction of activity/property of untested chemicals can be exploited for the prioritization plan of synthesis and experimental testing. Validation of QSAR models plays a crucial role for the selection of robust and best predictive models that can be utilized for future activity/property prediction of new molecules. There exists a number of metrics to express the performance of a model but traditionally QSAR models are validated based on classical metrics for internal (Q^2) and external validation (R^2_{pred}). But being primarily dependent on the mean activity data of the training set compounds, both the metrics tend to achieve acceptable values (>0.5) whenever a data set with a wide range of activity/property data is considered. However, such values may not truly reflect the quality of predictions. Therein lies the utility of the r_m^2 metrics developed by Roy *et al.*, which consider the actual difference between the observed and predicted response data without consideration of training set mean, thereby serving as a more stringent measure for the assessment of model predictivity compared to the traditional validation metrics. The r_m^2 metrics depend chiefly on the difference between the observed and predicted activity data and convey more accurate information regarding the quality of predictions. Thus, the r_m^2 metrics strictly judge the ability of a QSAR model to predict the activity/property of untested molecules. We herein focus to have an overview of evolution of different r_m^2 metrics and the software tools for their calculation followed by their successful applications in QSAR modeling.

3.1   INTRODUCTION

A great amount of recent chemical research has been oriented worldwide toward the modeling and design of new chemicals. *In silico* approaches are playing a crucial role in rational drug discovery, property prediction, toxicity, and risk assessment of new drug molecules as well as chemicals [1]. The quantitative structure–activity relationship (QSAR) methodology is one of the computational tools which deal with the correlation between biological activity/toxicity/property of a molecule and its structural features [1, 2]. In a QSAR study, the variation of biological activity within the compounds of a congeneric series is correlated with changes in measured or computed features of the molecules referred to as descriptors. A QSAR model is developed employing a series of molecules with a definite response and this may help in screening large databases of new molecules [3, 4]. It reduces the huge expenditure of money and time for the preliminary experimental studies. Moreover, the Registration, Evaluation and Authorization of Chemicals (REACH) guidelines for animal safety [5] and the 3R concept [6] which represents the three words, that is, reduction, replacement, and refinement of animal experiments restrict the extensive use of animals for initial screening of large databases. The QSAR technique thus provides an alternative pathway for the design and development of new molecules with improved activity profile.

The broad field of QSAR also encompasses studies related to quantitative structure–property relationship (QSPR) and structure–toxicity relationship (QSTR). The QSPR [7] study deals with the molecular features governing physico-chemical properties of compounds, while the QSTR [8] technique determines the structural attributes of the molecules responsible for their toxicity profile. The activity/property encoding features obtained from the developed QSAR models may also be utilized for virtual screening of large libraries of diverse chemicals for a definite response parameter [9]. Besides this, the identification of the prime features imparting improved activity or lower toxicity to the molecules under a particular study facilitates the *in silico* design of new molecules. Thus, a focused library may be developed by compiling the newly designed molecules with a specific response. The principle objectives of QSAR analysis are [10] (a) prediction of new analogue compounds with better property, (b) better understanding and exploration of the mode of action, (c) optimization of the lead compound with decreased toxicity, (d) rationalization of wet laboratory experimentation, and (e) reduction of the cost, time, and manpower requirement by developing more effective compounds using a scientifically less exhaustive approach.

QSAR is an interdisciplinary study involving chemistry, biology, and statistics. A QSAR/QSPR model describes the modeled activity or property as a mathematical function of the chemical attributes [11–13]. The models are particularly suitable for drug design, material design, molecular modeling, and chemical engineering problems. QSAR plays an important role in lead structure optimization and the methods are essential for handling the huge amount of data associated with combinatorial chemistry. The prime utility of a QSAR model lies in its application as a chief database screening tool. QSAR models utilizing appropriate global adsorption, distribution, metabolism, and excretion (ADME) and toxicity models may be helpful in assessing drug-likeness of compounds while designing target focused compound libraries. The descriptors collected based on a validated QSAR model are utilized to select structures and structural building blocks bearing desired chemical features which are included in creating a focused library for biological evaluation. Prediction of specific biological activity, based on the analysis of QSAR of the training set, enables to sort active molecules with similar response for the development of focused libraries [14,

15]. Correlation of the response profile of the molecules with their partition coefficient through QSAR analysis helps to identify the absorption and distribution pattern of the molecules prior to in vivo analysis. Theoretical descriptors for QSPR models being derived solely from the molecular structure have been widely used in predicting various physico-chemical properties, such as boiling point, melting point, vapor pressure, critical properties, water solubility, autoignition temperatures, octanol/water coefficients, and others.

A huge number of QSAR, QSPR, and QSTR models have been developed covering a wide variety of endpoints and statistical techniques to assess the fitness and validity of significant correlations since its early stages. Subsequently, guidance for the approved procedures for the development of QSAR/QSPR models has been given in different literatures [16–20]. In spite of extensive use of QSAR, only recently, noteworthy consideration has been directed toward the validation of the developed QSAR models. Stringent parameters have been employed for extensive validation of the selected QSAR models. The validity of a QSAR model is assessed based on four key tools [21]: (i) cross-validation, (ii) bootstrapping, (iii) randomization of the response data, and (iv) external validation by splitting of the total set of compounds into a training set and a test set followed by verification of the predictive quality of the model using a true external validation set derived from a different source. In order to have a sound scientific basis for implementation of QSAR models for regulatory use, the REACH [22–23] legislation enforced in the European Union inferred that QSARs need to be assessed in terms of their scientific validity. The QSAR models should be validated according to the principles of Organization for Economic Cooperation and Development (OECD) for reliable predictions. These principles were agreed by the OECD member countries, QSAR and regulatory communities at the 37th Joint Meeting of the Chemicals Committee and Working Party on Chemicals, Pesticides, and Biotechnology held in Setubal (Portugal) in March 2002 and were further modified in November 2004. These principles are the best possible summary of the most important points that necessitate to be addressed to find consistent, reliable, and reproducible QSAR models [24].

There has been a great deal of arguments regarding the choice of the most appropriate procedure for validation of a QSAR model among the QSAR modelers [25]. According to one group of authors [26], internal validation can serves as a sufficient criterion for selection of the statistically significant QSAR model provided that such internal validation is done properly. According to Hawkins (26), when the available sample size is small, holding a portion of it back for testing is wasteful, and it is much better to use cross-validation, but ensuring that this is done properly. Hawkins et al., [27] suggest that larger calibration samples give better models than smaller calibration samples, and validation with larger sets is more reliable than with smaller ones. Properly done cross-validation (which uses all available compounds) may be better than the traditional approach of the splitting of the data set into training and test sets [27]. The model developed based on the training set may lack significant information regarding the molecular properties of the total chemical entities. On the contrary, another group of authors states the acceptability of a QSAR model should be based on its ability to predict the activity/property of untested molecules. According to Golbraikh and Tropsha [28], a QSAR model developed using a known set of chemical entities must be validated based on a validation set (test set) of molecules that has not been included for the development of the QSAR model. They proposed several stringent parameters and only the QSAR models exceeding the threshold values for each of these parameters can be considered satisfactory for activity prediction of new molecules not employed in the model development.

According to us, both internal and external validation tools should be used for a statistically significant QSAR model. However, the external predictivity parameter (R^2_{pred}) is largely dependent on the selection of the training set compounds. Moreover, the selection of the most significant QSAR model often becomes difficult in cases where comparable models are obtained with different qualities for the internal (Q^2) and external (R^2_{pred}) predictive parameters. An alternative measure r_m^2 (modified r^2) was suggested to be a better and more stringent metric for selection of the best predictive QSAR models by Roy and co-workers [29–33]. Three variants of r_m^2 have been reported by Roy et al., [29, 30]: (i) $r_{m\,(LOO)}^2$, (ii) $r_{m\,(test)}^2$, and (iii) $r_{m\,(overall)}^2$. The first two parameters are used for judging the internal and external predictivity of the model using the training and test sets, respectively. The third parameter, $r_{m\,(overall)}^2$ may be effectively applied on the whole data set considering LOO-predicted values for the training set and predicted values of the test set compounds. Thus, the parameter $r_{m\,(overall)}^2$ analyzes the developed QSAR model based on both internal and external validation statistics thereby providing an overall measure of the model predictive ability. The parameter $r_{m\,(overall)}^2$ takes into consideration the whole data set; it thus penalizes models for differences between the values of Q^2 and R^2_{pred} enabling one to select the best predictive model. To measure the closeness between the order of the predicted activity data and that of the corresponding observed activity, the $r_{m\,(rank)}^2$ parameter has been introduced by Roy et al., (34). The aim of the $r_{m\,(rank)}^2$ metric is to incorporate information about the rank-order predictions of the analyzed molecules. Different variants of r_m^2 metric have been extensively used in diverse QSAR research for validation purpose. This chapter provides an outline of the work involving the development of the r_m^2 metrics, software tools for their calculation followed by their application for successful validation of QSAR models.

3.2   EVOLUTION OF THE r_m^2 METRICS

The success of any QSAR model depends on precision of the endpoint response, choice of appropriate descriptors, and statistical tools, and most importantly the validation of the developed model with the best possible validation metrics. The reliability and accuracy of QSAR models can be established through appropriate validation of the process involved in developing the QSAR model and thus the validation step plays the most important role in the QSAR model building process [35–40]. Hence, the models should be validated both internally and externally in order to check their robustness and predictive potential for testing new chemical entities in the near future.

Several metrics are used to check the predictivity of the QSAR models. For the validation of QSAR models, three strategies can be primarily adopted [41]: (i) internal validation using the training set molecules, (ii) external validation based on the test set compounds, and (iii) overall validation employing the total data set. Internal and external validation metrics constitute the primary tools for the validation of the developed QSAR models and both the methods have been widely used by different groups of researchers for assessing the predictive ability of the developed models. Another method employs fitting of the dependent X matrix to randomized response parameters.

3.2.1   INTERNAL MODEL VALIDATION

Internal validation deals with the validation of a QSAR model based on the molecules involved in the QSAR model building process (training set data) [42, 43]. Leave-one-out cross-validation is the mostly used algorithm in this regard. In this technique, one compound is eliminated from the data set in each cycle and another model is built using the rest of the compounds. The model thus formed is used for predicting the activity of the eliminated compound. The process is repeated until all the compounds are eliminated once. On the basis of the predicting ability of the model, the predicted residual sum of squares (PRESS) (Eq. 1), the value of standard deviation of error of prediction (SDEP) (Eq. 2), and the cross-validated R^2 (Q^2) metrics (Eq. 3) for the model are determined. The higher is the value of Q^2 (more than 0.5), the better is the model predictivity [44–46].

$$PRESS = \sum (Y_{obs(train)} - Y_{pred(train)})^2 \qquad (1)$$

$$SDEP = \sqrt{\frac{PRESS}{n}} \qquad (2)$$

$$Q^2 = 1 - \frac{\sum (Y_{obs(train)} - Y_{pred(train)})^2}{\sum (Y_{obs(train)} - \overline{Y_{train}})^2} \tag{3}$$

In the above equations, $Y_{obs(train)}$ and $Y_{pred(train)}$ refer to the observed activity and the predicted activity calculated based on the LOO technique for the training set molecules. From Eq. 3, it can be stated that the mean response value of the training set molecules and the distance of the mean from the response values of the individual molecules play a crucial role in determining the value of Q^2.

As the value of the denominator ($\sum (Y_{obs(train)} - \overline{Y_{train}})^2$) on the right-hand side of the equation increases, the value of Q^2 also increases. Thus, even for large differences in the predicted and observed response values, acceptable Q^2 values may be obtained if the molecules exhibit a significantly wide range of response data. Hence, a large value of Q^2 does not necessarily indicate that the predicted activity data lie in close proximity to the observed ones although there may exist a good overall correlation between the values. Thus to obviate this error and to better indicate the model predictive ability, the r_m^2 metrics [$\overline{r_{m\ (LOO)}^2}$ and $\Delta r_{m\ (LOO)}^2$] (Eqs. 4 and 5) for internal validation, introduced by Roy and co-workers [30, 32, 33] can be applied as follows:

$$\overline{r_{m\ (LOO)}^2} = \frac{(r_m^2 + r'_m{}^2)}{2} \tag{4}$$

$$\Delta r_{m\ (LOO)}^2 = | r_m^2 - r'_m{}^2 | \tag{5}$$

Here, $r_m^2 = r^2 \times (1 - \sqrt{(r^2 - r_0^2)})$ and $r'_m{}^2 = r^2 \times (1 - \sqrt{(r^2 - r'_0{}^2)})$. Squared correlation coefficient values between the observed and predicted values with intercept (r^2) and without intercept (r_0^2) were calculated for determination of r_m^2. Change of the axes gives the value of $r'_0{}^2$, and the $r'_m{}^2$ metric is calculated based on the value of $r'_0{}^2$. The parameters k and k' indicate the slopes in the former and latter cases, respectively. The values r^2, r_0^2, and $r'_0{}^2$ are calculated as per the following equations:

$$r^2 = \frac{[\sum (Y_{obs} - \overline{Y_{obs}})(Y_{pred} - \overline{Y_{pred}})]^2}{\sum (Y_{pred} - \overline{Y_{pred}})^2 \times \sum (Y_{obs} - \overline{Y_{obs}})^2} \tag{6}$$

$$r_0^{\,2} = 1 - \frac{\sum (Y_{obs} - k \times Y_{pred})^2}{\sum (Y_{obs} - \overline{Y_{obs}})^2} \tag{7}$$

$$r'_0{}^2 = 1 - \frac{\sum (Y_{pred} - k' \times Y_{obs})^2}{\sum (Y_{pred} - \overline{Y_{pred}})^2} \tag{8}$$

$$k = \frac{\sum (Y_{obs} \times Y_{pred})}{\sum (Y_{pred})^2} \tag{9}$$

$$k' = \frac{\sum (Y_{obs} \times Y_{pred})}{\sum (Y_{obs})^2} \tag{10}$$

Here, Y_{obs} and Y_{pred} are the observed and the predicted response data while $\overline{Y_{obs}}$ and $\overline{Y_{pred}}$ refer to the mean values of the observed and the predicted response, respectively. A sample plot showing the method of calculation of the r^2, $r^2{}_0$, and $r'_0{}^2$ for a hypothetical set of data points is shown in **Figure 1**. To make the method of calculation of $r_m{}^2$ metrics more clear to the readers, we have used the hypothetical data points mentioned in **Table 1** for the calculation of $r_m{}^2$ metrics using Eqns. 4 to 10 and the computed values are presented in **Table 2**.

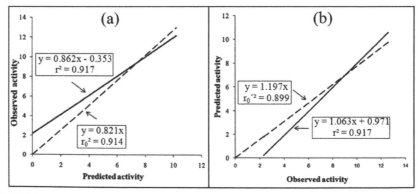

FIGURE 1   Regression plots obtained for a hypothetical set of data points with and without intercept: (a) predicted data is plotted along the *x*-axis while the observed data is plotted along the *y*-axis; (b) axes are interchanged.

TABLE 1 A hypothetical set of observed and predicted data for calculation of different variants of r_m^2 metrics

Compound No.	Observed Data	Predicted Data
1	2.30	1.2
2	4.60	2.10
3	5.10	3.50
4	6.20	4.20
5	7.80	5.60
6	8.60	6.70
7	9.20	7.90
8	10.50	8.10
9	11.40	9.56
10	12.58	10.20

TABLE 2 Calculation of r_m^2 metrics by using the hypothetical observed and predicted values from Table 1.

Metric	Value (from scaled data)
r^2	0.981
r_0^2	0.850
$r'_0{}^2$	0.910
K	1.34
k'	0.72
	0.627
$r_m^2 = r^2 \times (1 - \sqrt{(r^2 - r_0^2)})$	
	0.721
$r'_m{}^2 = r^2 \times (1 - \sqrt{(r^2 - r'_0{}^2)})$	
	0.674
$\overline{r_m^2} = \dfrac{(r_m^2 + r'_m{}^2)}{2}$	
	0.094
$\Delta r_m^2 = \mid r_m^2 - r'_m{}^2 \mid$	

3.2.2 EXTERNAL MODEL VALIDATION

Golbraikh and Tropsha [28] proposed that internal validation despite being the most popular technique for validation of a QSAR model is not the sufficient condition for the model to have a high predictive power. The cross-validation technique only provides a reasonable approximation of the ability of the model to predict the activity of new molecules. Thus, to precisely judge the external predictive potential of the developed model, a sufficiently large data set demands proper external validation by removing a portion of the whole data set as the test set. The R^2_{pred} (Eq. 11) parameter exclusively reflects the degree of correlation between the observed and predicted property data for the test set chemicals.

$$R^2_{pred} = 1 - \frac{\sum (Y_{obs(test)} - Y_{pred(test)})^2}{\sum (Y_{obs(test)} - Y_{training})^2} \qquad (11)$$

Here, $Y_{obs(test)}$ is the observed activity of the test set compounds and $Y_{pred(test)}$ is the predicted activity of the test set compounds. Analyzing Eq. 11, it is clear that R^2_{pred} is dependent on the mean activity value of the training set compounds and its distance from the activity values of the test set compounds. As the denominator term in the equations increases [$\sum (Y_{obs(test)} - \overline{Y}_{training})^2$], the value of the external validation parameter increases, apparently suggesting improved predictive ability of the developed QSAR model. Thus, a data set comprising of molecules exhibiting a wide activity range may show significantly acceptable values for the parameter, although large differences may exist between the predicted and corresponding observed activity values for the test set molecules. The R^2_{pred} value for an acceptable model should be greater than 0.5 (maximum value 1). Besides R^2_{pred}, Golbraikh et al., [28] also proposed several other parameters for analyzing the external predictive ability of the developed QSAR model. A real QSAR model should be close to an ideal one in order to exert high predictive ability. Thus, for an ideal model, the value of correlation coefficient (R) between the observed (y) and predicted (y') activities should be close to 1. However, it may be mentioned here that the work [28] did not consider the asymmetric feature of the least squares method. In case of least squares, the experimental versus fitted, and the fitted versus experimental plots are not always equivalent [47].

As already mentioned that similar to Q^2, the value of R^2_{pred} also depends on the mean response value of the training set compounds, high values of this parameter may be obtained when the test set compounds bear a wide range of response data; but this may not indicate that the predicted property values are very close to the corresponding observed ones. In order to determine the proximity between the observed and predicted response data, the r_m^2 metrics, viz. $\overline{r_m^2}_{(test)}$ and $\Delta r_m^2_{(test)}$ (similar to those employed for internal validation) are calculated for the test molecules [32, 33]. The calculation of this metric uses eqns. 4 to 10 for test set compounds.

3.2.3   OVERALL MODEL VALIDATION

More interestingly, the concept of r_m^2 metrics is not limited to the training and test set activity data separately [30]. It can be extended to the whole dataset considering the LOO predicted activity for the training set and predicted activity for the test sets. Subsequently, the parameters have been referred to as $\overline{r_{m}^{2}}_{(overall)}$ and $\Delta r_{m}^{2}_{(overall)}$ which reflect the predictive ability of the model for the entire data set (the calculation uses eqns. 4 to 10 for the total set of compounds). Advantages of such consideration include: (i) Unlike external validation parameters, the $r_{m}^{2}_{(overall)}$ metrics include both training and test set compounds and thus the statistic is based on prediction of comparably large number of compounds imparting greater reliability to the prediction capacity measured based on the whole data set. (ii) In many cases, comparable models are obtained using internal and external validation techniques, where some models may show greater reliability in terms of the internal predictive parameters, while others may exhibit superior external validation parameters. In such a case, selection of the best model becomes difficult. Since $r_{m}^{2}_{(overall)}$ uses the entire data set, the value of this parameter enables selection based on an overall contribution of both internal and external validation techniques.

Compiling the above knowledge, the average r_{m}^{2} metrics calculated for the training, test and overall sets are denoted as $\overline{r_{m}^{2}}_{(LOO)}$, $\overline{r_{m}^{2}}_{(test)}$, and $\overline{r_{m}^{2}}_{(overall)}$, while the difference in r_{m}^{2} and r'_{m}^{2} values calculated are represented as $\Delta r_{m}^{2}_{(LOO)}$, $\Delta r_{m}^{2}_{(test)}$, and $\Delta r_{m}^{2}_{(overall)}$. It has been suggested that for a model to be considered as predictive one, the value of all variants of $\overline{r_{m}^{2}}$ should be higher than 0.5 and the Δr_{m}^{2} values should be lower than 0.2 [33].

3.3   SCALING OF RESPONSE DATA FOR CALCULATION OF THE r_m^2 METRICS

Calculation of the r_m^2 metrics being dependent on the values of r^2 and r_0^2, the value of the intercept obtained for the regression line correlating the observed and the predicted response data influences the computation of the r_m^2 metrics. Thus, a change in the unit of measurement of the same response data results in a shift of the regression line with respect to the origin of the plot for the observed and the predicted response, and hence, alters the intercept of the corresponding plot. Thus, the extent of fitting of the regression line forcefully through the origin by setting the intercept to zero varies significantly due a change in the intercept which is reflected aptly in the value of the r_0^2 metric (or $r_0'^2$ metric). Although the value of r^2 remains unchanged when calculated for the same set of observed and predicted response measured in different units, the value of the r_m^2 metrics may change due to an alteration in the value of r_0^2. This may result in a difference in the values of the r_m^2 metrics thus calculated and may affect the reproducibility of the developed model. To obviate such discrepancy and for consistency in the calculated values of r_m^2 variants, a minor modification has been incorporated by Roy et al., [48]. The modified version involves calculation of the r_m^2 variants based on the scaled values of the observed and the predicted response data. Scaling is done based on the maximum and the minimum experimental (observed) values of the response parameter based on the following equation.

$$\text{Scaled } Y_i = \frac{Y_i - Y_{\min(\text{obs})}}{Y_{\max(\text{obs})} - Y_{\min(\text{obs})}} \tag{12}$$

Here, Y_i refers to the observed/predicted response for the ith $(1, 2, 3, \ldots\ldots n)$ compound in the training/test set. Besides these, $Y_{\max(\text{obs})}$ and $Y_{\min(\text{obs})}$ indicate the maximum and minimum values, respectively for the observed response.

3.3.1 $r_m^2{}_{(RANK)}$: RANK-ORDER PREDICTION

To measure the closeness between the order of the predicted activity data and that of the corresponding observed activity, the $r_m^2{}_{(\text{rank})}$ parameter is determined [34]. With the aim of incorporating information about the rank-order predictions of the molecules within the scheme of widely used r_m^2 metrics, the $r_m^2{}_{(\text{rank})}$ metric was introduced by Roy and co-workers [34]. Unlike other r_m^2 metrics, the $r_m^2{}_{(\text{rank})}$ metric is calculated based on the correlation of the ranks obtained for the observed and the predicted response data. For the calculation of the metric, the observed and predicted response data of the molecules are ranked and the squared correlation coefficients (Pearson's coefficient) of the corresponding ranks are determined with ($r^2{}_{(\text{rank})}$) and without intercept ($r_0^2{}_{(\text{rank})}$). The values of $r^2{}_{(\text{rank})}$ and $r_0^2{}_{(\text{rank})}$ thus calculated based on the rank order are used to determine the value of the $r_m^2{}_{(\text{rank})}$ metric. The values of $r^2{}_{(\text{rank})}$ and $r_0^2{}_{(\text{rank})}$ differ from each other based on the difference in ranking of the two variables. An ideal ranking where the observed and the predicted response data perfectly match with each other yields zero difference between the two values for each molecule, and the $r_m^2{}_{(\text{rank})}$ metric attains a value of unity. An increase in the difference between the two rank orders for different molecules is marked by a decrease in the value of this metric with the recommended threshold value for acceptance being 0.5. The calculation of the new $r_{m\ (rank)}^2$ metric serves as an extrapolation of the extensively used r_m^2 metric with the subsequent integration of the prediction of rank orders of the molecules.

3.4 SOFTWARE TOOLS FOR CALCULATION OF THE r_m^2 METRICS

For providing a platform to perform the calculation of the scaled r_m^2 metrics, various open source software tools have been developed by different QSAR groups. The available software tools are summarized hereunder:

1. r_m^2 **calculator**: A Web application known as "r_m^2 calculator" (http://apt-software.co.in/rmsquare) has been developed for the calculation of all variants of the r_m^2 metrics by Roy et al., [48]. The input data requires the observed and the predicted response data either imported from a comma-separated values (csv) file (saved in *.csv format) or entered manu-

   ally for the calculation. The output data provides the values of $\overline{r_m^2}$ and Δr_m^2 metrics for the respective set (training/test/overall) of compounds. The calculation of r_m^2 metrics involves the determination of values of r^2, r_0^2 and $r_0'^2$ parameters together with information of the intercept of the regression line correlating the observed and the predicted activity data. The values of r_m^2 metrics may vary significantly with an alteration of the unit of measurement of the response data. To obviate such confusion and to have uniformity in the values of the r_m^2 metrics calculated using different units of measurement for the same response data, a scaling (normalization) option is also included in the calculator.

2. **Cheminformatics tools from Drug Theoretics (DTC) Laboratory:** Roy and co-workers have also developed a series of cheminformatics tools for the QSAR fraternity. These tools are available in the Web page http://dtclab.webs.com/software-tools. To calculate the r_m^2 metrics, one needs to download the MLRplusValidation.jar file (it is platform-independent) and just click on it to run the program. As input, two csv files (saved in *.csv format) are required, one for the training set and the other for the test set compounds. After submitting the input files, one will get the output file consisting of internal, external, and overall r_m^2 metrics along with values of classical validation metrics as well as the results for Golbraikh and Tropsha's model acceptability criteria. To make it more user friendly, user manual and sample .csv files are provided in the mentioned Web site.

3. **CORAL:** The r_m^2 metrics has been implemented in the CORAL freeware available at http://www.insilico.eu/coral. The software is developed by the Istituto di Ricerche Farmacologiche "Mario Negri" of Italy by Toropov *et al.*, Toropov and co-workers successfully calculated r_m^2 metrics in various QSAR/QSPR models [49, 50].

4. **QSARINS:** QSARINS (QSAR-INSUBRIA) is a new software for the development and validation of multiple linear regression QSAR models with ordinary least squares (OLS) method and genetic algorithm for variable selection [51]. This program is mainly focused on the external validation of QSAR models. Along with the other classical external validation metrics, one can also calculate r_m^2 metrics by employing the QSARINS software. The detailed workflow of QSARINS is mentioned in the literature [51].

3.5 SUCCESSFUL APPLICATIONS OF THE r_m^2 METRICS FOR STATISTICALLY SIGNIFICANT QSAR MODELS

To ensure the predictive ability of the developed QSAR/QSPR models, the r_m^2 metrics have been widely used in several QSAR publications. The r_m^2 metrics analyze the models solely based on their ability to predict the activity of the training/test/overall set of compounds and thus it facilitates an improved screening of the most predictive *in silico* models. Different QSAR researchers reveal the significance of the r_m^2 metrics for the selection of the best QSAR models in their research work [52–79]. Here, we have presented a few successful applications of the r_m^2 metrics for the development of statistically significant QSAR models, though this list is not exhaustive.

Roy and Popelier [52] developed predictive QSAR models for hepatocyte toxicity of phenols using quantum topological molecular similarity (QTMS) descriptors. The QTMS descriptors were calculated at different levels of theory which include AM1, HF/3-21G(d), HF/6-31G(d), B3LYP/6-31+G(d,p), B3LYP/6-311+G(2d,p), and MP2/6-311+G(2d,p) and developed models based on these descriptors at each level. It was observed that the best model at each level was distinguished from others by a close proximity between the values of the two external predictive parameters, R^2_{pred} and $r_m^2{}_{(test)}$. The close correspondence between the two values of R^2_{pred} and $r_m^2{}_{(test)}$ demonstrated that the predicted activity data based on the respective models closely matched the observed activity values.

Roy and Popelier [53] also constructed predictive QSAR models using QTMS descriptors for the toxicity prediction of nitroaromatics to *Saccharomyces cerevisiae*. The results were analyzed based on different classical internal and external validation techniques. The selection of the best model was difficult due to a notable difference between the values of Q^2 and R^2_{pred} parameters. Thus, the value of $r_{m\ (test)}^2$ was calculated for all the models so as to enable the selection of the best developed QSAR model. The authors arrived at the conclusion that due to its ability to analyze the deviation between the observed and predicted activity data of the test set molecules more precisely, the $r_{m\ (test)}^2$ parameter is a stricter parameter for measuring external predictive ability of a QSAR model compared to R^2_{pred}.

Srivastava $et\ al.$, [54] proposed QSAR models for artemisinin derivatives and quantified the predictive ability of the best QSAR model based on an analysis of the r_m^2 metric. They derived a final quantitative relationship between antimalarial activity and structural properties based on robust validation parameters. The best reported QSAR model showed a notable difference in the values of R^2_{pred} (0.876) and $r_{m\ (test)}^2$ metrics (0.788). The difference in the values of the two parameters may be attributed to the increased residuals for the test set compounds, especially in case of compound nos. **34, 58, 137, 144,** and **161** which is well revealed in the calculation of $r_{m\ (test)}^2$. Thus, the $r_{m\ (test)}^2$ metric plays a prime role in selecting the best QSAR model with efficient predictive ability.

Liao $et\ al.$, [55] utilized all the three variants of r_m^2 metrics for assessing the predictive ability of the developed QSAR models for combretastatin A4 (CA-4) analogs as tubulin inhibitors. Although the values of Q^2 (0.666) and $r_{m\ (LOO)}^2$ (0.654) were close to each other, a marked difference was observed between the values of R^2_{pred} (0.806) and $r_{m\ (test)}^2$ (0.731). It can be explained by the fact that for the training set compounds, the observed and the predicted activity data lie in close proximity to each other. On the contrary, few compounds of the test set exhibit comparatively larger residual values which ultimately contribute to a lower value of $r_{m\ (test)}^2$. Moreover, the $r_{m\ (overall)}^2$ (0.713) parameter explains the overall predictive ability of the QSAR model and makes a balance between the values of the internal and external predictive parameters.

Roy $et\ al.$, [56] explored 2D and 3D QSARs of 2,4-diphenyl-1,3-oxazolines for ovicidal activity against $Tetranychus\ urticae$ and employed r_m^2 metrics for the selection of the best QSAR model. Due to the variation in the values of R^2_{pred} for the developed models by different statistical tools, selection of the best model was performed based on the $r_{m\ (overall)}^2$ parameter. As the $r_{m\ (overall)}^2$ metric takes into consideration the predicted and observed activity data of both the training and test sets and does not depend on the range of activity data like R^2_{pred}, it serves as a better measure for the selection of the best QSAR model from among comparable ones. So, despite bearing the maximum value for the R^2_{pred} (0.755) parameter, model 6 exhibits a lower value for the $r_{m\ (overall)}^2$ (0.526) parameter.

On the contrary, model 4 yielding the maximum value for the $r_m^2{}_{(overall)}$ (0.535) parameter was selected as the most significant QSAR model.

Toropov et al., [57] developed predictive models for bioconcentration factor using SMILES-based optimal descriptors and employed the r_m^2 statistics for the selection of the final best model. They obtained an $r_m^2{}_{(test)}$ value of 0.657 while an $R^2{}_{pred}$ value of 0.797 for a developed QSAR model and reported it to be the most satisfactory one. A lower value of $r_m^2{}_{(test)}$ compared to the $R^2{}_{pred}$ parameter occurred due to high predicted residual values for some compounds which were not considered in the case of the $R^2{}_{pred}$ parameter calculation.

Roy et al., [58] performed pharmacophore mapping, molecular docking and QSAR studies for structurally diverse compounds as cytochrome 2B6 (CYP 2B6) inhibitors. Among three equations obtained from the QSAR modeling, the first one developed using the genetic function approximation (GFA) with spline option yielded the maximum value for the $R^2{}_{pred}$ (0.843) parameter but a lower value for the $r_m^2{}_{(test)}$ (0.676) metric resulting in a reduced value for the $r_m^2{}_{(overall)}$ (0.754). Such difference between the values of $R^2{}_{pred}$ and $r_m^2{}_{(test)}$ was attributed to the fact that a difference of nearly one log unit existed between the observed and predicted activity data for some of the test set molecules. Thus, it was inferred that the poor predictive ability of this model was well reflected in the low value of $r_m^2{}_{(test)}$ parameter. Moreover, the size of the test set being small, the value of the $r_m^2{}_{(overall)}$ parameter was influenced to a greater extent by the variation of the predicted activity data of the training set compounds. On the contrary, the second equation developed using the GFA-spline option exhibited the maximum Q^2 (0.772) value together with maximum values for all the three r_m^2 [$r_m^2{}_{(test)}$ = 0.749, $r_m^2{}_{(LOO)}$ = 0.750, $r_m^2{}_{(overall)}$ =0.774] metrics. Thus it implied that the activity of the compounds predicted using this model closely coincided with the corresponding observed activity data. Hence, despite having a reduced value for the $R^2{}_{pred}$ (0.832) parameter, the second model was selected as the best one for activity prediction of untested molecules based on the value of $r_m^2{}_{(overall)}$ parameter.

Mitra et al., [59] performed QSAR studies of antilipid peroxidative activity of substituted benzodioxoles and employed the parameter $r_m^2{}_{(LOO)}$ as a measure for judging the predictive ability of the developed QSAR models. The model developed using the genetic partial least squares (G/PLS) technique based on the charge and physico-chemical descriptors capitulated a low value for $r_m^2{}_{(LOO)}$ (0.704) parameter although it showed a high value for LOO-Q^2 (0.825). On the contrary, a high value of $r_m^2{}_{(LOO)}$ [$r_m^2{}_{(LOO)}$ = 0.823, Q^2 = 0.784] was obtained for the GFA model developed with the molecular shape analysis (MSA) and spatial descriptors. This can be explained by the fact that among the two models, the residual values of compound nos. **11, 12,** and **15** in the case of the former model are much higher compared to those of the latter one. Thus, such a difference in the observed and predicted activity data is well reflected in the penalized value of $r_m^2{}_{(LOO)}$ (0.704) for the G/PLS model. The GFA model having the maximum $r_m^2{}_{(LOO)}$ value was selected as the best one for antioxidant activity prediction of benzodioxoles.

Kar et al., [60] developed QSAR models using the QTMS descriptors calculated at different levels of theory for prediction of toxicity of aromatic aldehydes to Tetrahymena pyriformis. Kar et al., developed several comparable models and more interestingly, the models with maximum Q^2 values yielded comparatively poorer $R^2{}_{pred}$ values and vice versa. Thus, the selection of the best model was done based on the value of $r_m^2{}_{(overall)}$ parameter. Since this parameter considers the prediction for both the training and test sets, it serves as a more stringent measure for judgment of the predictive potential of the developed QSAR models. In another study, while Kar et al., (61) developed QSAR models for toxicity of diverse organic chemicals to Daphnia magna using 2D and 3D descriptors and selected based model considering the value of the $r_m^2{}_{(overall)}$.

Dashtbozorgi et al., [62] predicted air-to-liver partition coefficient for volatile organic compounds using QSAR approaches based on PLS and artificial neural network (ANN). The ANN models with a large value of the $r_m^2{}_{(test)}$ (0.980) was selected, as this model could describe more accurately the relationship between the structural parameters and air-to-liver partition coefficients of volatile organic compounds. Moreover, an acceptable value of the $r_m^2{}_{(test)}$ parameter indicated that the difference between the observed and predicted activity data of the test set compounds was minimum.

Kar et al., [63] constructed interspecies toxicity correlation between toxicities to D. magna and fish to assess the ecotoxicological hazard potential of 77 diverse pharmaceuticals. A comparison of their models 6 and 7 for Daphnia toxicity revealed that model 6, despite bearing a maximum value for Q^2 (0.707), exhibited unacceptable value for the $r_m^2{}_{(overall)}$ (0.484) parameter. A difference of approximately 1 log unit between the observed and predicted activity data for some of the test set compounds accounts for such unacceptable values of the r_m^2 metrics for model 6. On the contrary, in the case of model 7, a little difference in the values of each of the internal (Q^2) and external ($R^2{}_{pred}$) predictive parameters with the respective r_m^2 metric signifies that the predicted and the observed activity data for both the whole training and test sets are located in close vicinity to each other and hence the model shows the maximum value for the $r_m^2{}_{(overall)}$ (0.543) parameter.

Arkan et al., [64] reported a QSAR analysis of diaryl substituted pyrazoles as CCR2 inhibitors. Amongst the different linear and nonlinear models, the model developed using the least squares support vector machine (LS-SVM) technique yielded the best results in terms of R^2 for both the training (0.911) and test sets (0.861), and acceptable values for the r_m^2 metrics [r_m^2 (LOO) = 0.638 and r_m^2 (test) = 0.564]. The results thus show that the observed and predicted activity data for the test set compounds closely coincide with each other indicating superior predictivity of LS-SVM models over the other models developed in the work. The other models, despite showing reported acceptable values of the internal predictive parameters, suffer from poor predictivity as reflected by the values of the r_m^2.

The metric r_m^2 (test) has been used by Khosrokhavar et al., [65] as the metric for selection of most predictive QSAR models for mycotoxins using multiple linear regression and SVM. However, among the two models, the model developed using the regression technique is more predictive compared to the SVM model. This can be inferred from the observation that in the case of the MLR model, a few compounds exhibit a difference of more than 2 log units between the observed and predicted activity data, while in case of the SVM model such a difference exists for a comparatively greater number of compounds. Hence the value of r_m^2 (test) is greater for the MLR (0.894) model than that for the SVM (0.833) model.

Lan et al., [66] used the r_m^2 metric for the development of molecular models for d-annulated benzazepinones as vascular endothelial growth factor receptor 2 (VEGF-R2) kinase inhibitors based on 3D-QSAR techniques. From the results, the authors inferred that both the comparative molecular field analysis (COMFA) and comparative molecular similarity analysis (COMSIA) models were well predictive in terms of their external predictive parameter (R^2_{pred}) but exhibited distinct variation when the r_m^2 (test) parameter was calculated. A higher value of the r_m^2 (test) parameter for the COMFA model signified that the activity of the test set molecules predicted by it closely matched the observed data. On the contrary, large residual values for the activity data predicted using the COMSIA model may be attributed to the reduced potential of this model for the activity prediction of untested molecules.

Mitra et al., [67] constructed various descriptor-based QSAR models, 3D-pharmacophore model and hologram quantitative structure–toxicity relationships (HQSAR) which have been utilized for identifying the essential structural attributes imparting a potential antioxidant activity profile of coumarin derivatives. The best GFA-spline model depicted highly acceptable values of r_m^2 metrics for internal, external as well as overall validation. The following values of r_m^2 (LOO) (0.796), r_m^2 (test) (0.725), r_m^2 (overall) (0.813), Δr_m^2 (LOO) (0.050), Δr_m^2 (test) (0.128), and Δr_m^2 (overall) (0.069) can explain that the observed and predicted values for the training, test, and overall set are quite close to each other and that the developed model is a robust and predictive one.

Kar and Roy [68] developed a classification and a regression-based QSTR as well as toxicophore models for the first time on basal cytotoxicity data of a diverse series of chemicals. The developed PLS model has a moderate R^2_{pred} value but the model is predictive enough as it showed an acceptable value of $\overline{r_m^2}_{(test)}$ (0.579) and $\Delta r_m^2_{(test)}$ (0.012). Again, the model is robust enough as the model had all acceptable values of r_m^2 metrics for the training and overall sets:

$\overline{r_m^2}_{(LOO)}$ (0.796), $\overline{r_m^2}_{(overall)}$ (0.813), $\Delta r_m^2_{(LOO)}$ (0.050), and $\Delta r_m^2_{(overall)}$ (0.069). Here, the $r_m^2_{(overall)}$ value considers predictions for both the training and test sets and provides a confidence for future predictions.

Quantitative structure-retention relationships (QSRRs) model was developed for predicting the gas chromatography retention indices of 169 constituents of essential oils by Qin et al., (69). The external validation of the models indicated that the final QSPR model M3 showed a good predictive power. The $\overline{r_m^2}_{(test)}$ metric value was equal to 0.810 and $\Delta r_m^2_{(test)}$ was 0.099 (lower than the cutoff value of 0.2). The author reported that the observed and predicted values of all the test set compounds were quite close to each other and the results of the external validation indicated the high predictive power of the model.

Five predictive computer models: ACD/PhysChem History, ADMET Predictor, T.E.S.T., EPI Suite-WSKOWWIN, and EPI Suite-WATERNT were used to predict water solubility of organic compounds by Cappelli et al., [70]. They have employed r_m^2 metrics as more stringent validation metrics for external validation. T.E.S.T. and ADMET confirm their better performance in prediction of compounds which are inside the applicability domain (AD) of the models. Two EPI Suite models are not acceptable considering these metrics, even excluding outlier compounds from the calculation. On the other hand, Δr_m^2 values are lower than 0.2 only for ACD and ADMET models.

The mixture toxicity of nonpolar narcotic chemicals was modeled by linear and nonlinear statistical methods naming forward stepwise MLR and radial basis function neural networks (RBFNNs) by Luan et al., [71]. The authors have employed r_m^2 metrics to select the most robust and predictive between two models. The values of $\overline{r_m^2}_{(LOO)}$ and $\Delta r_m^2_{(LOO)}$ for the training set of the MLR model are 0.928 and 0.046, respectively, while for the external test set, the corresponding metric values are 0.920 and 0.009, respectively. They have also calculated the r_m^2 values for the nonlinear model. When those values are compared, all of them are not only much higher than the threshold value, but also a little higher than the corresponding values of the linear model. For the nonlinear model, the

$\overline{r_m^2}_{(LOO)}$ is 0.967 and $\Delta r_m^2{}_{(LOO)}$ is 0.021 for the training set, while for the external test set, the values are 0.965 and 0.017, respectively. Based on the values obtained from r_m^2 metrics, superior prediction ability of the nonlinear model was concluded by Luan et al.,

Oral slope factors (OSFs) which are used to estimate quantitatively the carcinogenic potency of diverse chemicals have been modelled by Kar and Roy [72] employing classification and regression based QSAR models. Though the developed stepwise model had a higher Q^2 value than the PLS model and almost comparable R^2_{pred}, the PLS model was selected as the best model as the

values of $\overline{r_m^2}_{(test)}$ (0.624) and $\Delta r_m^2{}_{(test)}$ (0.155) were more acceptable than those of the stepwise model. It is interesting to point out that the differences between observed and predicted values for all the test compounds were quite smaller for the PLS model.

The interaction of 278 monocyclic and bicyclic pyrimidine derivatives with human A_{2A} adenosinereceptor (AR) was examined by utilizing molecular dynamics, thermodynamic analysis, and 3D-QSAR approaches by Zhang et al., [73]. The ligand-/receptor-based comparative molecular similarity indices analysis (CoMSIA) models of high statistical significance were generated and the constructed contour maps correlate well with the structural features of the antagonists essential for high A_{2A} AR affinity. Considering the r_m^2 values, receptor-based CoMSIA model was identified as superior to the ligand-based CoMSIA model while values of the other classical metrics were too close to identify the best one.

Das and Roy [74] attempted to develop classification and regression based QSAR models to capture specific structural information of ionic liquids responsible for their toxic manifestation to *Vibrio fischeri*. All the r_m^2 metric values were in the acceptable range for the best GFA-spline model. The average

r_m^2 value for external validation ($\overline{r_m^2}_{(test)}$ = 0.623) of this model was higher

than that for the internal validation ($\overline{r_m^2}_{(LOO)}$ =0.525) which could explain the

better external predictivity of the model. The $\overline{r_m^2}_{(overall)}$ value (0.554) was also acceptable for describing the overall predictive performance of the model. The

Δr_m^2 values for external ($\Delta r_m^2{}_{(test)}$= 0.156) and overall validation ($\Delta r_m^2{}_{(overall)}$ =0.195) were acceptable except that for the internal validation (=0.209), where it was just above the recommended tolerance limit of 0.2.

QSAR models have been performed on the cytotoxic activity in a human lung adenocarcinoma cell line (A549) for 43 cucurbitacin derivatives by Lang et al., [75]. Partial least squares with discriminant analysis (PLS-DA) and PLS tools were used to develop the models where variables were selected using the ordered predictor selection (OPS) algorithm. The authors computed r_m^2 metrics (along with classical validation parameters) as one of the stringent criteria to check the predictivity of the model for both internal as well as external validation tests. Finally, considering the small size of the data set used in the QSAR model, they have calculated $\overline{r_m^2}_{(overall)}$ and $\Delta r_m^2{}_{(overall)}$ for the overall validation.

The values of overall validation metrics (r_m^2 and Δr_m^2) were 0.673 and 0.139, respectively. The results were consistent with the threshold limits. As the test set compounds were very small in numbers for this data set, the overall validation metrics make the model more reliable for the purpose of future prediction.

Pramanik and Roy [76] used computational chemistry and statistical modeling to develop mathematical equations which can be applied to calculate toxicity of chemicals in *Escherichia coli*. The $\overline{r_m^2}_{(test)}$ and Δr_m^2 values have been considered for the selection of the best QSAR model. Acceptable values of these external parameters indicated that the observed and predicted toxicity values have a small difference. In another work, Pramanik and Roy [77] developed four quantitative predictive models for steady-state compartmental chemical mass concentrations from structural information, physico-chemical properties, degradation rate, and transport coefficients of 455 diverse organic chemicals using a quantitative structure-fate relationship (QSFR) study. Robustness and predictivity of the models were judged by different variants of r_m^2 metrics.

The impact of ligand conformation on the 3D-QSAR model of a series of 3-amino-6-arylpyrazines as ATR (ataxia telangiectasia and Rad3 related) kinase inhibitors was investigated by Luo et al., [78]. The authors have employed molecular dynamics (MDs) simulations to get the dynamic active conformations (DACs) of the compounds in the ATP binding site of ATR kinase. In their research work, along with classical validation metrics, r_m^2 metrics were employed to further validate the predictive ability of the best model. The $\overline{r_m^2}_{(test)}$ for the test set of model D2 was 0.548, which was higher than the required value (0.5). The Δr_m^2 for the test set also meets the criterion (0.196). In conclusion the authors have confirmed that the r_m^2 parameters of the test set of model D2 together with the classical approach of external validation suggest the reliability of the DACs model. Their results highlighted the importance of incorporating DACs of ligands using MD simulation in 3D-QSAR studies.

Ojha and Roy [79] presented a work that deals with QSAR modeling, pharmacophore mapping, and docking studies of a series of 35 thymidine analogues as inhibitors of *Plasmodium falciparum* thymidylate kinase (PfTMPK), an enzyme that catalyzes phosphorylation of thymidine monophosphate (TMP) to thymidine diphosphate (TDP). Based on the overall prediction, a model obtained from GFA followed by PLS was selected as the best model, though the R^2_{pred} of GFA model had a higher value. Here, the overall r_m^2 prediction is advantageous as it counts the difference between observed and predicted values of the training and test set compounds and thus makes a balance between robustness and predictivity. They have also employed $r_{m\,(rank)}^2$ for the model to check the rank order prediction.

In addition to the above presented, several other studies reported by different authors reveal the importance of the r_m^2 metrics for the selection of the best QSAR models. In a recent paper [32], it has been demonstrated that r_m^2 along with Δr_m^2 may serve as a more strict requirement for external validation in comparison to other available external validation metrics. Considering their stringency to identify the best robust and predictive model, increased uses of r_m^2 metrics may be expected in the near future.

3.6   CONCLUSION

The traditional internal and external validation metrics exhibit acceptable values as long as an overall good correlation is maintained between the observed and the predicted response data irrespective of the actual difference between the data. However, the r_m^2 metrics depend chiefly on the difference between the observed and predicted response data and convey more precise information regarding their difference. Therein lies the utility of the r_m^2 metrics. The $\overline{r_{m\,(LOO)}^2}$ and $\Delta r_{m\,(LOO)}^2$ parameters signify the internal predictive ability of the developed QSAR models. On the other hand, the $\overline{r_{m\,(test)}^2}$ and $\Delta r_{m\,(test)}^2$ metrics determine the proximity between the values of the observed and predicted response of the test set compounds. Thus, the r_m^2 parameters are stricter metrics for the validation of predictive models in comparison to the traditional ones. Moreover, the $\overline{r_{m\,(overall)}^2}$ metric gives a single value that considers predictions from both training and test set compounds and is not limited to the number of test set compounds as is the case for R^2_{pred}. Having the ability to reflect the predictive ability of the model in terms of both internal and external validation, the $\overline{r_{m\,(overall)}^2}$ parameter can be aptly utilized to identify the best QSAR model from among comparable models, especially when different models show different patterns in internal and external predictivity. The r_m^2 metrics have been utilized for the selection of the final QSAR models by various groups of QSAR modelers all over the world. It has been reported that several models bear unacceptable values of the r_m^2 parameters despite having statistically significant values for Q^2 and R^2_{pred}.

The $\overline{r_m^2}_{(overall)}$ parameter plays a crucial role for selecting the best model when comparable models present different patterns in Q^2 and R^2_{pred} values. The major concluding remarks are as follows:

The r_m^2 series of metrics have been used for internal as well as external validation tests in the recent QSAR literature, demonstrating their stringent requirements for models to pass with a true reflection of the quality of predictions from the models.

1. The r_m^2 series of metrics have been used for internal as well as external validation tests in the recent QSAR literature, demonstrating their stringent requirements for models to pass with a true reflection of the quality of predictions from the models.

2. The $r_m^2{}_{(rank)}$ metric determine the rank-order prediction of any QSAR model. Thus, in addition to the conventional validation metrics, an acceptable value of the $r_m^2{}_{(rank)}$ metric ensures that the predicted response data maintains a similar order as that of the observed response and thus improves the acceptability of the developed model.

3. Open source Web applications can be easily used for the computation of the r_m^2 metrics using the experimental (observed) and QSAR predicted data for a set of compounds.

4. The r_m^2 metrics may be used along with the classical validation metrics for the validation of QSAR/QSPR/QSTR models, especially when regulatory decisions are involved.

3.7 CONFLICT OF INTEREST

The authors declare no conflict of interest.

ACKNOWLEDGMENT

SK thanks the Department of Science and Technology, Government of India for awarding him a research fellowship under the INSPIRE scheme. KR thanks the Council of Scientific and Industrial Research (CSIR), New Delhi for awarding a major research project.

KEYWORDS

- **External validation**
- **Internal validation**
- **QSAR**
- **QSPR**
- r_m^2 **metrics**

REFERENCES

1. Helguera, A.M.; Combes, R.D.; Gonzalez, M.P.; Cordeiro, M.N. Applications of 2D descriptors in drug design: a DRAGON tale. *Curr. Top. Med. Chem.* **2008**, 8, 1628–1655.
2. Todeschini, R; Consonni, V. *Handbook of Molecular Descriptors*, Wiley-VCH: Weinheim, 2000.
3. Hoffman, B.T.; Kopajtic, T.; Katz, J.L.; Newman, A.H. 2D QSAR modeling and preliminary database searching for dopamine transporter inhibitors using genetic algorithm variable selection of Molconn Z descriptors. *J. Med. Chem.* **2000**, 43, 4151–4159.
4. Perkins, R.; Fang, H.; Tong, W.; Welsh, W.J. Quantitative structure-activity relationship methods: perspectives on drug discovery and toxicology. *Environ. Toxicol. Chem.* **2003**, 22, 1666–1679.
5. Worth, A.P.; Bassan, A.; De Bruijn, J.; Saliner, A.G.; Netzeva, T.; Patlewicz, G.; Pavan, M.; Tsakovska, I.; Eisenreich, S. The role of the European chemicals Bureau in promoting the regulatory use of (Q)SAR methods. *SAR QSAR Environ. Res.* **2007**, 18, 111–125.
6. Russell, W.M.S.; Burch, R.L. *The Principles of Humane Experimental Technique*, Methuen: London, **1959**.
7. Ferreira, M.M. Polycyclic aromatic hydrocarbons: a QSPR study. Quantitative structure-property relationships. *Chemosphere* **2001**, 44, 125–149.
8. Carlsen, L.; Kenessov, B.N.; Batyrbekova, S.Y. A QSAR/QSTR study on the human health impact of the rocket fuel 1,1-dimethyl hydrazine and its transformation products multicriteria hazard ranking based on partial order methodologies. *Environ. Toxicol. Pharmacol.* **2009**, 27, 415-423.
9. Tikhonova, I.G.; Baskin, I.I.; Palyulin, V.A.; Zefirov, N.S. Virtual screening of organic molecule databases. Design of focused libraries of potential ligands of NMDA and AMPA receptors. *Russ. Chem. B+* **2004**, 53, 1335–1344.
10. Cronin, M.T.D.; Jaworska, J.S.; Walker, J.D.; Comber, M.H.I.; Watts, C.D.; Worth, A.P. Use of QSARs in international decision-making frameworks to predict health effects of chemical substances. *Environ. Health Perspect.* **2003**, 111, 1391–1401.
11. OECD, Environment Directorate, Joint Meeting of the Chemicals Committee and The Working Party on Chemicals, Pesticides and Biotechnology. http://www.olis.oecd.org/olis/2004doc. nsf/ LinkTo/NT00009192/$FILE/JT00176183.PDF
12. Tropsha, A.; Gramatica, P.; Gombar, V.K. The importance of being earnest: validation is the absolute essential for successful application and interpretation of QSPR Models. *QSAR Comb. Sci.* **2003**, 22, 69–77.
13. Tropsha, A. In *Cheminformatics in Drug Discovery*; Oprea, T., Ed.; Wiley-VCH: Weinheim, 2005.
14. Leo, A. Calculating log P_{oct} from structures. *J. Chem. Rev.* **1993**, 93, 1281–1306.

15. Zheng, S.; Luo, X.; Chen, G.; Zhu, W.; Shen, J.; Chen, K.; Jiang, H. A new rapid and effective chemistry space filter in recognizing a drug like database. *J. Chem. Inf. Comput. Sci.* **2005**, 45, 856–862.

16. Walker, J.D.; Dearden, J.C.; Schultz, T.W.; Jaworska, J.; Comber, M.H.I. In: *QSARs for Pollution Prevention, Toxicity Screening, Risk Assessment, and Web Applications*, Walker, J.D., Ed.; SETAC Press: Pensacola, FL, **2003**, pp. 3–18

17. Walker, J.D.; Jaworska, J.; Comber, M.H.I.; Schultz, T.W.; Dearden, J.C. Guidelines for developing and using quantitative structure-activity relationships. *Environ. Toxicol. Chem.* **2003**, 22, 1653–1665.

18. Cronin, M.T.D.; Schultz, T.W. Pitfalls in QSAR. *J. Theoret. Chem. (Theochem)* **2003**, 622, 39–51.

19. Eriksson, L.; Jaworska, J.; Worth, A.P.; Cronin, M.T.D.; McDowell, R.M.; Gramatica, P. Methods for reliability and uncertainty assessment for applicability evaluations of classification- and regression-based QSARs. *Environ. Health Persp.* **2003**, 111, 1361–1375.

20. Tropsha, A.; Golbraikh, A. Predictive QSAR modeling workflow, model applicability domains, and virtual screening. *Curr. Pharm. Des.* **2007**, 13, 3494–3504.

21. Wold, S.; Eriksson, L. In: *Chemometrics Methods in Molecular Design*, van de Waterbeemd, H., Ed.; VCH: Weinheim, Germany, **1995**, pp. 309–318.

22. Zvinavashe, E.; Murk, A.J.; Rietjens, I.M.C.M. Promises and pitfalls of quantitative structureactivity relationship approaches for predicting metabolism and toxicity. *Chem. Res. Toxicol.* **2008**, 21, 2229–2236.

23. Gramatica, P. Principles of QSAR models validation: internal and external. *QSAR Comb. Sci.* **2007**, 26, 694–701.

24. OECD Principles for the Validation of (Q)SARs, http://www.oecd.org/dataoecd/33/37/37849783.pdf (Accessed December 29, 2013)

25. Roy, K. On some aspects of validation of predictive QSAR models. *Expert Opin. Drug Discov.* **2007**, 2, 1567–1577.

26. Hawkins, D.M.; Basak, S.C.; Mills, D. Assessing model fit by cross-validation. *J. Chem. Inf. Comput. Sci.* **2003**, 43, 579–586.

27. Hawkins, D.M.; Kracker, J.J.; Basak, S.C.; Mills, D. QSPR checking and validation: a case study with hydroxy radical reaction rate constant. *SAR QSAR Environ. Res.* **2008**, 19, 525–539.

28. Golbraikh, A.; Tropsha, A. Beware of q^2! *J. Mol. Graphics Mod.* **2002**, 20, 269–276.

29. Roy, P.P; Roy, K. On some aspects of variable selection for partial least squares regression models. *QSAR Comb. Sci.* **2008**, 27,302–313

30. Roy, P.P.; Paul, S.; Mitra, I.; Roy, K. On two novel parameters for validation of predictive QSAR models. *Molecules* **2009**, 14, 1660–1701.

31. Mitra, I.; Roy, P.P.; Kar, S.; Ojha, P.; Roy, K. On further application of r_m^2 as a metric for validation of QSAR models. *J. Chemometr.* **2010**, 24, 22–33.

32. Roy, K.; Mitra, I.; Kar, S.; Ojha, P.K.; Das, R.N.; Kabir, H. Comparative studies on some metrics for external validation of QSPR models. *J. Chem. Inf. Model* **2012**, 52, 396–408.

33. Ojha, P.K.; Mitra, I.; Das, R.N.; Roy, K. Further exploring r_m^2 metrics for validation of QSPR models. *Chemom. Intell. Lab. Sys.* **2011**, 107, 194–205.

34. Roy, K.; Mitra, I.; Ojha, P.K.; Kar, S.; Das, R.N.; Kabir, H. Introduction of $r_{m\ (rank)}^2$ metric incorporating rank-order predictions as an additional tool for validation of QSAR/ QSPR models. *Chemom. Intell. Lab. Sys.* **2012**, 118, 200–210.

35. Golbraikh, A.; Shen, M.; Xiao, Z.; Xiao, Y.D.; Lee, K.H.; Tropsha., A. J. Rational selection of training and test sets for the development of validated QSAR models. *Comput. Aided Mol. Design* **2003**, 17, 241–253.

36. Zheng, W.; Tropsha, A.A. novel variable selection quantitative structure property relationship approach based on the k-nearest-neighbor principle. *J. Chem. Inf. Comput. Sci.* **2000**, 40, 185–194.

37. Guha, R.; Jurs, P.C. Determining the validity of a QSAR model-a classification approach. *J. Chem. Inf. Model.* **2005**, 45, 65–73.

38. Aptula, A.O.; Jeliazkova, N.G.; Schultz, T.W.; Cronin, M. T. D. The better predictive model: High Q^2 for the training set or low root mean square error of prediction for the test set? *QSAR Comb. Sci.* **2005**, 24, 385–396.

39. Gramatica, P.; Giani, E.; Papa, E. Statistical external validation and consensus modeling: a QSPR case study for Koc prediction. *J. Mol. Graphics. Model.* **2007**, 25, 755–766.

40. Shen, M.; Beguin, C.; Golbraikh, A.; Stables, J. P.; Kohn, H.; Tropsha, A. Application of predictive QSAR models to identification and experimental validation of novel anticonvulsant compounds. *J. Med. Chem.* **2004**, 47, 2356–2364.

41. Wold, S. In: Chemometric Methods in Molecular Design. Van de Waterbeemd, H. (Ed.) VCH: Weinheim, 1995.

42. Stone, M. Cross-validatory choice and assessment of statistical predictions. *J. R. Stat. Soc. Ser. B* **1974**, 36, 111–147.

43. Wold, S. Cross-validatory estimation of the number of components in factor and principal components models. *Technometrics* **1978**, 20, 397–405.

44. Tichy, M.; Rucki, M. Validation of QSAR models for legislative purposes. *Interdisc. Toxicol.* **2009**, 2, 184–186.

45. Cruciani, G.; Baroni, M.; Bonelli, D.; Clementi, S.; Ebert, C.; Skagerberg, B. *QSAR Comb. Sci.* **2006**, 9, 101.

46. Debnath, A.K. In *Combinatorial library design and evaluation;* Ghose, A.K.; Viswanadhan, V.N., (Eds.); Marcel Dekker: New York, 2001.

47. Besalu, E.; De Julian-Ortiz, J.V.; Pogliani. L. Trends and plot methods in MLR studies. *J. Chem. Inf. Model* **2007**, 47, 751–760.

48. Roy, K.; Chakraborty, P.; Mitra, I.; Ojha, P.K.; Kar, S.; Das, R.N. Some case studies on application of "r_m^2" metrics for judging quality of QSAR predictions: Emphasis on scaling of response data. *J. Comput. Chem.* **2013**, 34, 1071–1082.

49. Toropov, A.A.; Toropova, A.P.; Benfenati, E. QSPR modelling of normal boiling points and octanol/water partition coefficient for acyclic and cyclic hydrocarbons using SMILES-based optimal descriptors. *Cent. Eur. J. Chem.* **2010**, 8, 1047–1052.

50. Toropova, A.P.; Toropov, A.A.; Lombardo, A.; Roncaglioni, A.; Benfenati, E.; Gini, G. A new bioconcentration factor model based on SMILES and indices of presence of atoms. *Eur. J. Med. Chem.* **2010**, 5, 4399–4402.

51. Gramatica, P.; Chirico, N.; Papa, E.; Cassani, S.; Kovarich, S. QSARINS: a new software for the development, analysis, and validation of QSAR MLR models. *J. Comput. Chem.* **2013**, 34, 2121–2132.

52. Roy, K.; Popelier, P.L.A. Exploring predictive QSAR models for hepatocyte toxicity of phenols using QTMS descriptors. *Bioorg. Med. Chem. Lett.* **2008**, 18, 2604–2609.

53. Roy, K.; Popelier, P.L.A. Exploring predictive QSAR models using quantum topological molecular similarity (QTMS) descriptors for toxicity of nitroaromatics to *Saccharomyces cerevisiae*. *QSAR Comb. Sci.* **2008**, 27, 1006–1012.

54. Srivastava, M.; Singh H.; Naik, P.K. Quantitative structure–activity relationship (QSAR) of artemisinin: the development of predictive in vivo antimalarial activity models. *J. Chemometr.* **2009**, 23, 618–635.

55. Liao, S.Y.; Chen , J.C.; Miao, T.F.; Shen, Y.; Zheng, K.C. Binding conformations and QSAR of CA-4 analogs as tubulin inhibitors. *J. Enzyme Inhib. Med. Chem.* **2010**, 25, 421–429.

56. Roy K.; Paul; S. Exploring 2D and 3D QSARs of 2, 4-Diphenyl-1,3-oxazolines for ovicidal activity against *Tetranychus urticae*. *QSAR Comb. Sci.* **2009**, 28, 406–425.
57. Toropov, A.A.; Toropova, A.P.; Benfenati, E. QSPR modeling bioconcentration factor (BCF) by balance of correlations. *Eur. J. Med. Chem.* **2009**, 44, 2544–2551.
58. Roy, P.P.; Roy, K. Pharmacophore mapping, molecular docking and QSAR studies of structurally diverse compounds as CYP2B6 inhibitors. *Mol. Simul.* **2010**, 36, 887–905.
59. Mitra, I.; Saha A.; Roy, K. QSAR of antilipid peroxidative activity of substituted benzodioxoles using chemometric tools. *J. Comput. Chem.* **2009**, 30, 2712–2722.
60. Kar, S.; Harding, A.P.; Roy K.; Popelier, P.L.A. QSAR with quantum topological molecular similarity indices: toxicity of aromatic aldehydes to *Tetrahymena pyriformis*; *SAR QSAR Environ. Res.* **2010**, 21, 149–168.
61. Kar, S.; Roy, K. QSAR modeling of toxicity of diverse organic chemicals to Daphnia magna using 2D and 3D descriptors. *J. Hazard. Mater.* **2010**, 177, 344–351.
62. Dashtbozorgi, Z.; Golmohammadi, H. Prediction of air to liver partition coefficient for volatile organic compounds using QSAR approaches. *Eur. J. Med. Chem.* **2010**, 45, 2182–2190.
63. Kar, S.; Roy; K. First report on interspecies quantitative correlation of ecotoxicity of pharmaceuticals. *Chemosphere* **2010**, 81, 738–747.
64. Arkan, E.; Shahlaei, M.; Pourhossein, A.; Fakhri, K.; Fassihi, A. Validated QSAR analysis of some diaryl substituted pyrazoles as CCR2 inhibitors by various linear and nonlinear multivariate chemometrics methods. *Eur. J. Med. Chem.* **2010**, 45, 3394–3406.
65. Khosrokhavar, R.; Ghasemi, J.B.; Shiri, F. 2D quantitative structure-property relationship study of Mycotoxins by multiple linear regression and support vector machine. *Int. J. Mol. Sci.* **2010**, 11, 3052–3068.
66. Lan, P.; Sun, J-R.; Chen, W-N.; Sun, P-H.; Chen, W-M. Molecular modelling studies on d-annulated benzazepinones as VEGF-R2 kinase inhibitors using docking and 3D-QSAR. *J. Enzyme Inhib. Med. Chem.* **2011**, 26, 367–377.
67. Mitra, I.; Saha, A.; Roy, K. Predictive modeling of antioxidant coumarin derivatives using multiple approaches: descriptor-based QSAR, 3D-pharmacophore mapping, and HQSAR. *Sci Pharm.* **2013**, 81, 57–80.
68. Kar, S.; Roy, K. First report on predictive chemometric modeling, 3D-toxicophore mapping and *in silico* screening of in vitro basal cytotoxicity of diverse organic chemicals. *Toxicol in vitro* **2013**, 27, 597–608.
69. Qin, L-T.; Liu, S-S.; Chen, F.; Xiao, Q-F.; Wu, Q-S. Chemometric model for predicting retention indices of constituents of essential oils, *Chemosphere* **2013**, 90, 300–305.
70. Cappelli, C.I.; Manganelli, S.; Lombardo, A.; Gissi, A.; Benfenati, E. Validation of quantitative structure-activity relationship models to predict water-solubility of organic compounds. *Sci. Total Environ.* **2013**, 463–464, 781–789.
71. Luan, F.; Xu, X.; Liu, H.; Cordeiro, M.N.D.S. Prediction of the baseline toxicity of non-polar narcotic chemical mixtures by QSAR approach. *Chemosphere* **2013**, 90, 1980–1986.
72. Kar, S.; Deeb, O.;Roy, K. Development of classification and regression based QSAR models to predict rodent carcinogenic potency using oral slope factor. *Ecotox. Environ. Saf.* **2012**, 82, 85–95.
73. Zhanga, L.; Liub, T.; Wanga, X.; Wanga, J.; Lic, G.; Lid, Y.; Yange, L.; Wanga, Y. Insight into the binding mode and the structural features of the pyrimidine derivatives as human A_{2A} adenosine receptor antagonists. *BioSystems* **2014**, 115, 13-22.
74. Das, R.N.; Roy, K. Development of classification and regression models for *Vibrio fischeri* toxicity of ionic liquids: Green solvents for the future. *Toxicol. Res.* **2012**, 1, 186–195.
75. Lang, K.L.; Silva, I.T.; Machado, V.R.; Zimmermann, L.A.; Caro, M.S.B.; Simões, C.M.O.; Schenkel, E.P.; Durán, F.J.; Bernardes, L.S.C.; de Meloe, E.B. Multivariate SAR and QSAR

of cucurbitacin derivatives as cytotoxiccompounds in a human lung adenocarcinoma cell line. *J. Mol. Graphics Modell.***2014**, 48, 70–79.

76. Pramanik, S.; Roy, K. Exploring QSTR modeling and toxicophore mapping for identification of important molecular features contributing to the chemical toxicity in *Escherichia coli*. *Toxicol in vitro.***2013**, 28, 265–272.

77. Pramanik, S.; Roy, K. Environmental toxicological fate prediction of diverse organic chemicals based on steady-state compartmental chemical mass ratio using quantitative structure-fate relationship (QSFR) models. *Chemosphere* **2013**, 92, 600–607.

78. Luo, H.; Shi, J.; Lu, L.; Wu, F.; Zhou, M.; Hou, X.; Zhang, W.; Ding, Z.; Li, R. Molecular dynamics-based self-organizing molecular field analysis on 3-amino-6-arylpyrazines as the ataxia telangiectasia mutated and Rad3 related (ATR) protein kinase inhibitors. *Med. Chem. Res.***2013**, 22, 1–12.

79. Ojha, P.K.;Roy, K. First report on exploring structural requirements of alpha and beta thymidine analogs for PfTMPK inhibitory activity using *in silico* studies. *Biosystems* **2013**,113, 177–195.

CHAPTER 4

CONSIDERING THE MOLECULAR CONFORMATIONAL FLEXIBILITY IN QSAR STUDIES

JAVIER GARCIA, PABLO R. DUCHOWICZ, and
EDUARDO A. CASTRO

Instituto de Investigaciones Fisicoquнmicas Teyricas y Aplicadas (INIFTA, CCT La Plata-CONICET), Casilla de Correo 16, Sucursal 4, 1900 La Plata, Argentina

CONTENTS

ABSTRACT

Conformational flexibility is a crucial aspect to be considered from the molecular structure for obtaining predictive quantitative structure–property relationships models. We develop two simple algorithms that are based in the stepwise inclusion procedure and the replacement method, which introduce conformational flexibility in two different ways: (i) by an iterative method and (ii) by taking into account the descriptor values of all the conformations at once. We apply such algorithms to predict the apparent second order inactivation rate constant for different serine protease inhibitors based on the 1,2,5-thiadiazolidin-3-one 1,1-dioxide scaffold, and also to structurally heterogeneous inhibitors of the angiotensin converting enzyme. Present approach improves the results obtained by both the stepwise inclusion technique and the replacement method.

4.1 INTRODUCTION

One of the most important goals of the theoretical chemistry field is to devise a proper way to predict the behavior of any substance within its environment. In order to achieve this goal, a very complex theory is needed; this theory would unify all the experimental observations done so far and it would also be able to predict any future observation.

Nowadays, the best effort involves the application of quantum mechanics to chemical systems composed by only a few small molecules; this allows gaining useful knowledge about their molecular structure in stationary states and also about their evolution in time. In order to do so, the best approach known so far is to solve Schrödinger's equation by taking into account 3 degrees of freedom for each particle that composes the system. However, the calculations needed to solve this kind of equations are extremely expensive when relatively small systems are considered, like heavy atoms or small molecules, and impossible when the systems involve a number of molecules close to Avogadro's number.

Nevertheless, a great deal of experimental research has been done in past years in order to understand the way that chemical systems work. These experiments result in a great amount of experimental data: entropies, enthalpies, free energies, biological activities, etc. So, it is possible to ask a simple but yet very difficult question to answer: is there any way to relate through simple calculations (or, in other words, the information that can be obtained from the molecular structure) the experimental observations that have been gathered over the years?

The quantitative structure–property relationships (QSPR) and quantitative structure–activity relationships (QSAR) theory provides a simple way to predict the properties of chemical substances and avoids the use of intensive calculations [1–3]. Within the framework of this theory, the problem of successfully modeling the complete system is translated into the necessity of finding an unknown relationship (model) between the molecular structure and the chemical or biological property of interest. Therefore, the molecular structure is represented through molecular descriptors which are the variables to be used in the model. There are descriptors of different types, and a straightforward criterion to classify them is by their *dimensionality*. The three-dimensional (3D) descriptors depend on the position of atoms in space (geometry); the 2D descriptors consider the molecular representation through a chemical graph; the 1D only depend on the functional groups types; and the 0D depend on the atom types that conform the molecule and their bonds.

At first sight, the prediction of biological activities in QSAR studies is considered more difficult than the prediction of physico-chemical properties, due to the known fact that biological systems usually involve more complex molecular environments. As a matter of fact, most of the biological activities of interest are related to the interaction between very complex molecules (usually these involve proteins). Evidently, this kind of interaction between an enzyme and its substrate takes a specific conformation of both molecules. This means that, in order to create a successful QSAR model, one should model the considered molecule while it interacts with the enzyme. Of course, this is a very demanding task, so a new challenge is to develop an algorithm with the ability of considering the conformational flexibility of molecules, in order to improve the predictions. We address this problem later, but first we have to introduce some useful notation.

4.1.1 NOTATION

We will assign the matrix to the total set of descriptors:

$$X = \begin{pmatrix} X_{11} & X_{12} & \cdots & X_{1N} \\ X_{21} & X_{22} & \cdots & X_{2N} \\ \vdots & \vdots & \ddots & \vdots \\ X_{D1} & X_{D2} & \cdots & X_{DN} \end{pmatrix} \tag{1}$$

where stands for the -th descriptor calculated for the -th molecule. stands for the number of molecules (including those of the training set and the test set) and D for the total number of descriptors. The matrix X has $D \times N$ size.

The matrix contains the chosen descriptors for the model. The element represents the -th descriptor of the model calculated for the i-th molecule. The vector will stand for the calculated values of the property. Its i-th element represents the calculated value of the property for the -th molecule. stands for the number of descriptors used in the model. Obviously, $d \leq D$; usually, $d \ll D$.

$$x = \begin{pmatrix} x_{11} & x_{12} & \cdots & x_{1N} \\ x_{21} & x_{22} & \cdots & x_{2N} \\ \vdots & \vdots & \ddots & \vdots \\ x_{d1} & x_{d2} & \cdots & x_{dN} \end{pmatrix} \tag{2}$$

It will prove useful to decompose the matrix x in several column vectors x_j. Each vector x_j contains all the descriptors in the model calculated for the j-th molecule.

The mathematical model obtained in a QSAR study can be expressed in the form:

$$Y = f(x_1, x_2, \cdots, x_N) \tag{3}$$

We can also define a vector which has the experimental value of the property for each molecule, Y_{Exp}.

4.1.2 LINEAR MODELS

Using the notation introduced earlier, we can express a linear model in the following way:

$$Y = a_0 + a_1 x_1 + a_2 x_2 + \ldots + a_D x_D = a_0 + ax \tag{4}$$

where $a = (a_1 a_2 \ldots a_D)$ and is a row vector which contains times the number . The are obtained using a least squares fitting [4].

Linear models are very popular in QSAR studies due to the fact that they are fairly easy to obtain, and also because they do not overfit the training set as much as other model types [5].

Among all the linear models that can be established, the best of them will be the one that yields the lowest standard deviations in both the training and the test sets [6].

$$S = \sqrt{\frac{1}{N-d-1} \sum_{N}^{i=1} \left(Y_i - Y_{exp,i}\right)^2} \tag{5}$$

In order to develop a linear model that leads to the best predictions, we should calculate several models (by choosing different descriptors sets and doing a least squares fitting), calculate S_{cal} and S_{val}, and then from all the obtained models, select the one which has the lowest S_{cal} and S_{val}. Of course, one would be tempted to try every possible combination of descriptors, but this number is very high. The methodology that involves calculating all possible regressions among variables is called the full search (FS) method. The total number of regressions involved in FS is:

$$\frac{D!}{d!(D-d)!} \tag{6}$$

Table 1 shows an estimate of the time that takes performing all the regressions using 1,500 descriptors on a modern mid-tier computer. It becomes evident that it would not be possible to perform an FS if we want to take into account models that involve more than three descriptors. For this reason, researchers have made a great effort for developing methodologies that are able to explore the descriptor space in a more efficient way (in other words, they try to find the best approximate combination of descriptors while performing a smaller number of regressions).

TABLE 1 Number of regressions and estimated time needed (1,500 descriptors and 100 molecules)

d	N_{reg}	Approx. time (h)
1	1.5×10^3	5×10^{-4} (2 s)
2	1.12×10^6	0.4
3	5.61×10^8	2×10^2 (9 days)
4	2.10×10^{11}	8×10^4 (9 years)
5	6.28×10^{13}	2×10^7 ((3×10^3 years)
8	6.24×10^{20}	2×10^{14} (3×10^{10} years)

4.1.3 THE CONFORMATIONAL PROBLEM

Earlier in this chapter we state that 3D descriptors take into consideration the special distribution of the atoms. These positions are usually chosen to be the ones that minimize the energy of the molecule. It is well known that most molecules have several equilibrium conformations (i.e., the nuclear positions are placed in a local minimum of the potential energy surface. See, for example, [7] and [8]). If we calculate a 3D descriptor for every conformation, its value will be different for each one of them. Therefore, the descriptors contained in the model and the quality of its predictions will depend on which conformation is chosen to represent each molecule in the model.

When we want to take into account the fact that a molecule can adopt several conformations, we should add a new index to the matrix X. Let us call this new "hypermatrix" as $\widehat{X}$. Its elements $\widehat{X}_{ijk}$ represent the i-th descriptor calculated for the k-th conformation of the j-th molecule. Indexes i, j, and k range from 1 to D, from 1 to N and from 1 to N, respectively, where D and N keep their meanings from previous sections, and M is the number of conformations considered for each molecule. Although it would not be necessary to include the same amount of conformations for each molecule, we do so in order to simplify our algorithms. We can also split $\widehat{X}$ into vectors $\widehat{X}_{ij}$: these vectors contain the i-th descriptor calculated for all the conformations of the -th molecule.

Other two useful variables will be the matrix $\widehat{Y}$, whose elements $\widehat{Y}_{ij}$ represent the predicted value of the property for the j-th conformation of the i-th molecule, and $\widehat{E}$, whose elements $\widehat{E}_{ij}$ are the energies of the i-th conformation of the j-th molecule. Both matrices have $N \times M$ size.

Obviously, the new index from matrix $\widehat{X}$ introduces a new difficulty: in the process of creating a QSAR model, we cannot directly use a simple formula like (4), that involves the mentioned matrix. Now we need to come up with a procedure that transforms the matrix $\widehat{X}$ into another matrix X, that possesses only two indexes. We call this new difficulty the conformational problem. There are several ways in which this problem could be solved. The easiest one would be to pick for every molecule the conformation which has the lowest energy. However, in case we try to predict the activity of some group of molecules in relation to a certain ligand (e.g., if we want to predict the inactivation constant of several molecules in relation to the activity of an enzyme), then we could model every molecule taking into account its interaction with the enzyme in the simulation. Simulations of this kind are very demanding and we will not dig any further into such procedures. Therefore, our main goal in the present chapter is to solve the conformational problem in an alternative and efficient way.

4.1.4   MATHEMATICAL ALGORITHMS

In this section, we propose three algorithms intended to provide a solution to the conformational problem. As we see, each one of these alternatives represents a completely different approach to the problem: the first of them is an FS adapted to explore the complete $\widehat{X}$ matrix (we see that this kind of procedure is not adequate for establishing a predictive model); the second of them is an iterative method which creates a matrix $X^{(l)}$ in each step, while the third alternative creates descriptors that take into account several conformations at once.

CONFORMATIONAL FS

The conformational FS (CFS) consists of performing all the possible regressions, including all the descriptors from $\widehat{X}$, instead of using a reduced matrix X. This method is extremely demanding as it needs to calculate a great number of linear regressions. It is very straightforward to realize that the number of regressions is:

$$M^N \frac{D!}{d!(D-d)!} \tag{7}$$

This number is huge even for very small sets. For example, using a set of 700 descriptors, 5 conformations per molecule and 10 molecules to obtain a 4-descriptor model, it would be necessary to complete 9.69×10^{16} linear regressions. This task would take $\sim 10^6$ years.

Besides, this method is not able to distinguish between training and test sets, because it must try every possible conformation, so it does not have a criterion to choose conformations in the test set. For this reason, its results are not possible to use it for predicting unknown values of the property. Nevertheless, it will be useful to show that one can create a model that fits much better the experimental data when the best conformations are chosen.

CONFORMATIONAL STEPWISE METHOD

CS is an iterative method which can be described by the following algorithm:
1. Given $\widehat{X}$, use some criterion to obtain a matrix $X^{(0)}$ with one conformation per molecule. For example, one could pick the lowest energy conformations.
2. Set $l = 0$
3. Use the Stepwise Inclusion Method[4] to obtain a model:
   $Y^{(l)} = a_0^{(l)} + a_1^{(l)} x_1^{(l)} + \ldots + a_d^{(l)} x_d^{(l)}$
4. Use the expression for $Y^{(l)}$ to obtain $\widehat{y}^{(l)}$. (i. e., calculate the value of the property for every conformation of every molecule by using the model created in step 3.)

5. For each, compare the elements $\widehat{Y}_{jk}$ and use a criterion based on the predicted values of the model created in this iteration to pick a conformation for each molecule. In other words, create a mapping $k = \mu(j)$

6. Set $l = l + 1$.

7. Build $X^{(l)}$ using $X_{ij}^{(l)} = \widehat{X}_{ij\mu(j)}$

8. If $l < niter$ go to 3. Else STOP.
    niter is a parameter that states the number of iterations that will be performed.

It should be noted that CS constructs a matrix $\widehat{X}^{(l)}$ for each step. Each one of these matrices should be different to the rest of them because different conformations are picked in each step (although the method could choose the same set of conformations every time, but this is very unlikely). We have chosen the stepwise inclusion method in order to generate a model in each step, because we want a computationally cheap way to do so. In case a more precise method is chosen (like the replacement method, for instance), we would not be able to calculate as many iterations as we want. Besides, most methods give as a result several models and the user has to pick one of them. Contrarily, the stepwise inclusion method provides only one model; this property makes it very straightforward to include in our algorithm, because we do not need to think which model we should choose in each step.

CONFORMATIONAL REPLACEMENT METHOD

The idea behind this method and the one behind the CS method is completely different. In this case, instead of picking one conformation per molecule in each step, we define new descriptors that take into account those from all the conformations. To do so, the following matrices are defined:

- $X^{min} : X_{ij}^{min} = min(\widehat{X}_{ij})$

- $X^{mean} : X_{ij}^{mean} = \dfrac{1}{M}\sum_{k=1}^{M}\widehat{X}_{ijk}$

- $X^{max} : X_{ij}^{max} = max : (\widehat{X}_{ij})$

- $X^{range} : X_{ij}^{range} : max(\widehat{X}_{ij}) - min((\widehat{X}_{ij}))$

- $X^{(0)}$ matrix with the lowest-energy conformations

Note that the first four matrices we define here contain information about several conformations in the molecule: X^{min} and X^{max} choose for every descriptor the conformation with its lowest value (note that for each descriptor, it chooses a different conformation). X^{range} is the subtraction between X^{max} and X^{min}, and X^{mean} contains information about all the conformations. On the other hand, $X^{(0)}$ only contains the descriptors calculated for the conformations with the lowest energy.

After calculating such matrices mentioned before, they are included in a larger matrix:

$$X = \begin{pmatrix} X^{min} & X^{max} & X^{mean} & X^{range} & X^{(0)} \end{pmatrix} \tag{8}$$

This matrix has $5 \times N \times D$ elements and obviously contains information about all the conformations. The final step is to explore this greater matrix using the replacement method [6],[9]. Hence, we call our new method the conformational replacement method (CRM).

4.2 MATHERIALS AND METHODS

4.2.1 CONFORMATIONAL SEARCH AND GEOMETRY OPTIMIZATION

Unless otherwise stated, for all our molecules we keep the S-configuration for the sp3 carbon atoms (including racemic mixtures). The initial conformations of the compounds are drawn with the aid of the "model build" modulus of Hyper-Chem 6.03 program for Windows [10]. Later, we scan the conformational space of the molecules by means of the molecular dynamics module of HyperChem. We use the MM+ molecular mechanics force field to heat the starting geometries from 0 to 900 K in 0.1 ps. After that, the temperature is kept constant by coupling the system to a simulated bath with a relaxation time of 0.5 ps. After an equilibration period of about 5 ps, a 500 ps simulation is carried out and we save the coordinates every 10 ps. The simulation time step is 1 fs. The saved geometries are then optimized to an energy gradient smaller than 0.01 kcal mol–1 Å–1 by means of the semiempirical method PM3 with the Polak–Ribiere algorithm. The simulation is continued in every case until we get 50 conformations per molecule.

4.2.2 MOLECULAR DESCRIPTORS CALCULATION

For each set of molecules plus conformations plus property values we compute by using E-DRAGON [11] via the virtual platform vcclab [12]. This program can calculate more than 1,500 0D–3D descriptors including descriptors of various types such as constitutional, topological, geometrical, charge, GETAWAY, WHIM, 3D-MoRSE, molecular walk counts, BCUT descriptors, 2D-Autocorrelations, aromaticity indexes, randic molecular profiles, radial distribution functions, functional groups, atom-centered fragments, empirical, and properties [13]. Nevertheless, we only use the 3D descriptors as these are the only ones whose values vary from one conformation to another.

4.3 EXPERIMENTAL DATA SETS

In order to test the algorithms proposed in the previous sections, we resorted to four molecular sets which have already been studied elsewhere[14, 15]. For simplicity, we called these as HLE, CatG, PR3, and Angio. The molecules are shown in **Tables 3–6**, and in **Figures 1** to 4. In order to increase the number of numerical runs performed, from each one of the four sets we created two additional sets by (i) exchanging molecules from the training and test sets (HLE-b, CatG-b, PR3-b, and Angio-b) and by (ii) only considering the 20 first conformations obtained by the molecular dynamics in the original set (HLE-20, CatG-20, PR3-20, and Angio-20). This led to a total of 12 sets. We also added to these 12 sets a small one (CatG-R), which was obtained from CatG. **Table 2** summarizes the main characteristics of these sets. In what follows, we provide a brief description of the properties we studied for each set and their relevance.

4.3.1 1,2,5-THIADIAZOLIDIN-3-ONE 1,1-DIOXIDE COMPOUNDS AS SELECTIVE INHIBITORS OF HUMAN SERINE PROTEASES

The proteolytic enzymes human leukocytes elastase (HLE), cathepsin G (Cat G), and proteinase 3 (PR 3) are chymotripsin-like proteases with implications in the etiology and/or pathophysiology of several inflammatory diseases, such as pulmonary emphysema, chronic bronchitis, and adult respiratory distress syndrome [16–19]. Depressed levels of physiological protein inhibitors usually lead to protease–antiprotease imbalance; therefore, there has been great interest in developing highly selective and potent irreversible inhibitors of serine proteases [20].

It has been observed that HLE and Cat G resist the inhibition by proteins, although they are inhibited by low molecular weight compounds. Furthermore, not all the efficient inhibitors are useful for treatment because some of them present poor absorption when orally administered. The 1,2,5-thiadiazolidin-3-one 1,1-dioxide structural scaffold has been proved useful for the synthesis of

several inhibitors due to its high versatility for appending peptidyl or nonpep-
tidyl recognition elements, which favors the optimization of multiple binding
interactions to several enzyme subsites that allow suppressing their activities.

The sets HLE, CatG, and PR3 contain inhibitors based on the 1,2,5-thiadia-
zolidin-3-one 1,1-dioxide structural scaffold with several different substituents,
such as sulfones, sulfides, sulfonamides, phosphates, carboxylates, etc. Each set
has the value of the apparent second order inactivation rate constant [M-1 s-1]
of each molecule against the correspondent enzyme measured with the progress
curve method [21]. For modeling purposes, the values are converted into loga-
rithmic form .

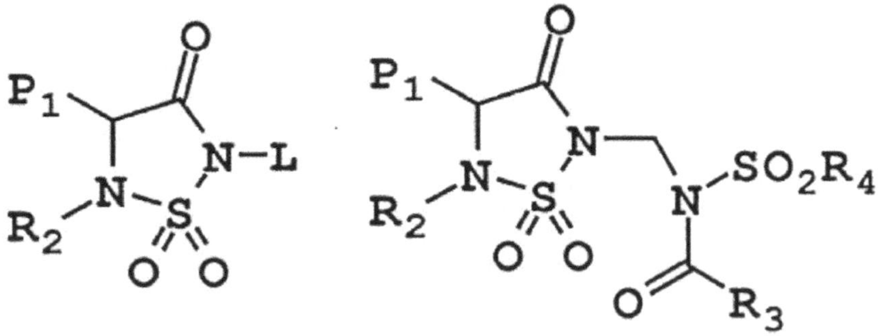

FIGURE 1   1,2,5-tiadiazolidine-3-one 1,1-dioxide scaffold. To the left the general scaffold,
to the right the scaffold to molecules 97-113.

4.3.2   *ANGIOTENSIN CONVERTING ENZYME INHIBITORS*

Angiotensin is a peptide hormone that causes vasoconstriction and a subsequent
increase in blood pressure. Its activity is mainly due to its angiotensin II form,
which is derived from angiotensin I. This reaction is catalyzed by the angio-
tensin-converting enzyme (ACE). Therefore, there has been a great interest in
synthesizing ACE inhibitors due to their potential application as pharmaceutical
drugs for the treatment of hypertension and congestive heart failure [22].

The set of molecules we have chosen is equal to that in Ref. [15]. As the
authors claim in their article, most of the experimental data on ACE inhibitors is
confidential, and therefore has not been published, so this set contains very old
information and the molecular structures are very different from each other. We
expect this set of molecules to lead to poor statistics.

The biological property measured in this case is , defined as , where IC_{50}
refers to the concentration of inhibitor which would be necessary to decrease the
enzymatic activity to half of its original value.

TABLE 2   Summary of the main characteristics for each tested data set

Ncal	N	M	N_{cal}	N_{val}	D	Taken from
CatG-R	10	3	10	0	20	CatG
HLE	132	50	90	42	692	[14]
HLE-b	132	50	74	58	692	HLE
HLE-20	132	20	90	42	692	HLE
CatG	120	50	84	36	692	[14]
CatG-b	120	50	70	50	692	CatG
CatG-20	120	20	84	36	692	CatG
PR3	100	50	70	30	692	[14]
PR3-b	100	50	53	47	692	PR3
PR3-20	100	20	70	30	692	PR3
Angio	72	50	51	21	688	[15]
Angio-b	72	50	40	32	688	Angio
Angio-20	72	20	51	21	688	Angio

TABLE 3   Molecules belonging to the datasets HLE, CatG and PR3

Molecule	R_1	R_2	$L(R_3)$	R_4
001	isobutyl	n-butyl	SO_2Ph	
002	isobutyl	(p-COOCH$_3$)Bzl	SO_2Ph	
003	isobutyl	(p-COOH)Bzl	SO_2Ph	
004	isobutyl	(m-COOCH$_3$)Bzl	SO_2Ph	
005	isobutyl	(m-COOH)Bzl	SO_2Ph	
006	isobutyl	(o-COOCH$_3$)Bzl	SO_2Ph	
007	isobutyl	(o-COOH)Bzl	SO_2Ph	
008	isobutyl	(p-CH$_2$COOH)Bzl	SO_2Ph	
009	isobutyl	CH$_2$COO-t-Bu	SO_2Ph	
010	isobutyl	CH$_2$COO-Bzl	SO_2Ph	
011	isobutyl	CH$_2$COOH	SO_2Ph	
012	isobutyl	methyl	SO_2CH_3	
013	isobutyl	methyl	SO_2(p-Cl phenyl)	
014	isobutyl	benzyl	SO_2(p-Cl phenyl)	
015	isobutyl	methyl	SO_2Ph	
016	isobutyl	benzyl	SO_2Ph	

TABLE 3   (*Continued*)

017	isobutyl	CH_2CH_2Ph	SO_2Ph
018	isobutyl	Methyl	SO_2CH_2Ph
019	isobutyl	Methyl	SO_2CH_2(p-Cl phenyl)
020	isobutyl	Benzyl	SO_2CH_2(p-Cl phenyl)
021	isobutyl	Methyl	$SO_2(CH_2)_3Ph$
022	isobutyl	Benzyl	$SO_2(CH_2)_3Ph$
023	isobutyl	Methyl	SO_2(m-CF_3 phenyl)
024	isobutyl	Benzyl	SO_2(m-CF_3 phenyl)
025	benzyl	H	SO_2Ph
026	benzyl	Methyl	SO_2Ph
027	benzyl	Benzyl	SO_2Ph
028	(D) benzyl	Benzyl	SO_2Ph
029	benzyl	n-butyl	SO_2Ph
030	benzyl	t-cinnamyl	SO_2Ph
031	benzyl	CH_2COO-t-Bu	SO_2Ph
032	(D) benzyl	CH_2COO-t-Bu	SO_2Ph
033	benzyl	(p-CH_2COOH)Bzl	SO_2Ph
034	n-propyl	Methyl	SO_2Ph
035	n-propyl	Benzyl	SO_2Ph
036	$(CH_2)_4NH_2$	Methyl	SO_2Ph
037	$(CH_2)_4NH_2$	Benzyl	SO_2Ph
038	CH_2CO_2H	Benzyl	SO_2Ph
039	DL-ethyl	Methyl	SO_2Ph
040	DL-ethyl	Benzyl	SO_2Ph
041	isopropyl	Methyl	SO_2Ph
042	isopropyl	Benzyl	SO_2Ph
043	n-butyl	Methyl	SO_2Ph
044	n-butyl	Benzyl	SO_2Ph
045	benzyl	Benzyl	$OOCCH_3$
046	benzyl	Benzyl	$OOCCH_2COOH$
047	benzyl	Benzyl	$OOCCH_2OH$
048	benzyl	Benzyl	$OOCCHOHCH_3$
049	benzyl	Benzyl	$OOCCHOHC_6H_5$
050	benzyl	Benzyl	SO_2CH_3
051	benzyl	Benzyl	SO_2CH_2COOH

TABLE 3   (*Continued*)

052	benzyl	Benzyl	$SO_2(CH_2)_2COOH$
053	benzyl	Benzyl	SO_2(o-carboxy)phenyl
054	benzyl	Benzyl	SO_2(m-carboxi)phenyl
055	benzyl	Benzyl	SO_2(p-carboxi)phenyl
056	benzyl	Methyl	2-benzoxazolylthio
057	benzyl	Benzyl	2-benzoxazolylthio
058	benzyl	Benzyl	6-amino-2-benzothia-zolylthio
059	benzyl	Benzyl	5-phenyl-1,3,4-oxadi-azolyl-2-thio
060	isobutyl	Methyl	3-phenyl-5-mercapto-1,2,4-oxadiazolyl
061	isobutyl	Benzyl	3-phenyl-5-mercapto-1,2,4-oxadiazolyl
062	isobutyl	Methyl	2-mercaptobenzothia-zolyl
063	isobutyl	Benzyl	2-mercaptobenzothia-zolyl
064	isobutyl	Methyl	2-mercaptobenzoxa-zolyl
065	isobutyl	Benzyl	2-mercaptobenzoxa-zolyl
066	isobutyl	Methyl	4,5-diphenyl-2-mer-capto-oxazolyl
067	isobutyl	Benzyl	4,5-diphenyl-2-mer-capto-oxazolyl
068	isobutyl	Methyl	5-phenyl-2-mercapto-1,2,4-oxadiazolyl
069	isobutyl	Benzyl	5-phenyl-2-mercapto-1,2,4-oxadiazolyl
070	isobutyl	Methyl	5-phenyl-2-mercapto-benzoxazolyl
071	isobutyl	Benzyl	5-phenyl-2-mercapto-benzoxazolyl
072	benzyl	Methyl	5-phenyl-2-mercapto-1,3,4-oxadiazolyl
073	benzyl	Benzyl	5-phenyl-2-mercapto-1,3,4-oxadiazolyl

TABLE 3 (*Continued*)

074	benzyl	Methyl	2-mercaptobenzoxa-zolyl
075	benzyl	Benzyl	2-mercaptobenzoxa-zolyl
076	benzyl	Benzyl	6-amino-2-mercapto-benzoxazolyl
077	(S) isobu-tyl	H	BocGly
078	(S) isobu-tyl	H	Gly (HCl)
079	(S) isobu-tyl	Methyl	BocGly
080	(S) isobu-tyl	Methyl	Gly (HCl)
081	(S) isobu-tyl	H	Boc-L-Phe
082	(S) isobu-tyl	H	L-Phe (HCl)
083	(S) isobu-tyl	Methyl	Boc-L-Phe
084	(S) isobu-tyl	Methyl	Boc-D-Phe
085	(S) isobu-tyl	Benzyl	Boc-L-Phe
086	(S) isobu-tyl	Benzyl	Boc-D-Phe
087	(S) isobu-tyl	Methyl	Cbz-L-Phe
088	(S) isobu-tyl	Methyl	Cbz-D-Phe
089	(S) isobu-tyl	Methyl	L-Phe (HCl)
090	(S) isobu-tyl	Methyl	D-Phe (HCl)
091	(S) isobu-tyl	Methyl	Boc-L-Met
092	(S) isobu-tyl	Methyl	L-Met (HCl)
093	(S) isobu-tyl	Methyl	Boc-L-Met(O)$_2$

TABLE 3   (*Continued*)

094	Benzyl	Benzyl	Boc-L-Phe	
095	Benzyl	Benzyl	L-Phe (HCl)	
096	Benzyl	Benzyl	Boc-D-Phe	
097	Isobutyl	Methyl	Isobutyloxy	Methyl
098	Isobutyl	Methyl	n-butyloxy	Methyl
099	Isobutyl	Methyl	Benzyloxy	Methyl
100	Isobutyl	Methyl	Methoxy	Phenyl
101	Isobutyl	Methyl	n-butyloxy	Phenyl
102	Isobutyl	Benzyl	Phenyl	Methyl
103	Isobutyl	Methyl	Benzyloxy	Methyl
104	Isobutyl	Methyl	Methyl	(p-NH$_2$)phenyl
105	Isobutyl	Methyl	CH$_2$NHBoc	Methyl
106	Isobutyl	Benzyl	CH$_2$NHBoc	Methyl
107	Isobutyl	Methyl	CH$_2$NHCbz	Methyl
108	Isobutyl	Benzyl	CH$_2$NHCbz	Methyl
109	Isobutyl	Methyl	CH$_2$NHCbz	Phenyl
110	Isobutyl	Benzyl	NHCH$_2$COOEt	Methyl
111	Benzyl	Benzyl	Methoxy	Phenyl
112	Benzyl	Benzyl	n-butyloxy	Phenyl
113	Benzyl	Benzyl	n-butyloxy	Methyl
114	Ethyl*	H	OOCCMe$_3$	
115	Ethyl*	Methyl	OOCCMe$_3$	
116	Ethyl*	Benzyl	OOCCMe$_3$	
117	Ethyl*	H	2,6-Dichlorobenzoate	
118	n-Propyl	H	OOCCMe$_3$	
119	n-Propyl	(p-HOOCCH$_2$) benzyl	OOCCMe$_3$	
120	Isopropyl	H	OOCCMe$_3$	
121	Isobutyl	H	OOCCMe$_3$	
122	Isobutyl	Methyl	OOCCMe$_3$	
123	Isobutyl	Benzyl	OOCCMe$_3$	
124	Isobutyl	(p-CH$_3$OOC) Benzyl	OOCCMe$_3$	
125	Isobutyl	Benzyl	OOCCH$_3$	
126	Isobutyl	H	Benzoate	

TABLE 3   (*Continued*)

127	Isobutyl	Methyl	Benzoate
128	Isobutyl	Benzyl	Benzoate
129	Isobutyl	H	2,6-Dichlorobenzoate
130	Isobutyl	Methyl	2,6-Dichlorobenzoate
131	Isobutyl	Benzyl	2,6-Dichlorobenzoate
132	Isobutyl	($HOOCCH_2$) Benzyl	2,6-Dichlorobenzoate
133	Isobutyl	H	*trans*-Cinnamate
134	Isobutyl	Methyl	*trans*-Cinnamate
135	Isobutyl	H	(alfa)-Flourocinna-mate
136	Isobutyl	Methyl	(alfa)-Flourocinna-mate
137	Isobutyl	Methyl	Dihydrocinnamate
138	Isobutyl	Benzyl	Dihydrocinnamate
139	Isobutyl	Methyl	Phenylacetate
140	Isobutyl	Benzyl	Phenylacetate
141	Isobutyl	Methyl	3-Nicotinate
142	Isobutyl	Methyl	Phenylthioacetate
143	Isobutyl	Methyl	Phenylsulfonyl acetate
144	Isobutyl	Methyl	(4-Pyridylthio) acetate
145	Isobutyl	Methyl	4-(N-Methyl-4-pyri-dyl) acetate
146	Isobutyl	Methyl	(S) Mandelate
147	Isobutyl	Methyl	$CH_3OCH_2CH_2OCH_2COOH$
148	Isobutyl	Methyl	$CH_3OCH_2CH_2OCH_2CH_2OCH_2COOH$
149	Benzyl	Benzyl	2,6-Dichlorobenzoate
150	Benzyl	Benzyl	$OOCCH_3$

TABLE 4　Experimental value of for the molecules from the HLE data set. * Indicates that the molecule belongs to the validation set in HLE and HLE-20, whereas ** indicates that the molecule belongs to the validation set in HLE-b

Molecule	k^*_{inact}	Molecule	k^*_{inact}	Molecule	k^*_{inact}	Molecule	k^*_{inact}
001**	8230	034	780	082	49500	117	3700
002**	67800	035	7260	083**	358100	118	1300
003	7800	036*	Inactive	084*	613200	119	4500
004**	63600	037**	Inactive	085**	652400	120**	Inactive
005**	38700	038*	Inactive	086**	752500	121**	4100
006**	25800	039**	190	087*	637900	122	42700
007*	7690	040*	810	088**	1056800	123*	60500
008*	26700	041**	Inactive	089*	95000	124	13700
009*	2020	042**	Inactive	090	187700	125*	163300
010*	1710	043**	1080	091*	304400	126	91600
011**	1050	044*	8060	092**	69800	127*	267500
012	4590	060**	153460	093*	157500	128**	335900
013**	32200	061*	67840	094**	Inactive	129*	711800
014**	219000	062*	67300	095**	Inactive	130**	4928300
015	9490	063*	22360	096**	Inactive	131	2381000
016	95200	064**	80580	097**	11900	132**	1220000
017*	6590	065**	174440	098*	40500	133**	31300
018**	22300	066**	1540	099*	22000	134**	318200
019*	47500	067*	560	100**	51100	135**	56400
020	165000	068*	25280	101	70500	136	628200
021	15400	069*	168130	102*	71000	137	296300
022*	9990	070	22630	103**	28300	138**	3200
023	38200	071**	Inactive	104	9900	139*	357100
024**	240000	072*	Inactive	105	140500	140	63800
025**	inactive	073**	Inactive	106**	148900	141**	105100
026**	inactive	074*	Inactive	107	229400	142	395400
027**	inactive	075**	Inactive	108*	134000	143*	753200
028*	inactive	076*	Inactive	109**	92700	144	161300
029**	Inactive	077**	62600	110	14100	145**	108300
030*	Inactive	078	5000	113**	1970	146**	308100
031**	Inactive	079**	117000	114*	300	147**	71100
032	Inactive	080**	16900	115**	400	148*	79700
033**	Inactive	081	70100	116*	1500	149*	3600

TABLE 5 Experimental value of of the molecules from the PR3 data set. * Indicates that the molecule belongs to the validation set in PR3 and PR3-20, whereas ** indicates that the molecule belongs to the validation set in PR3-b

Molecu-leele	$k^*_{inactive}$	Molecu-leele	$k^*_{inactive}$	Molecu-leele	$k^*_{inactive}$	Molecu-leeee	$k^*_{inactive}$
001**	430	035*	4960	075**	Inactive	109**	29200
002	1280	036	Inac-tiveee	076*	Inactive	110*	5200
003**	840	037**	Inactive	077*	1700	111**	Inac-tive
004**	7080	038**	Inactive	079*	28000	112**	Inac-tive
005*	10300	039*	200	081*	1800	113	Inac-tiveve
006**	2440	040**	80	083*	64600	114	900
007	1050	041*	Inacti-vee	085**	11900	115**	300
008**	1770	042**	Inactive	087**	126200	116	400
009*	1830	043*	Inactive	088*	157300	117	3400
011	310	044**	inactive	090	13500	118	5100
012*	370	060*	16350	094*	330	119**	2000
013	6280	061**	1510	095**	2320	120*	inac-tive
014**	16200	062**	5990	096**	240	121	2400
015	2250	063*	1070	097*	1200	122**	5900
016**	5240	064	10350	098**	3400	123**	1800
018**	9580	065**	9130	099*	3000	126**	2600
019**	16900	066	1560	100*	6100	127	12800
020**	20300	067**	340	101**	6400	128	26000
021*	8020	068*	12630	102*	16000	129	88200
022*	3250	069*	3590	103**	10100	130**	33400
023**	4780	070*	11100	104	3200	131	14400
024*	2250	071**	1090	105	27500	132**	196400
027**	Inac-tiveeve	072**	Inac-tiveeee	106**	2400	133**	9500
033*	inac-tive	073	Inactive	107	27400	134*	9700
034**	1830	074**	inactive	108**	30100	149**	3500

TABLE 6 Experimental value of of the molecules from the CatG data set. * Indicates that the molecule belongs to the validation set in CatG and CatG-20 while ** indicates that the molecule belongs to the validation set in CatG-b. Underlined molecules also belong to the CatG-R data set.

Molecule	k^*_{inact}	Molecule	k^*_{inact}	Molecule	k^*_{inact}	Molecule	k^*_{inact}
001**	0	031	1130	065	60	112	80
002**	790	032±̲	280	071*	50	1̲1̲3̲±**	5400
003**	70	033**	3760	072	490	114*	inactive
004*	80	034	Inactive	073*	17460	115	inactive
005**	350	035**	130	074**	430	116**	inactive
006**	60	036**	inactive	075*	17130	117	inactive
007*	150	037*	inactive	076	15740	118*	inactive
008**	290	038**	inactive	077	150	119**	200
009**	30	039**	inactive	078**	70	120	Inactive
010*	inactive	040	inactive	079**	60	121*	70
011**	inactive	0̲4̲1̲±	inactive	0̲8̲0̲±	20	122**	Inactive
012	inactive	042	inactive	0̲8̲1̲±**	Inactive	123*	200
013**	inactive	043**	inactive	082*	100	124**	300
0̲1̲4̲	180	044**	610	083*	Inactive	126**	1100
015*	Inactive	045	10600	084	40	1̲2̲7̲	300
0̲1̲6̲	110	046*	22700	085**	400	128**	90
017	Inactive	047*	12800	0̲8̲6̲	60	129	500
018**	100	048**	12680	087**	140	130**	60
019*	160	049*	12330	088**	50	131**	30
020*	70	050*	8500	089	50	132	2300
021	20	051*	25230	090	40	133*	1200
022*	60	052**	17370	091**	Inactive	134**	100
023	Inactive	053**	350	092	10	136	100
024	inactive	054	20710	093*	60	139	200
025**	30	055	66680	103	200	141*	90
026	120	056*	430	107	60	142**	70
027	11200	057**	17130	108**	70	145**	inactive
028	1580	058	15740	109**	inactive	146	100
029*	320	059**	490	110**	70	149*	2200
030*	760	0̲6̲4̲±	30	111	90	150**	10600

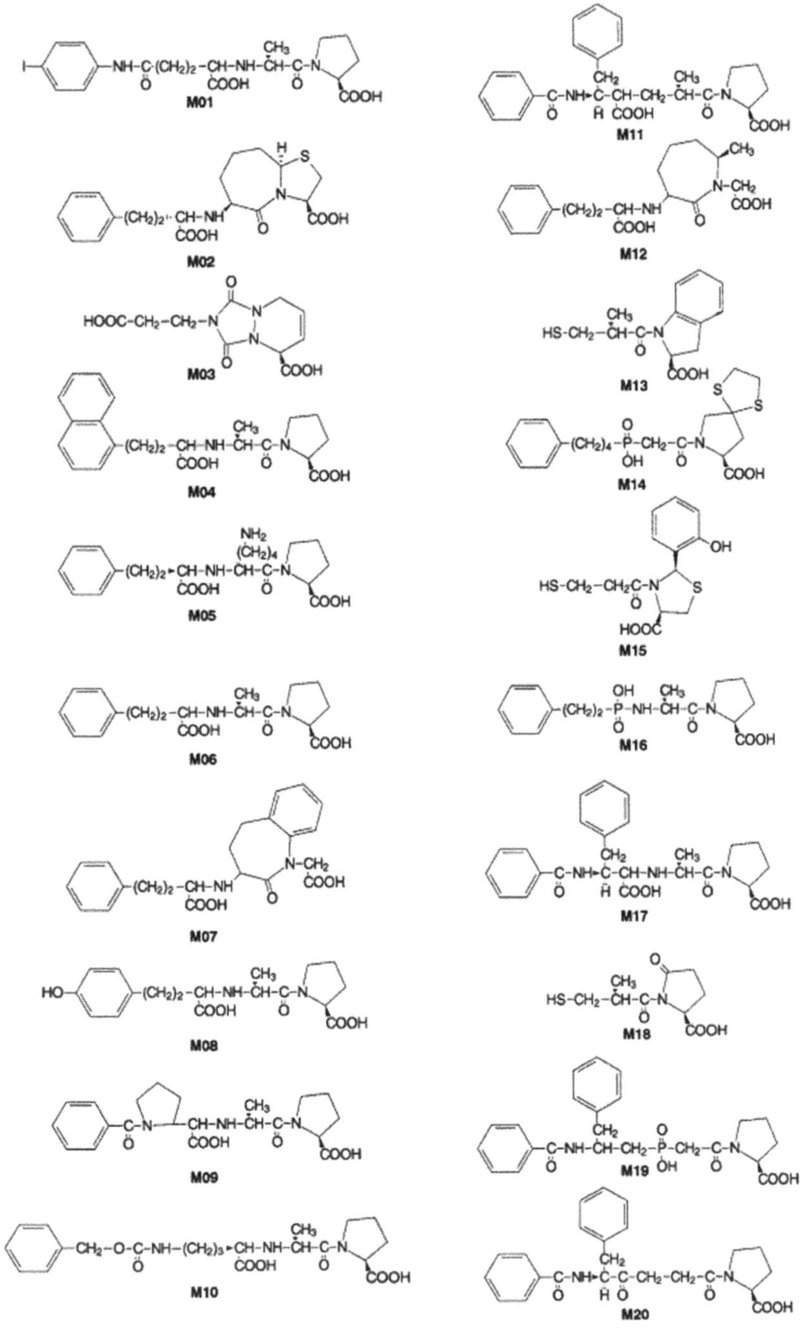

FIGURE 2   The first 20 molecules from the Angio data set.

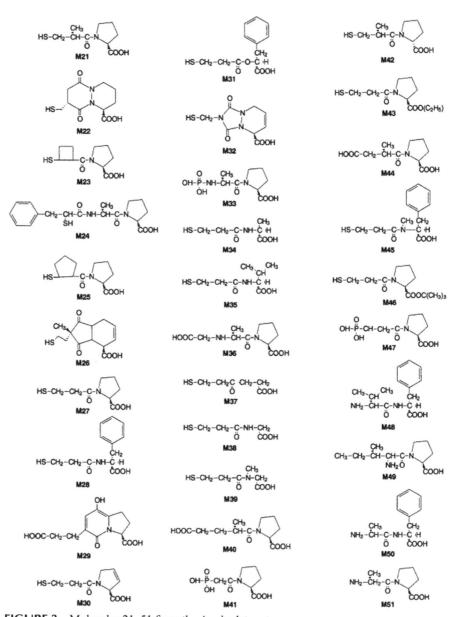

FIGURE 3   Molecules 21–51 from the Angio data set.

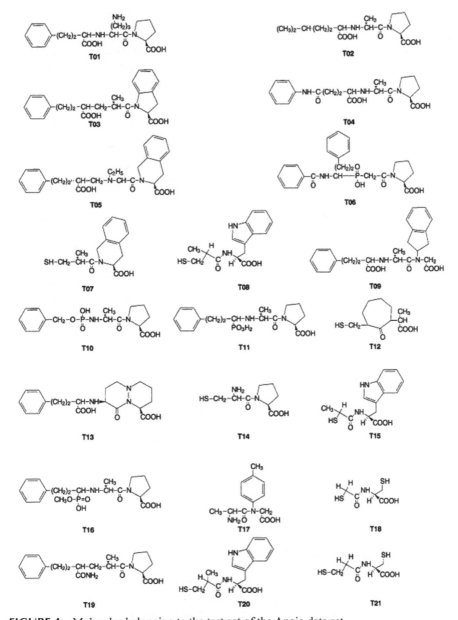

FIGURE 4 Molecules belonging to the test set of the Angio data set.

TABLE 7   Experimental value of pIC_{50} of the molecules from the Angio data set. * Indicates that the molecule belongs to the validation set in Angio and Angio-20.

Molecule	pIC_{50}	Molecule	pIC_{50}	Molecule	pIC_{50}
M01	9.64	M18*	8.05	M35*	5.8
M02*	9.22	M19*	8	M36*	5.62
M03*	9	M20*	7.92	M37*	5.62
M04	8.96	M21	7.64	M38*	5.55
M05*	8.92	M22*	7.42	M39*	5.52
M06	8.92	M23*	7.31	M40	5.31
M07	8.77	M24	7.3	M41	5.08
M08	8.55	M25*	7.19	M42*	4.96
M09*	8.54	M26*	7	M43	4.77
M10*	8.54	M27	6.7	M44*	4.66
M11*	8.52	M28*	6.37	M45*	4.51
M12*	8.52	M29*	6.34	M46	4.41
M13*	8.43	M30*	6.19	M47	4.32
M14	8.4	M31*	6.15	M48	4.28
M15*	8.22	M32	6.15	M49	3.89
M16*	8.15	M33	6.11	M50*	3.72
T01	8,66	T08	7,46	T15	7,19
T02	8,59	T09	7,4	T16	6,36
T03	8,32	T10	7,39	T17	5,59
T04	8,28	T11	7,29	T18	4,72
T05	8,19	T12	7,28	T19	4,59
T06	7,92	T13	7,25	T20	4,48
T07	7,7	T14	7,2	T21	4,17
T01	8,66	T08	7,46	T15	7,19

4.4   RESULTS AND DISCUSSION

We tested our three algorithms by applying them to the sets that were described earlier in this chapter. Also applying the stepwise inclusion method [4] and the replacement method [9] by choosing the conformations with the lowest energy for each molecule. The replacement method provides several models, with varying S_{cal} and S_{val}, so in order to avoid models that overfit the test set we took a 20% criterion: from all the available models, we first considered the one with lowest S_{cal}; let us call this value S_{min}. Then, we only took into account the models from the [S_{min}, 20% greater than S_{min}] interval. Within all the models that meet this requirement, we picked the one with the lowest S_{val}. Note that this criterion allowed us to automatically pick the models without the need of user's intervention.

In the CS algorithm, we used the following criteria: 300 iterations for picking the conformations with the lowest value of the predicted property; 300 iterations for picking the conformations whose predicted value is closest to the mean of the predicted values for all the conformations of the molecule; and 300 iterations for picking the conformations whose predicted values are the largest value.

In the following tables, we show the best models obtained with each algorithm for the different data sets, and in addition, the relative percentage improvement between our algorithms and the ones they are based on. The relative percentage improvement was calculated as $\%imp = 100\left(S_{val}^{reg} - S_{val}^{conf}\right) / S_{val}^{reg}$ where stands for (SI, RM) and stands for the conformational variants (CS, CRM).

TABLE 8 Standard deviation of the best models obtained for the CatG-R data set

Method	S_{cal} $d=2$	%imp	S_{cal} $d=4$	%imp
SI (minimum energy)	0,49	34,69	0,37	67,57
CS	0,32		0,12	
RM (minimum energy)	0,46		0,16	
FS (minimum energy)	0,46	73,91	0,16	87,50
CFS	0,12		0,02	

TABLE 9 Standard deviation of the models provided by the different algorithms for the data sets based on HLE

Data Set Variant	Method	$d=2$ S_{cal}	S_{val}	%imp	$d=4$ S_{cal}	S_{val}	%imp	$d=6$ S_{cal}	S_{val}	%imp
HLE	SI	1.19	1.07	0.00	0.99	1.12	16.96	0.89	1.09	18.35
	CS	1.19	1.07		1.09	0.93		0.95	0.89	
	RM	1.19	1.07	4.67	1.03	0.92	10.87	0.95	0.87	5.75
	CRM	1.26	1.02		1.04	0.82		0.87	0.82	
HLE-20	SI	1.23	1.15	0.00	1.06	1.00	12.00	0.96	1.03	9.71
	CS	1.23	1.15		1.09	0.88		0.94	0.93	
	RM	1.23	1.15	7.83	1.09	0.91	6.59	1.02	0.89	3.37
	CRM	1.23	1.06		1.06	0.85		0.98	0.86	

TABLE 9   (*Continued*)

HLE-b	SI	1.06	1.61	9.94	0.89	1.71	23.39	0.77	1.51	19.87
	CS	1.04	1.45		0.89	1.31		0.75	1.21	
	RM	1.00	1.35	0.00	0.91	1.25	3.20	0.76	1.15	2.61
	CRM	1.00	1.35		0.92	1.21		0.75	1.12	

TABLE 10   Standard deviation of the models provided by the different algorithms for the data sets based on CatG.

Data Set Variant	Method	$d = 2$		%imp	$d = 4$		%imp	$d = 6$		%imp
		S_{cal}	S_{val}		S_{cal}	S_{val}		S_{cal}	S_{val}	
CatG	SI	0.74	0.91	18.68	0.68	0.91	28.57	0.63	0.80	16.25
	CS	0.76	0.74		0.63	0.65		0.49	0.67	
	RM	0.78	0.75	9.33	0.72	0.68	25.00	0.62	0.67	14.93
	CRM	0.78	0.68		0.64	0.51		0.61	0.57	
CatG-20	SI	0.75	0.83	4.82	0.68	0.89	29.21	0.61	0.95	31.58
	CS	0.71	0.79		0.63	0.63		0.59	0.65	
	RM	0.78	0.71	5.63	0.71	0.73	23.29	0.66	0.72	33.33
	CRM	0.78	0.67		0.68	0.56		0.55	0.48	
CatG-b	SI	0.73	0.92	21.74	0.65	0.83	15.66	0.57	0.91	20.88
	CS	0.70	0.72		0.60	0.70		0.52	0.72	
	RM	0.86	0.77	10.39	0.69	0.72	12.50	0.61	0.72	2.78
	CRM	0.73	0.69		0.68	0.63		0.48	0.70	

TABLE 11   Standard deviation of the models provided by the different algorithms for the data sets based on PR3

Data Set Variant	Method	$d = 2$		%imp	$d = 4$		%imp	$d = 6$		%imp
		S_{cal}	S_{val}		S_{cal}	S_{val}		S_{cal}	S_{val}	
PR3	SI	0.92	1.24	12.10	0.78	1.21	22.31	0.69	1.12	11.61
	CS	0.95	1.09		0.70	0.94		0.61	0.99	
	RM	1.05	1.05	13.33	0.80	0.96	11.46	0.72	0.91	2.20
	CRM	0.97	0.91		0.80	0.85		0.67	0.89	
PR3-20	SI	0.96	1.19	18.49	0.81	1.11	18.02	0.74	1.10	11.82
	CS	0.66	0.97		0.72	0.91		0.66	0.97	
	RM	1.03	1.03	6.80	0.81	1.01	12.87	0.66	0.99	14.14
	CRM	1.01	0.96		0.77	0.88		0.65	0.85	

TABLE 11   (*Continued*)

	SI	0.89	1.05	10.48	0.76	1.16	25.86	0.68	1.14	18.42
	CS	0.93	0.94		0.81	0.86		0.75	0.93	
PR3-b										
	RM	0.88	0.89	5.62	0.71	0.87	6.90	0.59	1.03	24.27
	CRM	0.88	0.84		0.76	0.81		0.74	0.78	

TABLE 12   Standard deviation of the models provided by the different algorithms for the data sets based on Angio

Data Set Variant	Method	$d = 2$		%imp	$d = 4$		%imp	$d = 6$		%imp
		S_{cal}	S_{val}		S_{cal}	S_{val}		S_{cal}	S_{val}	
	SI	1.03	1.73	19.65	0.88	1.85	32.43	0.78	2.42	45.87
	CS	1.05	1.39		0.85	1.25		0.79	1.31	
Angio										
	RM	1.12	1.26	4.76	1.02	1.32	5.30	0.83	1.52	2.63
	CRM	1.16	1.20		0.99	1.25		0.80	1.48	
	SI	1.04	1.42	2.82	0.88	1.67	14.97	0.79	1.96	19.39
	CS	1.04	1.38		0.87	1.42		0.66	1.58	
Angio-20										
	RM	1.17	1.19	0.00	0.98	1.38	4.35	0.83	1.54	-7.14
	CRM	1.20	1.19		0.92	1.32		0.86	1.65	
	SI	1.09	1.66	28.31	0.94	1.83	31.69	0.83	1.84	2.17
	CS	1.15	1.19		0.66	1.25		0.55	1.80	
Angio-b										
	RM	1.15	1.15	12.17	0.99	1.29	21.71	0.78	1.34	3.73
	CRM	1.25	1.01		1.06	1.01		0.72	1.29	

We can see that the algorithms that take into account the conformational flexibility build better models than the simpler algorithms they are based on. (i.e., CS gives better results than SI and CRM gives better results than RM). There are some cases in which the improvement is remarkable; for example, S_{val} becomes 45% smaller when we use CS instead of SI in one of the data sets of **Table 11** with $d = 6$, and also we can get a 33% improvement by using CRM instead of RM in one of the data sets of **Table 9**.

Moreover, the most remarkable result is that when we performed an FS on the small data set CR we found out that by taking into account a very small number of conformations, only five per molecule, the best model showed a reduction in it standard deviation of up to 88%!

In one of our examples the model we obtained by using CRM was worse than the one obtained with RM (the only result with negative %*imp*, data set Angio-20, with $d = 6$ in **Table 12**). This does not mean that for this case $\widehat{X}$ is a worse representation of the problem than $X^{(0)}$ because at least they should be equally good (this holds true because X contains $X^{(0)}$). Instead, it means that $X^{(0)}$ is too large of a matrix for RM to find the best available models.

4.5   CONCLUSIONS

The 88% improvement in the exact search of **Table 7** is a very important result that indicates, at least for the studied data set, that the lowest energy conformation is not the most representative of the property under study. This shows that it is mandatory to take into account the conformational flexibility of the molecules.

In most cases, the proposed methods were able to take into account the conformational flexibility and, hence, provide better results than those in which the conformations are not considered. More precisely, CS always gives better (or equal) results than SI, and CRM gives better (or equal) results than RM.

The CS method (conformational stepwise; compute several stepwise inclusions picking different conformations by using a specific criterion in each one of them) is computationally very cheap, so its good results are very promising. Besides, one could implement different criteria in order to choose the set of conformations for each step. The main disadvantage of this method is that in order to predict a property value, one should perform all the iterations with any molecule.

The fact that CRM (conformational replacement method; construct a greater matrix with descriptors that take into account all the conformations and then perform a RM search) gives better (or equal) results than RM implies that the matrix $\widehat{X}$ describes the system in a better way than $X^{(0)}$. This is not surprising, because the former contains the latter. Although the better results seem promising, one should always keep in mind that $\widehat{X}$ is five times larger than $X^{(0)}$, so the computational cost of finding the best linear models becomes much more demanding.

The least favorable case of **Table 12** gives us the hint that the results of CRM can be further improved if we utilize a better search method.

The main conclusion that can be reached from the concepts exposed in this chapter is that the conformational flexibility consideration is very important when QSAR models improvement is wanted, and that it is possible to develop simple algorithms for this purpose.

ACKNOWLEDGMENTS

PRD acknowledges the financial support from the National Research Council of Argentina (CONICET) PIP11220100100151 project and to Ministerio de Ciencia, Tecnología e Innovación Productiva for the electronic library facilities. JG has a PhD fellowship from CONICET. PRD is a member of the scientific researcher career of CONICET.

KEYWORDS

- **Algorithms**
- **Molecules**
- **QSAR**
- **Replacement method**
- **Stepwise inclusion technique**

REFERENCES

1. Hansch C., L.A., *Exploring QSAR. Fundamentals and Applications in Chemistry and Biology*. 1995: American Chemical Society.
2. Karitzky, A.R., V.S. Lobanov, and M. Karelson, *QSPR: the correlation and quantitative prediction of chemical and physical properties from structure*. Chemical Society Reviews, 1995. **24**: p. 279–287.
3. Kubinyi, H., *QSAR: Hansch Analysis and Related Approaches*. 2008: Wiley-Interscience.
4. Rawlings, J.O., S.G. Pantula, and D.A. Dickey, *Applied Regression Analysis: A Research Tool*. 2nd edition ed. 1998: Springer.
5. Vicente, E., *et al.,, Exploring 3-arylquinoxaline-2-carbonitrile 1,4-di-n-oxides activities against neglected diseases with QSAR*. Chemical Biology and Drug Design, 2010. **76**: p. 59–69.
6. Mercader A.G., D.P.R., Fernández F.M., Castro E.A., *Advances in the replacement and enhanced replacement method in QSAR and QSPR theories*. Journal of Chemical Information and Modelling, 2011. **51**: p. 1575–1581.
7. Badawi, H.M., *et al.,, Conformational properties and vibrational analyses of monomeric pentafluoropropionic acid CF_3CF_2COOH and pentafluoropropionamide $CF_3CF_2CONH_2$*. Canadian Journal of Analytical Sciences and Spectroscopy, 2007. **5**: p. 252–269.
8. Cutín, E.H., *et al.,, Conformation and gas-phase structure of difluorosulphenylimine cyanide, $F_2S(O)NCN$*. Journal of Molecular Structure, 1995. **354**: p. 165–168.
9. Ibezim, E., *et al.,, QSAR on aryl-piperazine derivatives with activity on malaria*. Chemometrics and Intelligent Laboratory Systems, 2012. **110**: p. 81–88.
10. *Hyperchem v6.0*. Available from: http://www.hyper.com/News/PressRelease/Release-60Feb2000/tabid/411/Default.aspx.
11. *E-dragon*. Available from: http://www.vcclab.org/lab/edragon.

12. Tetko, I.V., *et al.,*, *Virtual computational chemistry laboratory - design and description.* Journal of Computer-Aided Molecular Design, 2005. **19**: p. 453–463.
13. Todeschini, R., *et al.,*, *Weighted holistic invariant molecular descriptors. Part 2. Theory development and applications on modeling physicochemical properties of polyaromatic hydrocarbons.* Chemometrics and Intelligent Laboratory Systems, 1995. **27**: p. 221–229.
14. Garcia, J., *et al.,*, *A comparative QSAR on 1,2,5-thiadiazolidin-3-one 1,1-dioxide compounds as selective inhibitors of human serine proteinases.* Journal of Moecular Graphics and Modelling, 2011. **31**: p. 10–19.
15. Bersuker, I.B., S. Bahçeci, and J.E. Boggs, *Improved electron-conformational method of pharmacophore identification and bioactivity prediction. Application to angiotensin converting enzyme inhibitors.* Journal of Chemical Information and Computational Science, 2000. **40**: p. 1363–1376.
16. Groutas, W.C., *et al.,*, *Structure-based design of a general class of mechanism-based inhibitors of the serine proteinases employing a novel amino acid-derived heterocyclic scaffold.* Biochemistry, 1997. **36**: p. 4739–4750.
17. Dhami, R., *et al.,*, *Acute cigarette smoke-induced connective tissue breakdown is mediated by neutrophils and prevented by 1-antitrypsin.* American Journal of Respiratory Cell and Molecular Biology, 2000. **22**: p. 244–252.
18. Stockley, R.A., *The role of proteinases in the pathogenesis of chronic bronchitis.* American Journal of Respiratory and Critical Care Medicine, 1994. **150**: p. S109–S113.
19. Barnes, P.J., *Novel approaches and targets for treatment of chronic obstuctive pulmonary disease.* American Journal of Respiratory and Critical Care Medicine, 1999. **160**: p. S72–S79.
20. Brouwer, A.J., *et al.,*, *Synthesis and biological evaluation of novel irreversible serine protease inhibitors using amino acid based sulfonyl fluorides as an electrophilic trap.* Bioorganic & Medicinal Chemistry, 2011. **7**: p. 2397–2406.
21. Morrison, J.F. and C.T. Walsh, *The behaviour and significance of slow-binding enzyme inhibitors.* Advanced Enzymology, 1988. **61**: p. 201–301.
22. Kierszenbaum, A.L., *Histology and cell biology: an introduction to pathology.* 2007: Mosby Elsevier.

CHAPTER 5

PRACTICAL ASPECTS OF BUILDING, VALIDATION, AND APPLICATION OF 3D-PHARMACOPHORE MODELS

ELUMALAI PAVADAI[1] and KELLY CHIBALE[1, 2]

[1]Department of Chemistry, South African Medical Research Council Drug Discovery and Development Research Unit, University of Cape Town, Rondebosch 7701, South Africa

[2]Institute of Infectious Disease and Molecular Medicine, University of Cape Town, Rondebosch 7701, South Africa

Corresponding authors: *pelumalai@gmail.com (Dr. Elumalai Pavadai)*
kelly.chibale@uct.ac.za (Prof. Kelly Chibale)

CONTENTS

ABSTRACT

A pharmacophore is a specific three-dimensional arrangement of essential chemical features of molecules that mediates biological activity and thus plays a critical role in the hit identification and lead optimization stages of the drug discovery and development process. A pharmacophore can be derived either from the binding site of a target or a set of active ligands. In this chapter, we describe practical aspects of building of pharmacophore models and their validation. In addition, limitations and issues associated with pharmacophore models are also presented along with some practical applications of these models.

5.1   INTRODUCTION

Drug discovery is an inventive process of finding new small molecules, which can be used to prevent and/or treat diseases with minimum undesirable side effects. It involves several common tasks to identify hit molecules including chemical synthesis and biological screening of a large number of compounds. Once found, hits need to be optimized to generate leads, which require additional synthesis. The whole process takes ~7–15 years at an approximate cost of ~$1.2 billion to bring a new drug to the market[1]. Additionally, the success rate is extremely low. For example, only 5 out of 40,000 drugs tested in animals reach human testing and finally only 1 in 5 drugs reaching clinical studies is approved[2]. This all indicates that finding a new therapeutic drug is difficult, time consuming, expensive, and needs consideration of many aspects. To meet these challenges, new approaches are needed to facilitate, accelerate, and streamline the drug discovery and development processes[2]. These challenges may in part be addressed using computer-aided drug design (CADD) or *in silico* drug design methods. CADD uses high computational power and computational techniques in conjunction with three-dimensional (3D)-structures of proteins and their binding interactions with ligands, etc. It has been estimated that CADD approaches account for ~10% of pharmaceutical R&D expenditure and this is expected to rise to 20% by 2016[3].

   CADD is an exciting and diverse discipline based on the various aspects of applied and basic research[4]. It is widely used to speed up and facilitate hit identification and hit-to-lead selection, optimize the absorption, distribution, metabolism, excretion and toxicity profile (ADMET) and potentially avoid safety issues[2]. The frequently used CADD approaches can be differentiated, based on the methodologies applied, into receptor/target/structure- and ligand-based drug design methods. The structure-based methods include homology modeling, drug–target docking and protein–protein docking, etc., whereas ligand-based drug design methods include 3D pharmacophore, quantitative structure–activity/property relationships (QSAR/QSPR), similarity search, etc. Academic institutions and pharmaceutical companies are actively involved in the development of new CADD tools that will further improve the effectiveness and efficiency of the drug discovery and development processes with attendant increase in the predictability of drug toxicity[2]. In this chapter, one of the well-established ligand-based drug design approach, 3D-pharmacophore models, is covered in detail.

5.1.1 3D-PHARMACOPHORE

A pharmacophore is a 3D representation of structural or chemical features of a set of ligands, which is responsible for their biological activities. According to IUPAC, a pharmacophore is defined as "an ensemble of steric and electronic features that is necessary to ensure the optimal intermolecular interactions with a specific biological target and to trigger (or block) its biological response"[5]. However, a pharmacophore does not mean a real molecule, but an abstract description of common molecular interactions of structurally diverse ligands to a common binding site of a defined target. Thus a pharmacophore is a common descriptor shared by a set of active ligands or from the protein binding site. Therefore, the pharmacophore model is able to accurately explain the nature and location of the functional groups of a ligand with the binding site of a target protein. It also provides information of various types of noncovalent interactions and their characteristics.

A pharmacophore model is comprised of features that are moieties or regions with specific atoms or bond types in a molecule. These features include hydrophobic, aromatic, hydrogen bond acceptor, hydrogen bond donor, positive and negative ionizable moieties, etc. Generally two types of pharmacophore feature representations are used: vectors (e.g., hydrogen bond acceptors) and single points (e.g., hydrophobic features). The vector features represent the location on the ligand, and another point represents the location of the complimentary feature on the protein required for the interaction. The characteristic 3D locations of these features are often specified using different types of constraints such as location, distance, angle, torsion, and shape. A typical pharmacophore model and its mapping onto the active compound are shown in **Figure 1(A)** and **(B)**, respectively. The model has three types of chemical features and their 3D-location constraints. The hydrophobic, hydrogen-bond donor and hydrogen-bond acceptor regions are shown in cyan, purple, and green colour, respectively.

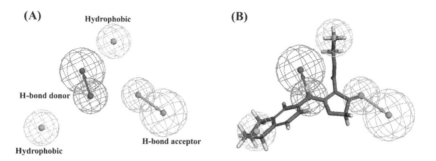

FIGURE 1(A) A 3D-Pharmacophore model. **(B)** The model mapping with an active compound. Pharmacophore features are color-coded with green for hydrogen-bond acceptor, light-blue for hydrophobic feature, and purple for hydrogen-bond acceptor features.

In recent years, pharmacophore approaches have been increasingly employed in modern medicinal chemistry to identify hit molecules in the drug discovery and development processes, due to the low hit rates in high-throughput bioassays [6]. Significantly, the pharmacophore model has been proven to be successful in understanding the binding or key interactions between target and ligand and in identification of novel hit molecules with 3D-database searching or virtual screening. One major advantage of pharmacophore models is the ability to discover very diverse structural scaffolds, because the same chemical features of a pharmacophore model can map onto the multiple structural elements of the functional groups of compounds. In addition to these, 3D-restraints of pharmacophore models are used in molecular docking to guide structure-based virtual screening and to generate virtual compound libraries. Therefore, building a pharmacophore model for a set of active ligands or for a target protein will effectively be used to perceive the interactions between ligand and protein and to facilitate the hit identification process. Various tools are available for building different pharmacophore models, for example: Catalyst (Accelrys), MOE (Chemical Computing Group), Phase (Schrodinger), LigandScout (Inte:Ligand), etc. The history and the development of the pharmacophore concept in the past century have been extensively reviewed by Gund[7], Wermuth[5], Van Drie[8], and Langer and Wolber[9]. This chapter covers some practical aspects of building ligand- and structure-based pharmacophore models and their application in the drug discovery and development process. The chapter also discusses the validation of these models.

5.2 BUILDING OF PHARMACOPHORE MODELS

Building an accurate pharmacophore model for a given set of ligands or protein binding site is a relatively difficult task. The available methods for building pharmacophore models can generally be divided into two categories, ligand- and structure-based pharmacophore models, and the schematic representations for building both pharmacophore model categories is shown in **Figure 2** and **3**, respectively. The building of these two groups of pharmacophore model is discussed in detail in the following sections.

5.2.1 LIGAND-BASED PHARMACOPHORE MODELS

Ligand-based pharmacophore models play key roles in facilitating the drug discovery and development processes in the absence of 3D-structures of biological targets when a series of compounds with biological activity is known. This can especially be a method of choice for membrane proteins such as efflux pump proteins and G protein-coupled receptors (GPCR), etc. There are two approaches in building ligand-based pharmacophore models, viz. common-feature and 3D-QSAR pharmacophore models. Both approaches are aimed at identifying a common 3D arrangement of chemical features from 3D structures of a set of ligands, which is essential for ligand molecules to interact with a specific binding site of a target protein. Generally, modeling of pharmacophore models for a given set of active ligands, also known as a training set, involves two important steps. Generating a diverse conformational space for each ligand in the training set to represent the conformational flexibility of ligands and aligning those generated multiple conformations to identify the best overlay of the pharmacophore features. Then, determining the essential chemical features to establish pharmacophore models. Modeling the conformational flexibility of ligands and overlaying conformations are key techniques but also main challenges in ligand-based pharmacophore modeling, as the active conformations of the molecules are usually unknown[10]. Several automated academic and commercial pharmacophore modeling software have been developed for building ligand-based pharmacophore models[11] for instance Hip-Hop [12] and HypoGen[7,13] of Catalyst (http://www.accelrys.com/products/catalyst/), DISCO[14] (http://www.tripos.com/data/SYBYL/DISCOTech_072505.pdf), GASP[15] (http://www.tripos.com/data/SYBYL/GASP_072505.pdf), GALAHAD[16] (http://www.tripos.com/data/SYBYL/GALAHAD_9-7-05.pdf), PHASE[17] (http://www.schrodinger.com/productpage/14/13/), and MOE (http://www.chemcomp.com/MOE-Pharmacophore_Discovery.htm). However, all these programs only differ in the algorithms used for modeling the flexibility of ligands and for the alignment of molecules, and the definitions of pharmacophore features[18a]. Detailed discussion and comparison of these programs have been published elsewhere[10, 18b, 19a–d] and the overview of building of ligand-based pharmacophore model is shown in **Figure 2**. Some important practical aspects relevant to the both 3D-QSAR pharmacophore and common-feature models are discussed hereunder.

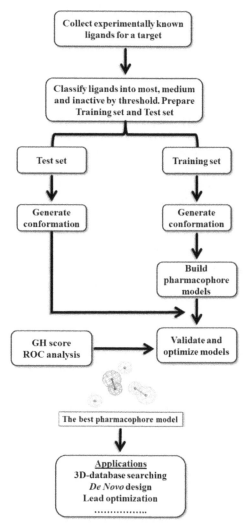

FIGURE 2   Overview of building of ligand-based pharmacophore models.

5.2.1.1   3D-QSAR PHARMACOPHORE MODEL

The 3D-QSAR pharmacophore model, also known as predictive pharmaco-phore model, is widely employed to quantitatively explore the common essen-tial chemical features among a considerable number of structures of ligands with great diversity. This pharmacophore model is derived from a set of ligands with known activity values against a given target, and thus could serve as a mod-el in assessing other ligands for their ability to map the essential features and predicting their activities. However, the building of 3D-QSAR models needs the correct alignment of ligands for reliable activity prediction, which limits their application in virtual screening. Although a variety of programs are available for building 3D-QSAR pharmacophore models, HypoGen of Catalyst from Accelrys Inc. (www.accelrys.com) is the mostly used program because it provides flexible options during pharmacophore generation. To build 3D-QSAR pharmacophore models using HypoGen, a minimum of 16 structurally diverse ligands of the training set with corresponding IC_{50}, K_i, or EC_{50} values spanning over four orders of magnitude, including several most active, moderately active, and some least active ligands are required (http://accelrys.com/resource-center/case-studies/training-set-selection.html). The biological activity of ligands should have been obtained with similar experimental conditions and procedures. Since the training set ligands play a very important role in determining the quality of the pharmacophore models, they must have a large range of activities to obtain critical information on the pharmacophoric requirements.

After carefully selecting the training set ligands, the 3D conformational search for the bioactive conformation of each ligand is modeled by making multiple conformers within a specific energy range. For this, several conformational search algorithms have been developed, which have strengths and weaknesses. The conformational search algorithms should usually address two main issues: sufficient coverage of the energy landscape and diversity of the representation among the conformational models of the ligand under consideration[20]. The Catalyst program offers different conformation selection and torsion search strategies for generating diverse ligand conformations such as Fast, Best, CAESAR, Systematic search, Random search, and Boltzmann jump. The comparisons of various conformation search algorithms-implemented in several widely used molecular modeling packages, including Catalyst, MacroModel (http://www.schrodinger.com/MacroModel/), Omega (http://www.eyesopen.com/omega), MOE, and Rubicon (http://www.daylight.com/dayhtml/doc/rubicon/) as well as stochastic proximity embedding (SPE)-suggest that Catalyst may relatively be more effective in sampling the full range of the conformational space of ligands[21]. In addition, the capabilities of the Catalyst's conformational generation algorithm have been studied with 510 pharmaceutically relevant protein–ligand complexes extracted from the protein data bank (PDB) and the results revealed that Catalyst is capable of producing high-quality conformers[22]. Moreover, the analysis of specific settings for Catalyst recommended that generation of 255 conformers using the BEST option and a 20 kcal/mol produces conformations with RMS of less than 1 Å to the X-ray structure of the ligand. This program's functions are supported by the generalized CHARMm force field[23]. The Hypo-Gen algorithm generates predictive pharmacophore models using three phases-constructive, subtractive, and optimization-based on the given training set, conformational models, and pharmacophore features. The conformational options, interfeature distance, input features, and training set ligands are the main parameters, which affect the pharmacophore modeling.

5.2.1.2   COMMON-FEATURE PHARMACOPHORE

A common-feature pharmacophore model is useful when few active ligands are available with different structures. This model is built with a set of a minimum of two or three active ligands, also called training set. From different chemical scaffolds, the training set is assumed to have similar binding modes with the binding site of a target. Programs such as Hip-Hop, Phase, MOE, etc., are commonly used to derive 3D spatial arrangements of chemical features that are common to the training set ligands; these programs do not require biological activity during the process of building models. The Hip-Hop, for example, evaluates the training set ligands on the basis of the types of chemical features they contain, along with the ability to adopt a conformation that allows those features to be superimposed on a particular configuration[12]. Thus, the choice of training set ligands influences the quality of the pharmacophore models. Several parameters may also be controlled in order to build diverse pharmacophore models. One example of such parameters is how many pharmacophore features need to be mapped or missed to molecules, which may be determined based on the activity of the training set molecules. Additionally, the quality of the pharmacophore models may optionally be enhanced by adding exclusion volume (steric) constraint features to an input pharmacophore model, for example, the excluded volumes is placed in the regions of inactive ligands but not in the active ligands. The output models are ranked as they are built and also the ranking could be a measure of how well the ligands map onto the built pharmacophore, as well as the rarity of the pharmacophore model. The rank can be higher as the pharmacophore model is less likely to map to the inactive ligands and the reverse is also true. Usually, the top ranked model is expected to have the hypothetical orientation of the active molecules, albeit the first model may not necessarily be the best pharmacophore model.

5.2.2   STRUCTURE-BASED PHARMACOPHORE MODELS

The structural genomics consortium rapidly generates numerous 3D structures of proteins and of protein–ligand complexes[24a–c]. In addition, several computational algorithms and tools are available for the prediction of ligand-binding sites on proteins[25]. The availability of 3D structures of protein and protein–ligand complexes and the information of predicted binding sites of proteins can effectively be used for building pharmacophore models. Several programs are available, which are used to build pharmacophore models from protein–ligand complex and protein-binding sites, including Catalyst/Discovery Studio (www.accelrys. com), Chemogenomics[26], FLAP[27a,b], GBPM[28], HS-Pharm[29], LigandScout[30], MOE (http://www.chemcomp.com/software.htm, 2011), MUSIC[31], Pocket v2[32], Schrodinger (Schrodinger, http://www.schrodinger.com/), Snooker[33], and Sybyl (Tripos, http://tripos.com/). The methodology of these programs usually follows subsequent steps including preparing the protein, detecting/predicting the binding site, generating pharmacophore features, and selecting important features (**Figure 3**)[34]. The methods for building structure-based pharmacophore models may be classified based on the availability of protein structures into two categories: protein-based (without ligand) and protein–ligand complex based pharmacophore models. The choice of the method depends on the availability of protein structure with or without ligand. The overview of building of structure-based pharmacophore model is shown in **Figure 3**. In the following sections, we cover the building of both structure-based pharmacophore methods.

5.2.2.1 PROTEIN-BASED PHARMACOPHORE MODEL

The protein-based pharmacophore modeling uses a protein structure (without ligand), which is comparable to the protein–ligand complex. If the experimental structure of the target protein is not available, a protein model can be built by homology modeling approaches, which use the sequence and 3D structure of homolog proteins[35a, b]. In the building of protein-based pharmacophore models, the protein preparation is an essential step, as it cleans and optimizes some common problems present in the protein structures such as removing unnecessary water molecules, standardizing atoms, and protonating residues. Then, the ligand-binding site is predicted on protein structure. For this, many computational algorithms are available to predict ligand-binding sites. These are classified into evolutionary-, geometry-, energy-, and combined or knowledge-based methods. All these methods have been reviewed in detail elsewhere[36a–d]. This is an important step as structure-based pharmacophore modeling relies on the accurate prediction of the ligand-binding site. Subsequently, the pharmacophore modeling programs are used to construct the pharmacophore features on the predicted binding site, which analyze the possible complementary chemical features of the binding-site residues and their spatial relationships, finally establishing a pharmacophore model. For example, the interaction protocol implemented in Discovery Studio (Accelrys Software Inc.) is the commonly used one, the protocol uses LUDI algorithm which first generates the LUDI[37] interaction maps within the protein-binding site and the map is then converted into best fitting pharmacophore features such as hydrogen bond acceptors, hydrogen bond donors, and hydrophobes. The derived pharmacophore features from this method generally consist of a large number of unprioritized features; thus, they need to be reduced to fit to the ligand molecules. This is a major difficulty in the protein-based pharmacophore model. Various strategies are used to reduce features including clustering of features, deleting the inaccessible/unnecessary features, comparing of docking poses of known ligands, and site-directed mutagenesis results. Finally, the important features are carefully selected based on the most frequent features from the comprehensive pharmacophore map, which would be necessary for the biological activity. Some target proteins have multiple binding modes[38a, b] that may thus require constructing different pharmacophore models.

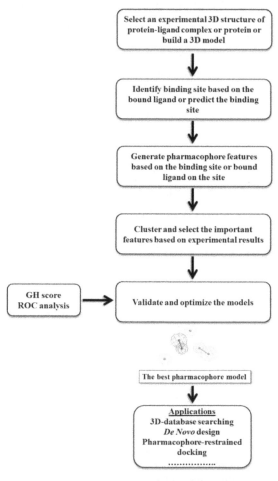

FIGURE 3   Overview of building of structure-based pharmacophore models.

5.2.2.2   *PROTEIN–LIGAND COMPLEX-BASED PHARMACOPHORE MODEL*

Protein–ligand complex-based pharmacophore models involve determining the key interaction points between protein and ligand. The limitation of this method is the need for structures of protein–ligand complexes, indicating that this approach may not be used when the ligand is not available within the binding site of the target protein of interest. All the above-mentioned programs can be used for this purpose. However, LigandScout, available from Inte: Ligand GmbH (http://www.inteligand.com/) is frequently preferred to automatically derive pharmacophore models from protein–ligand complexes. This program first hybridizes and characterizes bonds of a ligand using a heuristic approach together with template-based numeric analysis, which is not present in the PDB (http://www.rcsb.org/pdb/) structures. The pharmacophore features, such as hydrogen bond acceptor and donor, charge, and hydrophobicity, are then constructed from interactions between ligand and protein atoms. According to the binding information, the model can finally be refined or a common model may be derived by overlaying all models into one.

The building of structure-based pharmacophore models is mainly affected by protein flexibility, which is due to induced-fit effects; in addition, the conformational flexibility plays an important role in ligand binding. This flexibility should be considered in building both protein and protein–ligand complex-based pharmacophore models. This flexibility could be handled by building and aligning pharmacophore models from the different snapshots of protein or protein–ligand complexes of molecular dynamics (MD) simulations[39]. In addition to this, protein flexibility may be modeled by docking different flexible ligands and using the docking complexes for building pharmacophore models[40a,b]. The pharmacophore feature assigning schemes of the most programs considers only common interactions and ignores other interactions such as the halogen interactions and C–H bonding[41]. Additionally, the desolvation energy due to the entropic contributions to ligand binding is not considered completely[42]. The limitations and recent advances of structure-based pharmacophore model have been reviewed elsewhere[10, 29, 34, 43a, b].

5.3   VALIDATION

The pharmacophore-based methods are a well-established technology. However, the challenging problem in many cases of pharmacophore-based screening is the selection of false positives and negatives. This is mainly due to the quality of the pharmacophore models. It also indicates that the models have to be extensively validated prior to virtual screening, for example, checking whether the model is capable of predicting the activities of external compounds of the test set and classifying them correctly as actives or inactives. Usually the quality of the pharmacophore model, such as statistical significance, accurate-predictive power, and capability to identify active compounds from a given database, is verified with different methods, namely test set prediction, cost analysis, Fischer's randomization test and statistical analysis, for instance goodness of hit (GH), and receiver operating characteristic (ROC) curve. The cost analysis and Fischer's randomization validations are part of the HypoGen program. Some frequently used validation methods are briefly discussed hereunder.

5.3.1   TEST SET

A test set is a group of external compounds, which is commonly used to check the predictive pharmacophore model in terms of whether or not the model can predict the experimental activity of structurally diverse external molecules. The test molecules should be prepared in the same way as the training set molecules. In this validation, the performance of a pharmacophore model is examined by a regression against the test set compounds. If the model shows reasonably good correlation (correlation >0.70) between the pharmacophore model predicted activity and experimental activity, the model is believed to be of good quality[44]. In addition, in this validation, the compounds' activities are symbolically classified, as most active (+++), moderately active (++), and as inactive (+), to easily understand the predictive power of the model. This validation method provides quantitative information about the discriminative power of the pharmacophore model for distinguishing between active and inactive compounds, particularly in the selection of highly active compounds for pharmacophore-based virtual screening.

5.3.2   COST ANALYSIS

This statistical method is available within the HypoGen program, which is used to understand the statistical significance of the predictive pharmacophore model described in terms of fixed cost, null cost, and total cost[44-45]. The fixed cost is the simplest model that fits all data perfectly. The null cost is the highest cost of a pharmacophore with no features, which estimates activity to be the average of the activity data of the training set compounds. The total cost of any pharmacophore model should be close to the fixed cost to provide valuable models. Additionally, the pharmacophore model is considered significant when the difference between null and fixed cost value is big. It has also been shown that the cost difference value should be 40–60 bits for a pharmacophore model, which may indicate that the model has 75–90% probability of correlating the data. Besides, the other two parameters-configuration cost and error cost-are also used to determine the quality of any pharmacophore model. The configuration cost represents the complexity of the pharmacophore model space and should have a value lower than 17^{44}. The error cost dependents on the root-mean-square deviations (RMSDs) between the estimated and the experimental activities of the training set molecules. The RMSD represents the quality of the correlation between the experimental and the predicted activity data. The best pharmacophore model should have the highest cost difference, the lowest RMSD, and the best correlation.

5.3.3 FISCHER'S RANDOMIZATION TEST

The randomization test is performed to evaluate the statistical significance or reliability of the predictive pharmacophore model[46], which is available within HypoGen program. This validation uses the CatScramble program of Catalyst to generate random spreadsheets for training set molecules and arbitrarily reassign the activity values to each compound. Subsequently, different pharmacophore models are generated with exactly the same features and parameters employed in generating the original pharmacophore model. At a given 95% confidence level, 19 randomized pharmacophore models are generated and the cost value of these models should not be better than the original pharmacophore model[44]. This cross-validation can signify that there is a 95% chance for the model to represent a true correlation in the training set, thus providing strong confidence in an accurate and reasonable pharmacophore model with statistical significance.

5.3.4 GUNER-HENRY (GH) METHOD

GH is a frequently employed validation protocol to check whether the best pharmacophore model can be capable of selecting the active compounds during virtual screening[47a, b]. This statistical method evaluates the effectiveness and discriminative ability of pharmacophore models in the screening of active compounds from inactive or decoy compounds. For this validation, a decoy set, inactive compounds database, is prepared from the literature or hypothetical decoys may be prepared using DUD-E tools (Directory of Useful Decoys-Enhanced (http://dude.docking.org/)[48.] The decoys have similar physical properties compared to active compounds, such as molecular weight, hydrogen bond donors and acceptors, and log P. However, as their chemical structures and topologies are different they might not be active molecules to target. The prepared decoy data set is spiked with active (IC_{50}<1 µM) molecules, which are not used for building pharmacophore model. Then the pharmacophore model is used as a 3D query to screen the database containing active and decoy compounds. Statistical parameters like hit list (*Ht*), number of active percent of yields (%Y; Eq. 1), percent ratio of actives in the hit list (%*A*; Eq. 2), enrichment factor (EF, Eq. 3), false negatives, false positives, and goodness of hit score (GH; Eq. 4) are calculated using the following equations. The GH score ranges from 0, which indicates the null model, to 1, which indicates the ideal model.

$$\text{Percent yield of actives (\% Y)} = \frac{Ha}{Ht} \times 100 \tag{1}$$

$$\text{Percent ratio of actives (\%A)} = \frac{Ha}{A} \times 100 \tag{2}$$

$$\text{Enrichment factor (EF)} = \frac{Ha/Ht}{A/D} \tag{3}$$

$$\text{Goodness of Hit-list (GH)} = \left(\frac{Ha}{4HtA}\right) \times (3A + Ht) \times \left(1 - \frac{Ht - Ha}{D - A}\right) \tag{4}$$

where D and A are the total number of molecules and total number of active molecules in a database, respectively; Ht and Ha are the total number of hit molecules from a database and total number of active molecules in the hit list, respectively.

5.3.5   ROC CURVE

The ROC, is often utilized to assess the pharmacophore models as it reports a visual plot as well as numerical summary of the models' performance. The plot can be used as a quantitative measure to test whether the model distinguishes correctly a list of compounds as actives or inactives, which is determined by the area under the curve (AUC) of the corresponding ROC as well as other parameters namely true positives (TP), true negatives (TN), false positives (FP), and false negatives (FN)[49a, b]. The ROC curve is generated by plotting (1-specificity) on the "x-"axis against the sensitivity on "y". A random guess, that cannot discriminate actives from inactives, gives a straight line from (0, 0) to (1, 1). The curve moves toward the ideal situation (0, 1), as the accuracy of the model improves. The accuracy of the model can also be evaluated by measuring the AUC. The AUC ranges from 0.5, which indicates the random model, to 1, which indicates the perfect model.

Sensitivity, also known as positive true rate, is a measurement of a model to correctly identifying positives, for example, how well the model can pick the actives from the inactives. The sensitivity is defined by Eq. 5.

$$\text{Sensitivity (Se)} = \frac{TP}{TP + FN} \tag{5}$$

where TP and FP are true positives (actives that are correctly predicted as actives) and false positives (inactives that are incorrectly predicted as active), respectively. Specificity, also known as true negative rate, is a measurement of a model for correctly determining negatives, which is defined by Eq. 6.

$$\text{Specificity (Sp)} = \frac{TN}{TN + FP} \tag{6}$$

where TN and FP are true negatives (inactives that are correctly predicted as inactives) and false positives (inactives that are incorrectly predicted active), respectively. The overall performance and concordance rate of a model is calculated by Eq. 7, which is defined as the fraction of correctly classified both positives and negatives in the prediction.

$$\text{Concordance} = \frac{TP + TN}{TP + TN + FP + FN} \tag{7}$$

5.4 APPLICATIONS

Despite some limitations in the building of pharmacophore models, they are widely employed to quantitatively perceive the chemical features among a substantial number of structures with great diversity. Thus, the model is useful in elucidating a clear picture of interacting atoms between a ligand and a target. Additionally, the pharmacophore model can not only be used as a powerful search tool for virtual screening, but it can also serve as a tool in assessing other compounds for their ability to map the essential features and predicting their activities. Importantly, the pharmacophore-based virtual screening approaches accelerate the drug discovery process and increase its efficiency. It is affordable, fast, and an alternative to high-throughput screening (HTS) for finding new and novel hit molecules. Besides, it has been recently demonstrated that pharmacophore-based virtual screening could be an efficient technique in the search for natural product hit molecules[50]. In the following sections, we discuss some key applications of pharmacophore models.

5.4.1 PHARMACOPHORE-BASED VIRTUAL SCREENING

The computational technique of virtual screening or 3D database screening is considered one of the main techniques and complementary approaches to HTS in identifying hits molecules[51]. This technique is classified into two subcategories: structure- (also called docking-based) and ligand-based (also known as pharmacophore-based) virtual screening. Both methods are currently employed in drug discovery and development. However, it has been shown that pharmacophore-based virtual screening minimizes the issues that arise from structure-based virtual screening such as protein flexibility and insufficient scoring functions[52]. The recent advances and limitations have been reviewed[13, 41, 53a–c].

After building a pharmacophore model by using either ligand-based or structure-based approaches, it is then used as a "3D-query search" to identify hits within 3D-chemical databases, which are referred to as pharmacophore-based virtual screening. The pharmacophore model serves as a template and thus the chemical features of hits obtained from pharmacophore-based virtual screening are similar to those of the template. A number of screened hits from virtual screening could be similar to known hits and some of them may be completely based on novel scaffolds. The virtual screening methods have two essential steps: handling the conformational flexibility of database molecules and pharmacophore mapping. The handling of flexibility of each molecule in the database for the virtual screening is very similar to that employed in pharmacophore modeling such as preenumerating multiple conformations for each molecule in the database. Then the pharmacophore mapping or pattern identification checks whether a query pharmacophore is present in a given conformer of a molecule of the database. If the query matches with compounds that could be hit molecules, two types of pharmacophore-fitting strategies are commonly used: rigid and flexible. In the rigid strategy, the conformations of molecules are held rigid and the best fit is calculated; whereas in the flexible, the conformation of the ligand is slightly modified to better fit the pharmacophore, for example minimizing, with a specific energy threshold, the distances between pharmacophore model features and mapping atoms on the molecule. The flexible fitting strategy yields more hits than the rigid. The hit molecules are ranked according to the fit value, or estimated activity that is chosen based on the most active compounds. Higher fit values of compounds represent a better mapping to the pharmacophore model and depend on how close the features of the molecules map to the pharmacophore model are. High scoring hit molecules are later tested in vitro or in vivo. Recently, it has been shown that the utilization of hybrid virtual screenings, combinations of pharmacophore- and docking-based virtual screening methods, increase the retrieval of hit molecules from databases[44, 54a, b].

5.4.2 PHARMACOPHORE-BASED DE NOVO DESIGN

Lead optimization is a very important step in the drug discovery and development process. It involves modification of active compounds in order to achieve the desired properties. The pharmacophore-based de novo design can guide medicinal chemists by suggesting chemical modification to the synthesized compounds during lead optimization. This is particularly employed in the absence of 3D structure of protein targets[55a–d]. In contrast to pharmacophore-based virtual screening, the de novo approach may result in completely new and/or novel chemotypes. In this approach, diverse and synthetically accessible fragments are first collected based on the pharmacophore. Then, new molecules are constructed by using fragments under the consideration of the 3D pharmacophore. The ligand-based pharmacophore de novo design program, such as NEWLEAD[55c], PhDD[55b] and Qsearch[56] and SkelGen[57], etc., are currently used to design and optimize new lead molecules.

If the 3D structures of target proteins are known, pharmacophore models are employed to introduce new functional groups or hop scaffolds in the binding site during the structure-based lead optimization process. In this approach, a fragment 3D pharmacophore is first derived from the bound crystal structure of a ligand and its interacting residues. A 3D pharmacophore search of a database is then performed in order to identify matching fragment hits. Finally the fragments are enumerated with the scaffold to propose new lead molecules. The structure-based pharmacophore de novo design program, for example LUDI[5] and BUILDER[58] are utilized to design and optimize new lead molecules.

5.4.3 PHARMACOPHORE-BASED DOCKING

The pharmacophore information, such as distance or location and feature or functional group constraints, is effectively used to guide docking ligands, which is termed as pharmacophore-based or restrained docking. This kind of pharmacophore constraints could be good enough to reduce false positives during structure-based virtual screening. In this approach, the complementary features of a pharmacophore model, for example hydrogen bond donor and hydrogen bond acceptors, are first mapped onto the receptor, which were built by using structure- or structure-ligands complex based approaches. Then, the pharmacophore constraints are included in the scoring or matching stages of docking. It has been shown that the introduction of pharmacophoric constraints increases the efficiency of docking algorithms such as generating better conformations and reducing running time[59]. Two types of constraints could possibly be imposed, feature and 3D locations. The pharmacophore-based docking has been successfully integrated in FlexX-Pharm[60], an extended version of the FlexX program, which includes two different pharmacophore constraints: interaction constraints (interactions groups formed between receptor and ligand) and spatial constraints (a sphere that represents the ligand's atom position in the binding site). Other programs, for example Ph4Dock[61] and PhDOCK[62], are also employed for pharmacophore-based docking.

5.5   CONCLUSIONS

Since much progress in the CADD field has been made over the past decades, pharmacophore methods have become one of most successful tools in drug discovery. The 3D pharmacophore modeling approaches are now commonly used to perceive the structure–activity relationships of series compounds, and have been successfully and extensively applied in hit identification and lead optimization stages of the drug discovery and development processes. In this chapter, we have briefly summarized the building processes of four different pharmacophore models, common-feature, 3D-QSAR, protein-, and protein–ligand complex based pharmacophore models, by using commonly used programs like Hip-Hop, HypoGen, LigandScout, etc. Each of these programs has its own strengths and limitations. Additionally, we have briefly illustrated various frequently used model validation methods that could practically be employed to improve and understand their quality. The validated pharmacophore models could be useful in elucidating the receptor–ligand interactions, virtual screening, de novo design, and docking studies. Taken together, pharmacophore approaches are complementary tools to medicinal chemists and have become an integral part of hit identification and lead optimization in the drug discovery and development processes. Therefore, this chapter could serve as a helpful reference for computational and medicinal chemists.

ACKNOWLEDGEMENT

The University of Cape Town, South African Medical Research Council, and South African Research Chairs Initiative of the Department of Science and Technology administered through the South African National Research Foundation are gratefully acknowledged for support (K.C.).

KEYWORDS

- **3D-QSAR**
- **CADD**
- **Pharmacophore models**
- **Protein–ligand complexes**

REFERENCES

1. Shankar, R.; Frapaise, X.; Brown, B., LEAN drug development in R&D. *Drug Discov. Dev.* **2006**, 9, 57–60.
2. Kapetanovic, I. M., Computer-aided drug discovery and development (CADDD): *in silico*-chemico-biological approach. *Chem. Biol. Interact.* **2008**, *171*, 165–176.
3. van de Waterbeemd, H.; Gifford, E., ADMET *in silico* modelling: towards prediction paradise? *Nat. Rev.Drug Disv.* **2003**,*2* (3), 192–204.
4. Bajorath, J.; Klein, T.; Lybrand, T.; Novotny, J. In *Computer-aided drug discovery: from target proteins to drug candidates*, Pacific Symposium on Biocomputing, 1999, 4, pp 413–414.
5. Wermuth, C. G., Pharmacophores: historical perspective and viewpoint from a medicinal chemist. In *Pharmacophores and Pharmacophore Searches*; Langer, T and Hoffmann R. D., Eds.; Wiley-VCH Verlag GmbH & Co. KGaA, Weinheim, **2006**, Vol. 32; p 3.
6. Oprea, T. I., Current trends in lead discovery: are we looking for the appropriate properties? *J. Comput. Aided Mol. Des.* **2002**,*16* (5–6), 325–334.
7. Gund, P., Evolution of the Pharmacophore concept in pharmaceutical research. In *Pharmacophore Perception, Development and Use in Drug Design*; Güner O. F., Ed.; International University Line, La Jolla Calif., **2000**, pp.1.
8. Van Drie, J. H., History of 3D pharmacophore searching: commercial, academic and open-source tools. *Drug Discov. Today Tech.* **2011**,*7* (4), e255–e262.
9. Langer, T.; Wolber, G., Pharmacophore definition and 3D searches. *Drug Discov. Today Tech.* **2004**,*1* (3), 203–207.
10. Yang, S. Y., Pharmacophore modeling and applications in drug discovery: challenges and recent advances. *Drug Discov. Today* **2010**,*15* (11–12), 444–450.
11. Kurogi, Y.; Guner, O. F., Pharmacophore modeling and three-dimensional database searching for drug design using catalyst. *Curr. Med. Chem.* **2001**,*8* (9), 1035–1055.
12. Barnum, D.; Greene, J.; Smellie, A.; Sprague, P., Identification of common functional configurations among molecules. *J. Chem. Inform. Comput. Sci.* **1996**,*36* (3), 563–571.
13. Guner, O.; Clement, O.; Kurogi, Y., Pharmacophore modeling and three dimensional database searching for drug design using catalyst: recent advances. *Curr. Med. Chem.* **2004**,*11* (22), 2991–3005.
14. Martin, Y. C.; Bures, M. G.; Danaher, E. A.; DeLazzer, J.; Lico, I.; Pavlik, P. A., A fast new approach to pharmacophore mapping and its application to dopaminergic and benzodiazepine agonists. *J. Comput. Aided Mol. Des.* **1993**,*7* (1), 83–102.
15. Jones, G.; Willett, P.; Glen, R. C.; Gund P., Evolution of the pharmacophore concept in pharmaceutical research. In *Pharmacophore Perception, Development and Use in Drug Design*; Güner O. F., Ed.; International University Line, La Jolla Calif., **2000**, pp. 85.

16. Richmond, N. J.; Abrams, C. A.; Wolohan, P. R.; Abrahamian, E.; Willett, P.; Clark, R. D., GALAHAD: 1. Pharmacophore identification by hypermolecular alignment of ligands in 3D. *J. Comput. Aided Mol. Des.* **2006,***20* (9), 567–587.

17. Dixon, S. L.; Smondyrev, A. M.; Knoll, E. H.; Rao, S. N.; Shaw, D. E.; Friesner, R. A., PHASE: a new engine for pharmacophore perception, 3D QSAR model development, and 3D database screening: 1. Methodology and preliminary results. *J. Comput. Aided Mol. Des.* **2006,***20* (10–11), 647–671.

18. (a) Spitzer, G. M.; Heiss, M.; Mangold, M.; Markt, P.; Kirchmair, J.; Wolber, G.; Liedl, K. R., One concept, three implementations of 3D pharmacophore-based virtual screening: distinct coverage of chemical search space. *J. Chem. Inf. Model.* **2010,***50* (7), 1241–1247; (b) Wolber, G.; Seidel, T.; Bendix, F.; Langer, T., Molecule-pharmacophore superpositioning and pattern matching in computational drug design. *Drug Discov. Today* **2008,***13* (1), 23–29.

19. (a) Acharya, C.; Coop, A.; Polli, J. E.; MacKerell Jr, A. D., Recent advances in ligand-based drug design: relevance and utility of the conformationally sampled pharmacophore approach. *Curr. Comput. Aided Drug Des.* **2011,***7* (1), 10; (b) Evans, D. A.; Doman, T. N.; Thorner, D. A.; Bodkin, M. J., 3D QSAR methods: phase and catalyst compared. *J. Chem. Inf. Model.* **2007,***47* (3), 1248–1257; (c) Gao, Q.; Yang, L.; Zhu, Y., Pharmacophore based drug design approach as a practical process in drug discovery. *Curr. Comput. Aided Drug Des.* **2010,***6* (1), 37–49; (d) Patel, Y.; Gillet, V. J.; Bravi, G.; Leach, A. R., A comparison of the pharmacophore identification programs: catalyst, DISCO and GASP. *J. Comput. Aided Mol. Des.* **2002,***16* (8–9), 653–681.

20. Putta, S.; Landrum, G. A.; Penzotti, J. E., Conformation mining: an algorithm for finding biologically relevant conformations. *J. Med. Chem.* **2005,***48* (9), 3313–3318.

21. Agrafiotis, D. K.; Gibbs, A. C.; Zhu, F.; Izrailev, S.; Martin, E., Conformational sampling of bioactive molecules: a comparative study. *J. Chem. Inf. Model.* **2007,***47* (3), 1067–1086.

22. Kirchmair, J.; Laggner, C.; Wolber, G.; Langer, T., Comparative analysis of protein-bound ligand conformations with respect to catalyst's conformational space subsampling algorithms. *J. Chem. Inf. Model.* **2005,***45* (2), 422–430.

23. Brooks, B. R.; Bruccoleri, R. E.; Olafson, B. D.; States, D. J.; Swaminathan, S.; Karplus, M., CHARMM: a program for macromolecular energy, minimization, and dynamics calculations. *J. Comput. Chem.* **1983,***4* (2), 187–217.

24. (a) Berman, H. M.; Westbrook, J. D.; Gabanyi, M. J.; Tao, W.; Shah, R.; Kouranov, A.; Schwede, T.; Arnold, K.; Kiefer, F.; Bordoli, L., The protein structure initiative structural genomics knowledgebase. *Nucleic Acids Res.* **2009,***37* (suppl 1), D365–D368; (b) Chandonia, J.-M.; Brenner, S. E., The impact of structural genomics: expectations and outcomes. *Science* **2006,***311* (5759), 347–351; (c) Levitt, M., Growth of novel protein structural data. *Proc. Natl. Acad. Sci. U.S.A.* **2007,***104* (9), 3183–3188.

25. Campbell, S. J.; Gold, N. D.; Jackson, R. M.; Westhead, D. R., Ligand binding: functional site location, similarity and docking. *Curr. Opin. Struc. Biol.* **2003,***13* (3), 389–395.

26. Klabunde, T.; Giegerich, C.; Evers, A., Sequence-derived three-dimensional pharmacophore models for G-protein-coupled receptors and their application in virtual screening. *J. Med. Chem.* **2009,***52* (9), 2923–2932.

27. (a) Baroni, M.; Cruciani, G.; Sciabola, S.; Perruccio, F.; Mason, J. S., A common reference framework for analyzing/comparing proteins and ligands. Fingerprints for Ligands and Proteins (FLAP): theory and application. *J. Chem. Inf. Model.* **2007,***47* (2), 279–294; (b) Cross, S.; Baroni, M.; Carosati, E.; Benedetti, P.; Clementi, S., FLAP: GRID molecular interaction fields in virtual screening. validation using the DUD data set. *J. Chem. Inf. Model.* **2010,***50* (8), 1442–1450.

28. Ortuso, F.; Langer, T.; Alcaro, S., GBPM: GRID-based pharmacophore model: concept and application studies to protein–protein recognition. *Bioinformatics* **2006,***22* (12), 1449–1455.

29. Barillari, C.; Marcou, G.; Rognan, D., Hot-spots-guided receptor-based pharmacophores (HS-Pharm): a knowledge-based approach to identify ligand-anchoring atoms in protein cavities and prioritize structure-based pharmacophores. *J. Chem. Inf. Model.* **2008**,*48* (7), 1396–1410.

30. Wolber, G.; Langer, T., LigandScout: 3-D pharmacophores derived from protein-bound ligands and their use as virtual screening filters. *J. Chem. Inf. Model.* **2005**,*45* (1), 160–169.

31. Carlson, H. A.; Masukawa, K. M.; Rubins, K.; Bushman, F. D.; Jorgensen, W. L.; Lins, R. D.; Briggs, J. M.; McCammon, J. A., Developing a dynamic pharmacophore model for HIV-1 integrase. *J. Med. Chem.* **2000**,*43* (11), 2100–2114.

32. Chen, J.; Lai, L., Pocket v. 2: further developments on receptor-based pharmacophore modeling. *J. Chem. Inf. Model.* **2006**,*46* (6), 2684–2691.

33. Chen, Z.; Tian, G.; Wang, Z.; Jiang, H.; Shen, J.; Zhu, W., Multiple pharmacophore models combined with molecular docking: a reliable way for efficiently identifying novel PDE4 inhibitors with high structural diversity. *J. Chem. Inf. Model.* **2010**,*50* (4), 615–625.

34. Sanders, M. P.; McGuire, R.; Roumen, L.; de Esch, I. J.; de Vlieg, J.; Klomp, J. P.; de Graaf, C., From the protein's perspective: the benefits and challenges of protein structure-based pharmacophore modeling. *MedChemComm.* **2012**,*3* (1), 28–38.

35. (a) Elumalai, P.; Liu, H.-L., Homology modeling and dynamics study of aureusidin synthase—An important enzyme in aurone biosynthesis of snapdragon flower. *Int. J. Biol. Macromol.* **2011**,*49* (2), 134–142; (b) Friesner, R. A.; Abel, R.; Goldfeld, D. A.; Miller, E. B.; Murrett, C. S., Computational methods for high resolution prediction and refinement of protein structures. *Curr. Opin. Struct. Biol.* **2013**,*23* (2), 177–184.

36. (a) Ghersi, D.; Sanchez, R., Beyond structural genomics: computational approaches for the identification of ligand binding sites in protein structures. *J. Struct. Funct. Genomics* **2011**,*12* (2), 109–117; (b) Henrich, S.; Salo-Ahen, O. M.; Huang, B.; Rippmann, F. F.; Cruciani, G.; Wade, R. C., Computational approaches to identifying and characterizing protein binding sites for ligand design. *J. Mol. Recognit.* **2010**,*23* (2), 209–219; (c) Laurie, R.; Alasdair, T.; Jackson, R. M., Methods for the prediction of protein-ligand binding sites for structure-based drug design and virtual ligand screening. *Curr. Protein Pept. Sci.* **2006**,*7* (5), 395–406; (d) Pérot, S.; Sperandio, O.; Miteva, M. A.; Camproux, A.-C.; Villoutreix, B. O., Druggable pockets and binding site centric chemical space: a paradigm shift in drug discovery. *Drug Discov. Today* **2010**,*15* (15), 656–667.

37. Böhm, H.-J., The computer program LUDI: a new method for the de novo design of enzyme inhibitors. *J. Comput. Aided Mol. Des.* **1992**,*6* (1), 61–78.

38. (a) Taha, M. O.; Tarairah, M.; Zalloum, H.; Abu-Sheikha, G., Pharmacophore and QSAR modeling of estrogen receptor β ligands and subsequent validation and *in silico* search for new hits. *J. Mol. Graphics Modell.* **2010**,*28* (5), 383–400; (b) Wallach, I.; Lilien, R., Predicting multiple ligand binding modes using self-consistent pharmacophore hypotheses. *J. Chem. Inf. Model.* **2009**,*49* (9), 2116–2128.

39. Meagher, K. L.; Carlson, H. A., Incorporating protein flexibility in structure-based drug discovery: using HIV-1 protease as a test case. *J. Am. Chem. Soc.* **2004**,*126* (41), 13276–13281.

40. (a) Loving, K.; Salam, N. K.; Sherman, W., Energetic analysis of fragment docking and application to structure-based pharmacophore hypothesis generation. *J. Comput. Aided Mol. Des.* **2009**,*23* (8), 541–554; (b) Salam, N. K.; Nuti, R.; Sherman, W., Novel method for generating structure-based pharmacophores using energetic analysis. *J. Chem. Inf. Model.* **2009**,*49* (10), 2356–2368.

41. Horvath, D., Pharmacophore-based virtual screening. In *Chemoinformatics and Computational Chemical Biology*; Bajorath, J., Ed.; Springer, **2011**; pp 261.

42. Löwer, M.; Proschak, E., Structure–based pharmacophores for virtual screening. *Mol. Infom.* **2011**,*30* (5), 398–404.

43. (a) Oranit, D.; Alexandra, S.-P.; Ruth, N.; Wolfson, H. J., Predicting molecular interactions *in silico*: I. A guide to pharmacophore identification and its applications to drug design. *Curr. Med. Chem.* **2004,***11* (1), 71–90; (b) Pirhadi, S.; Shiri, F.; Ghasemi, J. B., Methods and applications of structure based pharmacophores in drug discovery. *Curr. Top. Med. Chem.* **2013,***13* (9), 1036–1047.

44. Elumalai, P.; Liu, H.-L.; Zhao, J.-H.; Chen, W.; Lin, D. S.; Chuang, C.-K.; Tsai, W.-B.; Ho, Y., Pharmacophore modeling, virtual screening and docking studies to identify novel HNMT inhibitors. *J. Taiwan Inst. Chem. Eng.* **2012,***43* (4), 493–503.

45. Debnath, A. K., Pharmacophore mapping of a series of 2, 4-diamino-5-deazapteridine inhibitors of Mycobacterium avium complex dihydrofolate reductase. *J. Med. Chem.* **2002,***45* (1), 41–53.

46. Fisher, R. A., *The Design of Experiments*. Oliver & Boyd, Oxford, England, **1935**; vol. xi; pp 251.

47. (a) Clement, O.; Kurogi, Y., Pharmacophore modeling and three dimensional database searching for drug design using catalyst: recent dvances. *Curr. Med. Chem.* **2004,***11* (22), 15p; (b) Guner, O. F.; Henry, D. R., Metric for analyzing hit lists and pharmacophores. In *Pharmacophore Perception, Development and Use in Drug Design*; Güner O. F., Ed.; International University Line, La Jolla Calif., **2000**; pp. 193.

48. Mysinger, M. M.; Carchia, M.; Irwin, J. J.; Shoichet, B. K., Directory of useful decoys, enhanced (DUD-E): better ligands and decoys for better benchmarking. *J. Med. Chem.* **2012,***55* (14), 6582–6594.

49. (a) Kirchmair, J.; Markt, P.; Distinto, S.; Schuster, D.; Spitzer, G. M.; Liedl, K. R.; Langer, T.; Wolber, G., The Protein Data Bank (PDB), its related services and software tools as key components for *in silico* guided drug discovery. *J. Med. Chem.* **2008,***51* (22), 7021–7040; (b) Triballeau, N.; Acher, F.; Brabet, I.; Pin, J.-P.; Bertrand, H.-O., Virtual screening workflow development guided by the "receiver operating characteristic" curve approach. Application to high-throughput docking on metabotropic glutamate receptor subtype 4. *J. Med. Chem.* **2005,***48* (7), 2534–2547.

50. Rollinger, J. M.; Stuppner, H.; Langer, T., Virtual screening for the discovery of bioactive natural products. In *Natural Compounds as Drugs Volume I*, Springer, **2008**; pp 211–249.

51. Walters, W. P.; Stahl, M. T.; Murcko, M. A., Virtual screening--an overview. *Drug Discov. Today* **1998,***3* (4), 160–178.

52. Kitchen, D. B.; Decornez, H.; Furr, J. R.; Bajorath, J., Docking and scoring in virtual screening for drug discovery: methods and applications. *Nat. Rev. Drug Discov.* **2004,***3* (11), 935–949.

53. (a) Hopfinger, A. J.; Duca, J. S., Extraction of pharmacophore information from high-throughput screens. *Curr. Opin. Biotechnol.* **2000,***11* (1), 97–103; (b) Langer, T.; Hoffmann, R., Virtual screening an effective tool for lead structure discovery. *Curr. Pharm. Des.* **2001,***7* (7), 509–527; (c) Sun, H., Pharmacophore-based virtual screening. *Curr. Med. Chem.* **2008,***15* (10), 1018–1024.

54. (a) Drwal, M. N.; Griffith, R., Combination of ligand-and structure-based methods in virtual screening. *Drug Discov. Today Tech.* **2013,***10* (3), e395–e401; (b) Elumalai, P.; Liu, H.-L.; Zhou, Z.-L.; Zhao, J.-H.; Chen, W.; Chuang, C.-K.; Tsai, W.-B.; Ho, Y., Ligand and structure-based pharmacophore modeling for the discovery of potential human HNMT inhibitors. *Lett. Drug Des. Discov.* **2012,***9* (1), 17–29.

55. (a) Hessler, G.; Baringhaus, K.-H., The scaffold hopping potential of pharmacophores. *Drug Discov. Today Tech.* **2011,***7* (4), e263–e269; (b) Huang, Q.; Li, L.-L.; Yang, S.-Y., PhDD: A new pharmacophore-based *de novo* design method of drug-like molecules combined with assessment of synthetic accessibility. *J. Mol. Graphics Modell.* **2010,***28* (8), 775–787; (c) Tschinke, V.; Cohen, N. C., The NEWLEAD program: a new method for the design of candidate structures from pharmacophoric hypotheses. *J. Med. Chem.* **1993,***36* (24), 3863–3870; (d)

Wang, W. J.; Huang, Q.; Yang, S. Y., Pharmacophore-based De Novo design. *De novo Mol. Design* **2013**, 201–214.

56. Lippert, T.; Schulz-Gasch, T.; Roche, O.; Guba, W.; Rarey, M., De novo design by pharmacophore-based searches in fragment spaces. *J. Comput. Aided Mol. Des.* **2011,**25 (10), 931–945.
57. Todorov, N. P., SkelGen. In *Scaffold Hopping in Medicinal Chemistry*; Brown, N., Ed.; and Hoffmann R. D., Eds.; Wiley-VCH Verlag GmbH & Co: KGaA, Weinheim, **2013**; p 231.
58. Roe, D. C.; Kuntz, I. D., BUILDER v. 2: improving the chemistry of a de novo design strategy. *J. Comput. Aided Mol. Des.* **1995,**9 (3), 269–282.
59. Schneidman-Duhovny, D.; Nussinov, R.; Wolfson, H. J., Predicting molecular interactions *in silico*: II. Protein-protein and protein-drug docking. *Curr. Med. Chem.* **2004,**11 (1), 91–107.
60. Hindle, S. A.; Rarey, M.; Buning, C.; Lengauer, T., Flexible docking under pharmacophore type constraints. *J. Comput. Aided Mol. Des.* **2002,**16 (2), 129–149.
61. Goto, J.; Kataoka, R.; Hirayama, N., Ph4Dock: pharmacophore-based protein-ligand docking. *J. Med. Chem.* **2004,**47 (27), 6804–6811.
62. Joseph–McCarthy, D.; Thomas, B. E.; Belmarsh, M.; Moustakas, D.; Alvarez, J. C., Pharmacophore–based molecular docking to account for ligand flexibility. *Proteins: Struct. Funct. Bioinf.* **2003,**51 (2), 172188.

CHAPTER 6

APPLICATION OF CONCEPTUAL DENSITY FUNCTIONAL THEORY IN DEVELOPING QSAR MODELS AND THEIR USEFULNESS IN THE PREDICTION OF BIOLOGICAL ACTIVITY AND TOXICITY OF MOLECULES

SUDIP PAN[1], ASHUTOSH GUPTA[2], DEBESH R. ROY[3], RAJESH K. SHARMA[2], VENKATESAN SUBRAMANIAN[*4], ANALAVA MITRA[*5], and PRATIM K. CHATTARAJ[*1]

[1]Department of Chemistry and Center for Theoretical Studies, Indian Institute of Technology Kharagpur, 721302, India

[2]Department of Chemistry, Udai Pratap Autonomous College, Varanasi, Uttar Pradesh, 221002 India.

[3]Department of Applied Physics, S.V. National Institute of Technology, Surat 395007, India

[4]Chemical Laboratory, Central Leather Research Institute, Council of Scientific and Industrial Research, Chennai 600 020, India

[5]School of Medical Science and Technology, Indian Institute of Technology Kharagpur, 721302, India

*Corresponding authors: subbu@clri.res.in,amitra@adm.iitkgp.ernet.in, pkc@chem.iitkgp.ernet.in

CONTENTS

ABSTRACT

The modeling of quantitative structure–activity relationships (QSAR) is a very useful approach in establishing a direct relationship between the physico-chemical properties and the biological activities of the studied species. They, therefore, act as trustworthy statistical tools in predicting the biological property of new species. The structural alteration, which causes the variation in biological properties, is the main driving force in building QSAR. In this chapter, we have reviewed the different approaches in constructing QSAR and their successful application in predicting biological activity and toxicity of different class of molecules. Their scope of applicability in medicinal chemistry toward drug design and the limitations therein have also been highlighted. Special attention has been drawn to represent the effective modeling of QSAR based on different global and local reactivity descriptors of conceptual density functional theory.

6.1   INTRODUCTION

Mankind, since time immemorial, has yearned for longevity, comfort, and worldly possession. Longevity requires good health which comes with deep knowledge of different biochemical and biophysical processes taking place within different living organisms. Only then a diagnosis of a disease and a possible drug for its treatment are formulated. Comfort can be on a level of physical, mental, or intellectual level. It is directly related to the state-of-the-art techniques of a particular era. Similarly worldly possession is related to advances made in material science and also on the biological sciences. In order to channelize the efforts of mankind toward the attainment of aforementioned aspirations, science and technology have been classified into different streams. Chemistry serves as a rivet across which all the branches of science revolve. Both the experimentalists and theoreticians understand very well that the mother earth is affluent with millions of molecules having different characteristics and properties. They tend to segregate them into two broad classes, namely organic and inorganic. Their primary objective deals with knowing the properties of these molecules and also their possible applications. At times, new molecules are formulated and their properties are explored. However, there are times when the syntheses of these molecules act as a big challenge, and, therefore, their properties are extrapolated on the basis of information available for known molecules. If the properties are thought to be of great significance to the humankind, only then the synthesis is attempted. Such a correlation technique to study the chemical behavior of such a mammoth number of molecules based on their closely related structures or properties is called structure–activity relationships (SAR) or structure–

property relationships (SPR). This approach helps in developing a fruitful activity or property relationships related to changes in molecular structure in order to predict the reactivity of an unknown compound. When a qualitative assessment is made then it is termed as qualitative structure–activity relationship, however, when a quantitative analysis is done, then the technique is called as quantitative structure–activity relationship (QSAR) or quantitative structure–property relationship (QSPR). Thus, QSAR/QSPR models are able to predict the activity/ property of a molecule both in qualitative and quantitative manner. It, therefore, helps in the prediction of a property of a molecule based on some correlation, and also, it provides solutions to different questions in a substantially reduced expenditure and time. These techniques are also employed to understand the toxicity caused due to overdose of food particle or drugs. Thus, the QSAR and QSPR techniques help in building up powerful mathematical regression models that efficiently predict the reactivity of an unknown molecule on the basis of behavior of an analogous set of chemically or structurally similar compounds. The toxicity criteria of a particular molecule toward a biological species are also analyzed through suitable equations that relate toxicity with molecular structure and hence a quantitative structure–toxicity relationship (QSTR) model.

In order to develop QSAR/QSPR/QSTR models, different mathematical tools have been utilized. Many different methods have been employed to design such models. Density functional theory (DFT) is a quantum-chemical theory which predicts the properties of a molecule on the basis of its electron density. Conceptual density functional theory (CDFT) is a manifestation of the application of DFT. It has been successfully and prominently employed in the prediction of different descriptors, which have further under the purview of QSAR, been able to assess the activity and toxicity of different molecules. CDFT is comparatively cheaper to other quantum-chemical tools such as ab initio methods. Therefore, its role in the development of QSAR models is tremendous.

In this chapter, we first of all outline the various theoretical tools and their role in knowing the biological activity and toxicity patterns in several molecules. **Section 6.2** describes various QSAR/QSPR/QSTR based methods. **Section 6.2.1** deals with the role, types, and applications of QSAR models toward the prediction of biological and medicinal activities. **Section 6.3** highlights CDFT method. **Section 6.3.1** describes the computational details employed in the prediction of QSAR/QSPR models. **Section 6.3.2** mentions about the application of CDFT in the prediction of toxicity with an approach called QSTR and also about QSAR/QSPR. In the subsequent sections, a few representative cases are highlighted. **Sections 6.3.3 and 6.3.4** contain the description about the utility of quantum chemical descriptors for the prediction of IC_{50} values of ACAT inhibitors and quantum chemical study on the synergistic effect induced by a mixture of different sets of antioxidants, respectively. **Section 6.4** concludes the chapter by highlighting the application of CDFT in developing QSAR models and their utility in predicting of biological activity and toxicity of molecules.

6.2   ROLE, TYPES, AND APPLICATIONS OF QSAR/QSPR/QSTR

QSAR is a technique which tries to predict the activity, reactivity, and properties of an unknown set of molecules based on analysis of an equation connecting the structures of molecules to their respective measured activities or reactivity and properties. Generally, at first the variation in activity and/or property and/ or toxicity of a known set of structurally analogue samples is studied with the changes in their molecular frameworks. The trends obtained from the study are then transformed into the form of equations, and, further they are applied to determine the reactivity, property, and/or toxicity of an unknown but structurally resembled set of systems. Since mathematical tools are utilized to develop equations, the quantification of different properties of a set of molecules is also easily carried out. Thus, the QSAR-based models become useful toward predicting chemical reactivity and toxicity of molecules. They act as a novel technique to build models correlating structure, activity, and toxicity of molecules. A proper rationale helps in finding the right answers.

Besides traditional QSAR techniques, other QSAR techniques have also been developed. Three-dimensional correlation models (3D-QSAR) for analyzing the structure–property relationships are now widely used. Using statistical correlation methods, their algorithm analyzes the relationship between the biological activity of a set of compounds and their 3D properties quantitatively. It involves the application of force field calculations. Based on the applied energy functions [1], it inspects both the steric fields (shape of the molecule) as well as the electrostatic fields.

The other type of QSAR involved *in silico* tools is the 3D Markovian electron delocalization negentropies (3D-MEDNEs) [2] for toxicity predictions. QSAR-based studies have shown their applications in many fields like ecotoxicology, drug discovery, antitumor, molecular modeling, biotoxicity, chemico–biological interactions, drug design, drug resistance, toxicity predictions, physico-chemical parameters, gastro-intestinal absorption, activity of peptides, data mining, drug metabolism, pharmacokinetics, determination of antihuman immunodeficiency virus (HIV) enzyme inhibitors, antitumor enzyme inhibitors, anticancer drugs, coinage metals, and in many other fields. Schultz *et al.,* [3] have highlighted the role of QSAR in chemical toxicology. Some other works have highlighted the development of the QSAR methodology and its application in the prediction of biotoxicity [4]. Articles on basics of QSAR regarding a predictive algorithm are also available in the literature [5]. Hammett [6] in his famous work on linear free-energy relationship based equations has highlighted the role of QSAR in predicting the reactivity of organic molecules involving substituted benzoic acid derivatives on the basis of the changes made in the substituent of the structures of such molecules. That led Taft to propose the mathematical equations for the structural changes in case of aliphatic compounds [7]. This was further extended to predict the biological activity of molecules with the aid of QSAR by Hansch and co-workers [8]. Other studies on the role of QSAR in the prediction of chemico–biological interactions [9] and drug design are well documented [10]. Various molecular descriptors within the purview of QSAR have been proposed to predict the medicinal properties of molecules [11]. QSAR has played a major role in biochemistry and in determination of other toxicological, physico-chemical, absorption, disposition, metabolism, and excretion (ADME) processes. It has helped in the development of various bioactive molecules from nondrug-like molecules [12] to drug resistance molecules [13]. It has further been able to predict molecules showing toxicological activity [14], different physico-chemical parameters [15], molecules having gastro-intestinal absorptive properties [16], activity of peptides [17], data mining [18], drug metabolism [19], prediction of pharmacokinetic, and ADME properties [20]. Other pertinent articles [21] and books [22] mentioning these qualities are also available in the literature. QSAR prediction strength lies in the information extracted from different databases. Some articles highlight various computational approaches for better correlative predictions [23]. There are studies in the literature dealing with the reaction between an electron-rich (nucleophile) and an electron-poor (electrophile) species. In fact with all these studies Schwöbel *et al.,* [24] built a database containing 3,000 quantitative and qualitative reactivity data for around 900 various compounds and their reaction toward almost 100 reference nucleophiles. There have been studies with a focus on the determination of properties of molecules based on QSAR techniques [25]. QSAR technique has been successfully applied in the designing and study of inhibitors to prevent the growth of HIV and hepatitis C virus (HCV) within living cells [26]. They have also been utilized in the prediction of antitumor enzyme inhibitors [27] and anticancer drugs [28]. Their utility in the prediction of the role of coinage metals in the design of antitumor drugs and tumor therapy has also been exhibited [29]. They have also been applied to study the toxicity of phenols [30], alkaloids [31], aliphatic ester [32], and modeling of antitubercular compounds [33]. They have played a significant role in the prediction of ecotoxicity. Different topological descriptors [34] have been developed to correlate the hazardous effect of chemical compounds on the ecosystem. The toxic effects of different compounds on marine life especially fishes have been made with the aid of specific absorption rate (SAR)-based regression analysis [35].

The role of QSPR in the correlation of the structure with various molecular properties (physical, chemical, biological, and technological) has been highlighted by Katrizky and co-workers [36]. Their application in the field of medicinal chemistry through the generation of different molecular descriptors was also reported [37]. It has been demonstrated that the data reduction methods such as principal component analysis (PCA) of matrixes which are formed by the assembly of related properties, provide information regarding the relationship among different properties of molecules. The applicability of QSPR is also important in pharmaceutical science. Grover *et al.,* [38] have summarized various studies regarding the role of QSPR in assessing various pharmacokinetic parameters for drug modeling in their reviews [38].

3D-QSAR comparative molecular field analysis (CoMFA) has also been applied extensively in the discovery and design of different molecules having desired properties. It has been used in the design of drugs and other applications [39]. CoMFA tries to predict the properties of a molecule by developing correlations between the structure and the pharmacological activity of compounds [39]. The potency of it in the design of effective enzyme inhibitors has also been explored [40], with the aid of molecular docking [40]. CoMFA has been applied for studying the interactions between different organic polychlorinated derivatives with aryl-hydrocarbon receptors [41].

6.2.1 ROLE OF DIFFERENT THEORETICAL METHODS IN THE DESIGN OF DIFFERENT QSAR MODELS

Since QSAR models have foundation laid on mathematical equations, over the years many different theoretical methods have been tried to construct efficient and reliable QSAR models. It is believed that answers to all the questions related to the universal forces can be deciphered with the aid of quantum chemistry (QC); however, the problem lies in the solution of the complex equations. Nevertheless, quantum chemistry has been utilized to design different QSAR models. It has been successfully tested for different biological systems [42]. Ab initio quantum chemistry provides better understanding of the electronic correlation effects than empirical methods, therefore different QC-based SAR models have been developed [43]. Different QC-based molecular descriptors have been developed which have provided answers to various enzyme-mediated processes and hallucinogenic activity [44] as well as the reactivity of several organic molecules, derivation of partition coefficients, and correlation of other physical parameters [45]. The influence of quantum chemical methods and the role of the various allied QC-based descriptors in the structure–activity/toxicity studies are discussed in detail elsewhere [46]. Applications of the SCF-MO [47] and various high level quantum chemical techniques toward modeling biomolecules and correlating their chemical reactivity with molecular structure are widely discussed topics. Sophisticated ab initio methods like localized perturbation theory and DFT are employed to understand the catalytic activity of enzymatic reactions, conformational energies, and nonbonded interactions [48]. Biological activity measures of large molecules like proteins, DNA, etc. from first principles quantum chemical approaches sometimes pose problems due to size and complexity of their structures. However, DFT and DFT-based molecular dynamics (MD) simulation studies [49] are found to be quite fruitful toward understanding the bond cleavage and bond formation processes of various biomolecular interactions. DFT and hybrid quantum mechanical/molecular mechanics (QM/MM) methods have been utilized in biological modeling and for studying the complex systems such as cytochrome P450 family of enzymes [50]. Their role in the field of medicinal chemistry [51] and in the prediction of toxicity measures for molecules acting as anticancer agents or as drugs are well known [52]. QC-based QSAR/QSPR models are also employed toward studying the biotoxicity of cisplatin complexes as effective anticancer drugs [53]. Sarmah and Deka [54] have further made a DFT-based 2D QSAR study on the anticancer activities of various nucleosides.

DFT as a powerful mathematical algorithm was exploited as a useful tool to provide sets of quantum chemical descriptors that help finding suitable correlations for enzymatic activities and toxicity of various classes of organic compounds and their derivatives [55]. Again Elstner and co-workers [56] have elaborated that the self-consistent charge density functional tight binding (SCC-DFTB) formalism, compared to DFT may appear as a better mathematical rationale for large biological systems, as the former method considers the phenomena of nonbonded interactions and charge transfer processes in a better way.

In order to handle large databases and descriptors for designing SAR model, spectral-SAR (S-SAR) has been proposed by Putz and co-workers. It considers the spectral norm in quantifying toxicity and reactivity with molecular structure. It has been utilized in the consideration of ecotoxicity, enzyme activity, and anticancer bioactivity [57]. The S-SAR model coupled with element specific influence paramater (ESIP) formulations [58] are also utilized for predicting ecotoxicity measures. QSAR studies on the anti-HIV-1 activity of HEPT (1-(2-hydroxyethoxy)methyl)-6-(phenylthio)thymine) [59] and further studies involving the minimum topological difference (MTD) method [60] were also reported [61].

Other methods to study biological and drug activities of molecules based on structure–activity-based regression models include different spectroscopic techniques like nuclear quadrupole resonance (NQR) [62], nuclear magnetic resonance (NMR), electron paramagnetic resonance (EPR), ultraviolet (UV), and infrared (IR) [63]. Other techniques such as variable selection and modeling method based on the prediction (VSMP) [64], quantitative structure-(chromatographic) retention relationships (QSRR) [65], topological quantum similarity index (TQSI) [66] models, and quantum topological molecular similarity (QTMS) descriptors [67] also have ample contributions toward ensuring refinements in the predictive nature of QSAR. Uses of soft electrophilicity and hydrophobicity [68] as descriptors have also become quite effective tools in predicting toxicity.

6.3   CONCEPTUAL DFT

Conceptual density functional theory (CDFT) [69] is a powerful tool to understand the molecular reactivity. It utilizes various global reactivity descriptors, which forecast reactivity trends for the whole molecule, like electronegativity [70] (χ), hardness [71] (η), and electrophilicity [72] (ω) along with closely related local descriptors like atomic charges [73] (Q_k), Fukui functions [74] $f(\mathbf{r})$ and their condensed-to-atom variants [75] (f_k) which determine the reactivity trends for each and every active site of the molecule. According to Mulliken [76], electronegativity (χ) can be defined as

$$\chi = \frac{IP + EA}{2} \tag{1}$$

where IP and EA are the ionization potential and electron affinity of a system, respectively.

The chemical potential (μ) of an atom/molecule is quantitatively determined by the theory of statistical ensembles and can be expressed as

$$\mu = \frac{\partial E}{\partial N}, \text{ at constant entropy} \tag{2}$$

where E be the energy and N be the number of electrons.

Gyftopoulos and Hatsopoulos [77] proposed electronegativity (χ) of a system as the negative of the electronic chemical potential (μ). Therefore, μ can also be expressed as

$$\mu_{\text{Mulliken}} = -\chi_{\text{Mulliken}} = -\frac{IP+EA}{2} = \left[\frac{\partial E(N)}{\partial N}\right]_{N=N_0} \tag{3}$$

The concept of "hardness" or "softness" in chemistry was first introduced by Ralph G. Pearson [78]. Global hardness (η) is described in terms of degree of tightness of the electron cloud encapsulating the nucleus/nuclei of an atomic/molecular system. Global softness (S) is considered as the reciprocal of global hardness, and, it describes the extent to which the electronic environment surrounding the nucleus/nuclei of an atomic/molecular species tends to loosen itself. Parr and Pearson [71] described hardness quantitatively in the form of a mathematical descriptor, and defined it to be the first derivative of the chemical potential (μ) or the second derivative of the energy (E) as a function of the number of electrons, N, at a fixed external potential $v(\mathbf{r})$:

$$\eta = \left(\frac{\partial \mu}{\partial N}\right)_{v(\mathbf{r})} = \left(\frac{\partial^2 E}{\partial N^2}\right)_{v(\mathbf{r})} \tag{4}$$

From the finite-difference approach, the corresponding curvature then equals $IP-EA$, which actually signifies hardness. Therefore:

$$\eta = \left(\frac{\partial \mu}{\partial N}\right)_{v(\mathbf{r})} = \left(\frac{\partial^2 E}{\partial N^2}\right)_{v(\mathbf{r})} \approx IP - EA \tag{5}$$

Global softness [79] (S) is defined as a reciprocal of the global hardness (η) for a molecular system, is expressed as

$$S = \frac{1}{\eta} = \left(\frac{\partial N}{\partial \mu}\right)_{v(\mathbf{r})} \tag{6}$$

A new descriptor called electrophilicity index (ω) was introduced by Parr and co-workers. The electrophilicity index (ω) as described by Parr et al., [72] is

$$\omega = \frac{\mu^2}{2\eta} = \frac{\chi^2}{2\eta} \tag{7}$$

Gazquez et al., [80], further showed that the electron-donating (ω^-) and the electron-accepting (ω^+) powers may be defined as

$$\omega^- = \frac{(\mu^-)^2}{2\eta^-}; \omega^+ = \frac{(\mu^+)^2}{2\eta^+} \tag{8}$$

where μ^- and μ^+ denote the chemical potential for electron donation and electron acceptance, respectively, whereas η^- and η^+ stand for the hardness for electron donation and electron acceptance, respectively.

Recently Chattaraj *et al.*, [81] proposed the concept of net electrophilicity ($\Delta\omega^{\pm}$) for a system to assess the resultant electron-accepting power shown by a molecule upon chemical response due to the combined attractive and repulsive effects as a result of the presence of both electrons and nuclei. The net electrophilicity ($\Delta\omega^{\pm}$) is defined as

$$\Delta\omega^{\pm} = \left\{\omega^{+} - \left(-\omega^{-}\right)\right\} = \left(\omega^{+} + \omega^{-}\right) \tag{9}$$

The Fukui function [74, 75, 82] ($f(\mathbf{r})$) is usually applied to quantitatively evaluate the extent of local response of a particular active site of a chemical system. It is widely applied as a popular local variant and is defined as the differential change in electron density due to an infinitesimal change in the number of electrons (N).

$$f(\mathbf{r}) = \left(\frac{\partial\rho(\mathbf{r})}{\partial N}\right)_{v(\mathbf{r})} = \left(\frac{\delta\mu}{\delta v(\mathbf{r})}\right)_{N} \tag{10}$$

Owing to a discontinuity in the derivative in Eq. (10) for integral values of N, three different types of Fukui functions can be defined for nucleophilic, electrophilic, and radical attacks by applying the finite difference and frozen core approximations [74,82]. A coarse-grained atom by atom representation of the Fukui function, called condensed-to-atom Fukui function, was put forward by Yang and Mortier [75] and it is based on a finite-difference approach in terms of the Mulliken population analysis (MPA) scheme.

The local softness $s(\mathbf{r})$ is related to the Fukui functions $f(\mathbf{r})$ through a chain rule as

$$s(\mathbf{r}) = \left(\frac{\partial\rho(\mathbf{r})}{\partial\mu}\right)_{v(\mathbf{r})} = \left(\frac{\partial\rho(\mathbf{r})}{\partial N}\right)_{v(\mathbf{r})} \cdot \left(\frac{\partial N}{\partial\mu}\right)_{v(\mathbf{r})} = f(\mathbf{r}).S \tag{11}$$

The CDFT-based global and local reactivity descriptors and their modes of influencing chemical reactivity are further appreciated in terms of the various allied molecular electronic structure principles like the maximum hardness principle [79, 83] (MHP), minimum polarizability principle [84] (MPP), minimum electrophilicity principle [85] (MEP), minimum magnetizability principle [86] (MMP), etc. Various reactivity descriptors theoretically justify the observed chemical behavior of a molecule. The variation of the conceptual DFT-based reactivity indices as a function of structural changes and/or substituent effects conveys invaluable insights into a quantitative correlation between chemical reactivity and toxicity. It is, however, pointed out that the magnitudes of the various reactivity descriptors are quite dependent on the used level of theory and the basis set [87]. Thus, for an effective theoretical benchmarking to provide a structure–activity/toxicity correlation at par with experimental values, proper knowledge regarding the selection of level of theory and/or basis set(s) is necessary. An appropriate choice indeed becomes new pathfinders toward building fruitful regression models for QSAR/QSPR/QSTR analyses.

6.3.1 COMPUTATIONAL DETAILS

The molecular geometries of the different classes of compounds studied by us as mentioned in t**Sections: 6.3.2, 6.3.3, and 6.3.4** are optimized at various levels (semiempirical and DFT) of theory using the Gaussian 98 or Gaussian 03 or Gaussian 09 [88] program packages. The stability of the optimized structures is characterized by their harmonic vibrational frequency values. The number of imaginary frequencies (NIMAG) is zero in every case, which corresponds to the existence of the given molecular geometry at a minimum on the potential energy surface. The IP and EA are computed through the Koopmans' theorem [89] or by using the energy difference between N and (N–1) electronic system or (N+1) and N electronic system called ΔSCF (Δ, a self-consistent field) technique. The atomic charges (Q_k) and Fukui functions [74] ($f(\mathbf{r})$) are computed from the Mulliken population analysis (MPA), natural population analysis (NPA), or Hirschfield population analysis (HPA) [90] schemes. The Hirschfield charges are computed with the BLYP/DND method using the DMOL3 package [91].

6.3.2 APPLICATIONS OF CONCEPTUAL DFT IN QSAR/QSPR/ QSTR

Conceptual DFT with its different parameters has been able to provide different models in order to assess the QSAR/QSPR/QSTR properties of different sets of molecules. Different parameters such as electrophilicity (ω), net atomic charges, HOMO-LUMO energies, frontier orbital electron densities, and superdelocalizabilities are some of the parameters which have been utilized to predict different models of QSAR/QSTR. Chattaraj *et al.,* have shown the applicability of electrophilicity index in the prediction of biological activity in many cases. A large number of testosterone derivatives and estrogen derivatives were shown to have biological activity defined and correlated in terms of mathematical equations containing electrophilicity index [92]. The regression values expressed in terms of R^2 were found to be in the range of 0.888–0.999 signifying the importance of such a chemical descriptor in the accurate prediction of biological activities of such molecules. The models have been developed by keeping the experimental values of relative binding affinity (RBA) as reference.

QSTR models have also been developed to determine the toxicity of benzidine derivatives and the series of polyaromatic hydrocarbons such as polychlorinated dibenzofurans (PCDF), polyhalogenated dibenzo-p-dioxins (PHDD), and polychlorinated biphenyls (PCB) by considering biological activity data (pIC_{50}) as the experimental value [93]. Their overall toxicity and probable site of reactivity were predicted in terms of their global and local electrophilicity parameters. Other terms such as Hartree–Fock (HF) energy were also shown to have their role in the prediction of such activities. These toxic molecules were further divided into classes of electron donors and acceptors and their interaction with biomolecules were assessed using Parr's charge transfer formula. Toxicity of some aliphatic amines was also predicted on the basis of global and local electrophilicities as well as HF energy. A good correlation in terms of R^2 values in the range of 0.800–0.993 were obtained in these cases. QSTR models to assess the toxicity of 252 aliphatic compounds on the *Tetrahymena pyriformis* for their 50% inhibitory growth concentration (IGC_{50}^{-1}) have also been developed by Chattaraj and co-workers [94]. They have found that global and local electrophilicity values could explain their toxicity through the QSTR models proposed by them. A good correlation was found in such models.

QSPR model for the lipophilic behavior (log K_{ow}) of a data set containing 133 PCB compounds were built using electrophilicity index, energy of lowest unoccupied molecular orbital (E_{LUMO}) and number of chlorine substituents (N_{Cl}) as descriptors [95]. The predicting ability of this model assessed in terms of R^2 was found to be in the range of 0.914. Similarly the toxicity analysis of 27 polychlorinated dibenzofurans by keeping activity values (pIC_{50}) as experimental quantities was performed by the generation of QSTR models [96]. Electrophilicity indices and local descriptors such as electrophilic power and local nucleophilicity were found to predict the toxicities in good correlation terms.

New descriptors based on the conceptual DFT have also been utilized in building up of QSAR models in some cases. Group philicity, which is obtained by the addition of local philicity of relevant atoms, has been shown to be an efficient descriptor in the prediction of toxic properties of chlorophenols (CPs) through QSAR/QSTR models, against *Daphnia magna*, *Brachydanio rerio*, and *Bacillus* [97]. In another study on the analysis of environmental effects of chloroanisoles, a multiphilic descriptor was calculated as the difference between nucleophilic and electrophilic condensed philicity functions and was employed in the design of appropriate QSAR/QSTR models [98]. It was found to be useful in the identification of active sites in the selected systems. However, the electrophilicity index (ω) descriptor performed better with R^2 value of 0.88. The same descriptor has been utilized in the design of QSAR/QSTR models for the complete series of chlorinated benzene in presence of solvent [99]; the dependent variable kept in this study was the median lethal concentration (LC_{50}) values of chlorobenzenes against *Rana japonica* tadpoles. It was observed that the solvent-derived ω produces a better correlation with toxicity than that of gas phase derived ω.

There have been a few QSAR/QSTR models in which simple and effective descriptors like the number of atoms (N_A) in a molecule have been employed. Roy *et al.,* have considered testosterone and estrogen derivatives to find out the potential of (N_A) in predicting the activities of those molecules [100]; good correlation with R^2 values of 0.80 was obtained in those cases. The same descriptor has also been tested for predicting the toxicity of 252 aliphatic compounds on *T. pyriformis*, however, better results were found when a combination of N_A and ω was utilized thereby highlighting the importance of electrophilicity descriptor [101]. The ability of a simple descriptor like the number of atoms (N_A) was also tested in the prediction of boiling point of alcohol, enthalpy of vaporization of PCB, *n*-octanol/water partition coefficient of PCB and chloroanisoles, pK_a values of carboxylic acids, phenols, and alcohols. A high value of regression coefficient (R^2) was obtained for this descriptor; however, the result was found to be improved further on the consideration of electrophilicity or of any other local variant in addition to the atom counting descriptor [102].

QSTR models employing conceptual DFT parameters like electrophilicity have been proposed for the determination of toxicity in arsenic derivatives [103]. It was found that the best model with R^2 value of 0.963 consisted of electrophilicity, atomic charge, and local philicity parameters. Other parameters such as atomic number and number of nonhydrogenic atoms were also explored to obtain the best QSTR model. There has been a benchmark study on the method of calculation of global reactivity descriptor and it was found that M05-2X method provided good results using the ΔSCF approach [87]. It was further observed that global reactivity descriptors, especially electrophilicity index, play an important role in the development of effective QSAR/QSPR/QSTR models, and their correlation coefficient obtained from the linear/multiple regression analysis of toxicity versus global reactivity index from different levels of theory did not change much. Thus, this study helped confirming the usefulness of global reactivity descriptors in QSAR/QSPR/QSTR models.

The importance of electrophilicity index as a descriptor was further proved in the QSTR model developed for the determination of toxicity of aliphatic compounds toward *T. pyriformis* wherein it was found to be better a descriptor in comparison to E_{LUMO} [104]. Other conceptual DFT descriptors like net electrophilicity index have been tested in the prediction of toxicity for halogen and sulfur compounds and were found to give good results, however, in the same study, electrophilicity index was found to be a good descriptor for the prediction of toxicity for chlorinated aromatic compounds [105].

Conceptual DFT descriptors like electrophilicity index and group philicity have been found to be good descriptor in the assessment of toxicity in aromatic compounds consisting of the set of electron-donor and electron-acceptor functional groups and also in the case of chlorophenols. The electron-donor and electron-acceptor aromatic compounds were studied for *T. pyriformis*, whereas chlorophenol compounds were studied for *D. magna*, *B. rerio*, and *Bacillus* [106]. The effectiveness of electrophilicity index was further shown in the QSPR models generated to predict the enthalpy of vaporization of 209 polychlorinated biphenyl congeners [107]. It was found that the combination of electrophilicity index, energy of lowest unoccupied molecular orbitals (E_{LUMO}), and the number of chlorine substituents (N_{Cl}) developed a QSPR model with R^2 values of 0.976.

6.3.3 *QUANTUM CHEMICAL DESCRIPTORS FOR THE PREDICTION OF IC$_{50}$ VALUES OF AMINOSULFONYL CARBAMATES*

The purpose of this section is to explain the biological activity of a series of acyl-CoA: cholesterol O-acyltransferase (ACAT) inhibitors [108], for example, aminosulfonyl carbamates in terms of a global reactivity descriptor, viz. electrophilicity index (ω) and a local parameter, viz. group charge on sulfonyl moiety ($\sum Q_{Sul}$). The biological activity of the considered ACATs was determined by incorporating them into cholesterol esters in microsomes isolated from rat liver, in terms of the micromolar drug concentration required to inhibit the enzymatic activity by 50% (IC$_{50}$) [109]. Since there was no report on the accurate estimation of error, we have used log (IC$_{50}$) to compress the range covered by the data between −1.00 and 2.21. A two-parameter (ω, $\sum Q_{Sul}$) regression model was developed for the carbamate derivatives (*training sets*). The predicted models were tested for the other similar compounds (~40–50% of training sets) of aminosulfonyl carbamates.

The electrophilicity index (ω), group charge on sulfonyl moiety ($\sum Q_{Sul}$) and experimental and calculated log (IC$_{50}$) values for the 25 aminosulfonyl carbamates (ID 1-25) are reported in Table 1. A total of 16 compounds (ID 1-16) are considered as the training set to perform a two parameter (ω, $\sum Q_{Sul}$) regression model. The regression model for the calculated log (IC$_{50}$) is as follows:

$$\log (IC_{50}) = 0.348 \times \omega + 36.860 \times \sum Q_{Sul} - 11.086$$

$$R = 0.903, \; SD = 0.208, \; N = 16 \tag{12}$$

Figure 1a presents the correlation plot between experimental and calculated log (IC_{50}). It can be noted that biological activity of the considered aminosulfonyl carbamates is explained successfully by using ω and $\sum Q_{Sul}$. The predicted regression model (Eq. 12) was tested to nine other homologous aminosulfonyl carbamates (ID 17–25) to check the efficiency of the predicted model. **Figure 1b** provides the correlation plot between experimental and calculated log (IC_{50}) for the test set. It was found that our predicted model can explain the biological activity of aminosulfonyl ureas with a comparable efficiency. Theoretical effort has been devoted to explain the experimental log (IC_{50}) values of the ACAT compounds considered in this study [110]. Patankar and Jurs [110a] have performed linear regression and nonlinear neural network models for a large number of ACAT compounds. Chhabria and co-workers [110b] used genetic function approximation for a QSAR study of some of the ACAT compounds considered in the present work. Both of those studies [110] have employed large number of structural descriptors. Predicted correlation between structure and activity was poor.

TABLE 1 Training and test sets of various aminosulfonyl carbamates along with their electrophilicity index (ω), group charge on sulfonyl moiety ($\sum Q_{Sul}$), and experimental and calculated log (IC_{50}) values.

Aminosulfonyl Carbamates

TRAINING SET

ID No.	R	R_1	R_2	R_3	ω (eV)	$\sum Q_{Sul}$	Obs. log (IC_{50})	Calc. log (IC_{50})
1	H				2.104	0.310	1.176	1.088
2	H				1.875	0.302	0.623	0.706

TABLE 1   (*Continued*)

3	H			2.061	0.320	1.079	1.412
4	H			2.269	0.324	1.763	1.642
5	H			2.093	0.317	1.301	1.343
6	H		H	1.979	0.318	1.581	1.315
7	H		H	2.096	0.324	1.412	1.598
8	H		H	2.477	0.324	1.716	1.712
9	H		H	2.064	0.314	1.279	1.214
10	H		H	1.987	0.303	1.057	0.769
11			H	2.070	0.307	0.663	0.955

TABLE 1   (*Continued*)

12	H			1.876	0.298	0.505	0.563
13	H			1.956	0.298	0.342	0.589
14	H			1.954	0.298	0.633	0.590
15	H			1.974	0.293	0.431	0.413
16	H		H	1.995	0.310	1.369	1.023

TEST SET

17	H			2.117	0.328	0.279	1.730
18	H			2.099	0.341	0.708	2.209
19	H			1.878	0.304	0.114	0.776

TABLE 1   (*Continued*)

No		Structure					
20	H		H	2.142	0.354	1.225	2.703
21	H			2.043	0.310	0.505	1.037
22	H		H	2.041	0.376	1.130	3.480
23	H		H	1.940	0.379	1.176	3.570
24	H		H	2.319	0.377	1.407	3.607
25	H	$CH_3-(CH_2)_{11}-$	H	2.010	0.376	1.519	3.455

The primary purpose of a successful QSAR study is the choice of less number of efficient descriptors (relevant with associated biomechanism), to avoid complex nature of the regression model as well as selection of useless descriptors without any scientific connection to the predictable property. A reasonable correlation between experimental and calculated bioactivity implies that the choice of descriptors in the present work is efficient. The electrophilicity index (ω) predicts the bioactivity and the toxicity of diverse classes of chemical compounds and drug molecules [92–106] where the electron transfer process is believed one of the most important factors in the interaction between inhibitors and biosystems. In a similar way the variation of local group charge on the sulfonyl moiety ($-S(=O)_2-$), that is, $\sum Q_{Sul}$ is expected to serve as a good descriptor in explaining the experimental IC_{50} values for ACAT inhibitors.

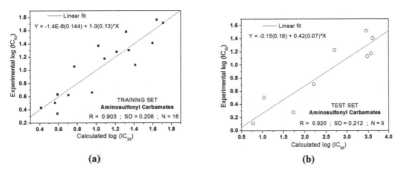

FIGURE 1   Experimental versus calculated biological activity (log IC_{50}) values using two-parameter ($\omega, \sum Q_{Sul}$) regression model (Equation 12) for the (a) training set and (b) test set of aminosulfonyl carbamates.

Therefore, quantum chemical descriptors were developed to explain the biological activity in terms of log (IC_{50}) of a series of 25 Acyl-CoA: cholesterol O-acyltransferase (ACAT) inhibitors, for example, aminosulfonyl carbamates. Electrophilicity index (ω) and group atomic charge on sulfonyl moiety ($\sum Q_{Sul}$) were found to be potent descriptors for more than 90% prediction of the observed log (IC_{50}) values. Predicted two-parameter regression models ($\omega, \sum Q_{Sul}$) for the training set of carbamates were applied to the respective unknown test sets, resulting in a favorable prediction of biological activities of those compounds with unknown experimental information. Therefore, the electrophilicity index (ω) and the group atomic charge on sulfonyl moiety ($\sum Q_{Sul}$) can be considered as two efficient descriptors in explaining bioactivity of ACAT inhibitors.

6.3.4   A QUANTUM CHEMICAL STUDY ON THE SYNERGISTIC EFFECT INDUCED BY A MIXTURE OF DIFFERENT SETS OF ANTIOXIDANTS FOR THE INHIBITION OF OXIDATION OF LINOLENIC ACID

In this section, an effort was made to understand the synergistic effect observed for combination of antioxidants. There are experimental reports on the synergistic effects observed for different combinations of phenolic compounds against the oxidation of linolenic acid (structure 1 in **Figure 2**) [111]. The antioxidants considered in the present study were gallic acid, ascorbic acid, and epicatechin, and, were shown as structures 2, 3, and 4, respectively in **Figure 2**. Stoichiometric mixture of epicatechin and ascorbic acid in 1:1 and 1:2 ratios were investigated for their synergistic effect. Antioxidant properties of the investigated molecules were compared with phenol on the basis of their bond dissociation energy (BDE). CDFT based reactivity descriptors, were also employed to unravel the synergistic effect.

6.3.4.1 THEORETICAL METHODOLOGY

The radical scavenging ability of any molecule is found to depend on three mechanisms. The first one deals with the gain of a hydrogen atom by a free radical. This mechanism is similar to the proton-coupled electron transfer (PCET).

$$ArO\text{-}H + R^{\cdot} \rightarrow ArO^{\cdot} + RH \tag{13}$$

The occurrence of such a hydrogen transfer (HAT) and PCET is determined by the BDE which measures the strength of the OH bond.

In the second mechanism the radical scavengers give an electron to the radical:

$$ArO\text{-}H + R^{\cdot} \rightarrow ArOH^{\cdot +} + R^{-} \tag{14}$$

$$ArOH^{\cdot +} + R^{-} \rightarrow ArO^{\cdot} + RH \tag{15}$$

This mechanism has been named electron transfer–proton transfer (ET–PT) mechanism. The third mechanism deals with sequential proton loss electron transfer (SPLET).

$$ArO\text{-}H + R^{\cdot} \rightarrow ArO^{-} + H^{+} \tag{16}$$

$$ArO^{-} + R^{\cdot} \rightarrow ArO^{\cdot} + R^{-} \tag{17}$$

$$R^{-} + H^{+} \rightarrow RH \tag{18}$$

The thermodynamic balance of the above mentioned three mechanisms appears to be the same since both the reactants and products are the same for all the cases. Therefore, the kinetic of the limiting step of each mechanism [112] is vital to decide through which mechanism it will proceed. It has been proven that in nonpolar environments (e.g., lipid bilayer membranes), PCET turns out as the only active process for polyphenols such as quercetin [113]. Therefore, in the present investigation only the HAT mechanism was considered.

HAT mechanism is thought to have a major effect on the antioxidant property of the molecules considered in the present study. Therefore, BDE values of different bonds especially O–H and C–H (in case of linolenic acid) of all the molecules are computed and their analysis for their antioxidant properties was made. Ionization energy, electron affinity, and reactivity descriptors like electronegativity, hardness, and electrophilicity also give an insight into the antioxidant property of a molecule. Along with that the energy differences between the reactants consisting of antioxidant and hydroxyl radical, and the products consisting of free radical and water molecule provide information about the antioxidant properties of a molecule. **Figure 2** depicts the optimized minimum energy structures of all antioxidants and their corresponding free radical molecules mostly involving O–H bonds (linolenic acid C–H bonds are also shown). Here we have considered that the O–H bond (linolenic acid C–H bond), which has the lowest BDE, breaks to form radical and the related results are displayed in **Table 2**.

6.3.4.1 BOND DISSOCIATION ENERGY

The BDE of an individual molecule was also compared with the BDE of phenol to assess its antioxidant property. It was seen that linolenic acid with C–H bonds at C-8 and C-5 possesses the lowest BDE (75.5 kcal/mol) among all the molecules, and, therefore, it accounts for its high oxidation tendency which is also observed experimentally. Structure 1a in **Figure 2** depicts the radical of linolenic acid for which the lowest BDE is obtained. Gallic acid was found to be a better antioxidant than the other considered antioxidants, viz. gallic acid, ascorbic acid, and epicatechin having BDE of 76.21 kcal/mol which shows its ease to form radicals (**Table 2** and structure 2a in **Figure 2**). Ascorbic acid was found to have BDE of 78.25 kcal/mol and epicatechin 79.78 kcal/mol. Their corresponding radicals responsible for these values of BDE are shown in structures 3a and 4a in **Figure 2**, respectively. Phenol (structure 5 in **Figure 2**) is known to react with agents like Fenton's reagent via a free radical mechanism, and, therefore, it was considered in the present study to assign BDE of individual species in a manner, which looks more comprehensible. Its BDE was found to be 89.64 kcal/mol and its corresponding radical is shown in structure 5a (**Figure 2**). The BDE values of linolenic acid, gallic acid, ascorbic acid, and epicatechin were found to be 14.13 kcal/mol, 13.43 kcal/mol, 11.39 kcal/mol, and 9.86 kcal/mol lesser than the BDE of phenol, respectively. The BDE values of the adducts made by the combinations of linolenic acid–gallic acid, linolenic acid–ascorbic acid in 1:1 ratio and ascorbic acid–gallic acid and epicatechin–ascorbic acid in 1:1 and 1:2 ratios, respectively are provided in **Table 2** (structures 6–10 in **Figure 2**). The bond responsible for the lowest BDE in case of linolenic acid–gallic acid combination was found to be the C–H bond at C-8 in structure 6a (**Figure 2**).

TABLE 2 Lowest BDE (D_e, kcal/mol) of different molecules computed at B3LYP/6-311G(d,p) level of theory. Values in parentheses depict relative BDE of a molecule with respect to BDE of phenol (D_{rel}, kcal/mol) studied at B3LYP/6-311G(d,p) level.

Molecule	No.	Radical	D_e (D_{rel})
Linolenic acid	1	Structure No. 1a	75.51 (14.13)
Gallic acid	2	Structure No. 2a	76.21 (13.43)
Ascorbic acid	3	Structure No. 3a	78.25 (11.39)
Epicatechin	4	Structure No. 4a	79.78 (9.86)
Phenol	5	Structure No. 5a	89.64 (0.00)
Linolenic acid–gallic acid	6	Structure No. 6a	80.30 (9.34)
Linolenic acid–ascorbic acid	7	Structure No. 7a	76.74 (12.90)
Ascorbic acid–gallic acid	8	Structure No. 8a	76.32 (13.32)
Epicatechin–ascorbic acid	9	Structure No. 9a	77.46 (12.18)
Epicatechin-2 (ascorbic acid)	10	Structure No. 10a	77.47 (12.17)

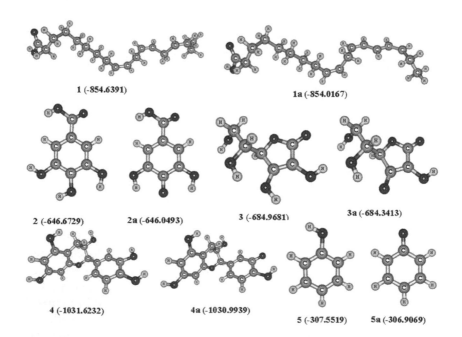

1 (-854.6391)   1a (-854.0167)

2 (-646.6729)   2a (-646.0493)   3 (-684.9681)   3a (-684.3413)

4 (-1031.6232)   4a (-1030.9939)   5 (-307.5519)   5a (-306.9069)

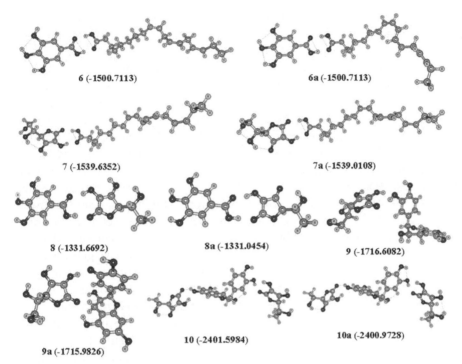

6 (-1500.7113)   **6a (-1500.7113)**

7 (-1539.6352)   **7a (-1539.0108)**

8 (-1331.6692)   **8a (-1331.0454)**

9 (-1716.6082)

9a (-1715.9826)

10 (-2401.5984)   **10a (-2400.9728)**

FIGURE 2   Optimized geometries at B3LYP/6-311G(d,p) level of different molecules and their corresponding free radical molecules involved in the generation of free radical with lowest bond dissociation energy. Values in parentheses are the electronic energy in arbitrary unit of different systems.

Note that the two units interact with each other through hydrogen bond between two COOH units of linolenic and gallic acids and the C–H bond at C-8 has the lowest BDE among all other bonds in individual linolenic acid and in the adduct. This implies that the value of BDE corresponding to the bond with the lowest BDE in case of individual linolenic acid (75.51 kcal/mol) gets increased to 80.30 kcal/mol when it combines with gallic acid. Clearly, gallic acid plays a substantial role in the prevention of oxidation of linolenic acid. In the adduct of linolenic acid and ascorbic acid (structure 7a in Figure 2) the lowest BDE value corresponds to the O–H bond of ascorbic acid and was found to be 76.74 kcal/mol which is higher than the BDE of linolenic acid (75.51 kcal/mol) but lower than the BDE observed for ascorbic acid (78.25 kcal/mol). Also the BDE of linolenic acid–ascorbic acid adduct for C–H at C-8 center of linolenic acid was found to be 80.03 kcal/mol.

It can be inferred that ascorbic acid individually is less easily oxidizable in comparison to linolenic acid, however, when it combines with linolenic acid, its BDE gets reduced which in other words implies the improvement of anti-oxidant property of ascorbic acid. In both cases corresponding to structures 6a and 7a, it is observed that the BDE value of C–H at C-8 position of linolenic acid increases and hence the propensity of the oxidation of linolenic acid gets reduced. This shows the role of antioxidants such as gallic acid and ascorbic acid in the prevention of the oxidation of linolenic acid. In the present study, we have also considered the combination of different antioxidants to assess their combined antioxidant properties. Structures 8 to 10 (in **Figure 2**) depict combination of ascorbic acid–gallic acid, epicatechin–ascorbic acid (1:1 ratio), and epicatechin–ascorbic acid (1:2 ratio), respectively. Their corresponding radicals with lowest BDE values compared to the other radicals are displayed in structures 8a–10a (**Figure 2**) and **Table 2**. It is worthwhile to compare the lowest individual BDE of these antioxidants with their combined set as it illustrates the synergistic effect reported by the experimental groups. Ascorbic acid, in the present study, is found to have BDE of 78.25 kcal/mol, whereas, gallic acid has BDE of 76.21 kcal/mol. The BDE in the adduct corresponding to structure 8a is 76.32 kcal/mol, which actually belongs to the O–H bond of ascorbic acid. Thus, it can be said that structure 8 does not show much increase in its antioxidant property vis-à-vis gallic acid, but it certainly predicts that the antioxidant property of ascorbic acid increases in the combined form. Similarly, it can be seen that BDEs of structure 9 (77.46 kcal/mol) and structure 10(77.47 kcal/mol) get lowered in comparison to the BDE (epicatechin: 79.78 kcal/mol and ascorbic acid: 78.25 kcal/mol) values of individual molecules. The combined units interact through the hydrogen bond. Since BDE of structure 10 does not differ much with that of structure 9, it can be inferred that 1:2 ratio of the epicatechin–ascorbic acid does not have much effect on BDE in comparison to its 1:1 combination ratio. Thus, the BDEs as observed for structures 9 and 10 clearly show that the synergistic effect of antioxidant occurs when two different antioxidants interact with each other.

6.3.4.3   USE OF CONCEPTUAL DFT BASED DESCRIPTORS

The IE, EA, χ, η and ω of different molecules are given in Table 3. The PCET mechanism as is shown in Eqs. 14 and 15 can be discussed on the basis of IE values. It is found that linolenic acid, gallic acid, ascorbic acid, epicatechin, and phenol have IE values (eV) of 8.006, 8.247, 8.790, 7.303, and 8.468, respectively. Clearly it implies that the propensity of linolenic acid to get oxidized does not follow PCET mechanism in comparison to other molecules.

   The combination sets are found to have lower IE values. Linolenic acid–gallic acid and linolenic acid–ascorbic acid have IE values of 7.429 eV and 7.594

eV, respectively. Similarly ascorbic acid–gallic acid (1:1) (IE=7.754 eV), epicatechin–ascorbic acid (1:1) (IE=7.323 eV) and epicatechin–ascorbic acid (1:2) (IE=7.270 eV) have lower IE in comparison to the IE values of the individual molecules. It implies that the combined set of molecules have more propensity to release electron in comparison to the individual molecules which further accounts for their better antioxidant properties. **Table 3** further highlights the hardness and electrophilicity values as observed for these molecules.

TABLE 3 Ionization energy (IE, eV), electron affinity (EA, eV), electronegativity (χ, eV), hardness (η, eV), and electrophilicity (ω, eV) of the studied molecules at B3LYP/6-311G(d,p) level

Structure No.	Molecules	IE	EA	χ	η	ω
1	Linolenic acid	8.006	−1.124	3.441	2.282	2.594
2	Gallic acid	8.247	−0.639	3.804	2.222	3.257
3	Ascorbic acid	8.790	−1.040	3.875	2.457	3.055
4	Epicatechin	7.303	−1.294	3.004	2.149	2.100
5	Phenol	8.468	−1.766	3.351	2.559	2.195
6	Linolenic acid–gallic acid	7.429	−0.189	3.620	1.905	3.440
7	Linolenic acid–ascorbic acid	7.594	−0.340	3.627	1.984	3.315
8	Ascorbic acid–gallic acid	7.754	−0.080	3.837	1.959	3.759
9	Epicatechin–ascorbic acid	7.323	−0.316	3.504	1.910	3.214
10	Epicatechin-2 (ascorbic acid)	7.270	0.224	3.747	1.762	3.985

It is found that the hardness and electrophilicity values of linolenic acid, gallic acid, ascorbic acid, epicatechin, and phenol are decreased and increased, respectively, in the adduct having different combination of individual molecules. In fact, the values obtained for the combinations of epicatechin and ascorbic acid are quite lower than those for their individual molecules which accounts for their more reactivity and less stability in comparison to individual molecules according to maximum hardness principle [84] and minimum electrophilicity principle [86]. This result is in line with the fact that synergistic effects are observed for the combination of antioxidants.

6.4 CONCLUSIONS

Chemists try hard to synthesize and understand the properties of different molecules. In order to cut the cost and the time and to know more about the properties of such molecules, molecular modeling is used as an advantageous tool. Different methods and models are designed to predict the properties, activities, reactivity, and toxicity. Conceptual density functional theory (CDFT) within the ambit of quantum chemistry has proven to be an important tool in the prediction of the properties of the molecules studied by us as mentioned in **Sections 6.3.2 to 6.3.4**. Its application along with the utilization of different statistical tools has provided different models such as QSPR, QSAR, and QSTR. In the present chapter, an analysis of different kinds of quantitative-structure–(property/activity/toxicity) relationship models was made. The role of different conceptual DFT based chemical reactivity descriptors such as hardness, electrophilicity, net electrophilicity, and philicity in the design of different QSAR/QSPR/QSTR models was highlighted. In addition, CDFT was employed to explain the synergistic effect shown by a mixture of antioxidants. Along with that, a simple descriptor like atom counting and its application in the prediction of various properties, reactivity, and toxicity of different molecules were discussed. It was found that these chemical descriptors within the purview of CDFT were able to predict accurately the desired properties of molecules.

ACKNOWLEDGMENTS

We are grateful to Professor Andrew Mercader for inviting us to contribute this chapter. PKC would like to thank the Department of Science and Technology, New Delhi for the J. C. Bose National Fellowship. SP thanks the Council of Scientific and Industrial Research, New Delhi for his fellowship. DRR is thankful to the Science and Engineering Research Board (DST), New Delhi for financial support by awarding FAST Track project grant (D.O. SR/FTP/PS-199/2011). We would also like to thank the reviewers for their help in improving this chapter.

KEYWORDS

- **Biological activity**
- **Conceptual DFT**
- **Structure–activity relationships**
- **Toxicity**

REFERENCES

1. a) Leach, A. R., Molecular Modelling: Principles and Applications, **2001**, ISBN 0-582-38210-6. (b) Puzyn, T.; Cronin, M. T.D.; Leszczynsk, J., Recent advances in QSAR studies methods and applications. In Challenges and Advances in Computational Chemistry and Physics, **2010**, vol.8.
2. a) Díaz, H. G.; Marrero, Y.; Hernández, I.; Bastida, I.; Tenorio, E.; Nasco, O.; Uriarte, E.; Castañedo, N.; Cabrera, M. A.; Aguila, E., *Chem. Res. Toxicol.* **2003**, *16*, 1318–1327. (b) Cruz-Monteagudo, M.; González-Díaz, H.; Borges, F.; Dominguez, E. R.; Cordeiro, M. N. D., *Chem. Res. Toxicol.***2008**, *21*, 619–632.
3. a) Schultz, T. W.; Cronin, M. T.; Walker, J. D.; Aptula, A. O., *J. Mol. Struct.* **2003**, *622*, 1–22. (b) Schultz, T. W.; Cronin, M. T.; Netzeva, T. I., *J. Mol. Struct.* **2003**, *622*, 23–38.
4. a) Nantasenamat, C.; Isarankura-Na-Ayudhya, C.; Naenna, T.; Prachayasittikul, V., *EXCLI J.***2009**, *8*, 74–88. (b) Selassie, C.; Verma, R. P., History of quantitative structure activity relationships. In Burger's Medicinal Chemistry, Drug Discovery and Development, Seventh Edition, Abraham, D. J.; Rotella, D. P. (eds.) John Wiley and Sons Inc.; New York, NY, **2010**. (c) Nandy, A.; Kar, S.; Roy, K., *SAR QSAR Environ. Res.* **2013**, DOI:10.1080/08927022.2013 .801076.
5. a) Selassie, C.; Mekapati, S.; Verma, R., *Curr. Top. Med. Chem.* **2002**, *2*, 1357–1379. (b) Roy, K.; Mitra, I., *Expert Opin. Drug Discov.* **2009**, *4*, 1157–1175.
6. Hammett, L. P., *Chem. Rev.* **1935**,*17*, 125-136.
7. Taft Jr, R., Separation of Polar, Steric and Resonance Effects in Reactivity in Steric Effects in Organic Chemistry. John Wiley and Sons, New York **1956**.
8. Hansch, C. *Acc. Chem. Res.* **1993**, *26*, 147–153.
9. a) Lien, E. J.; Hansch, C.; Anderson, S. M., *J. Med. Chem.* **1968**, *11*, 430–441. (b) Hansch, C.; Klein, T. E., *Acc. Chem. Res.* **1986**, *19*, 392–400. (c) Hansch, C.; Kim, D.; Leo, A. J.; Novellino, E.; Silipo, C.; Vittoria, A.; Bond, J. A.; Henderson, R. F., CRC *Crit. Rev. Toxicol.* **1989**, *19*, 185–226. (d) Hansch, C.; Gao, H., *Chem. Rev.* **1997**, *97*, 2995–3060.
10. a) Kubinyi, H., *Drug Discov. Today* **1997**, *2*, 538–546. (b) Martin, Y., Perspect. Drug Discov. Des. **1997**, 7, 1. (c) Norinder, U., Perspect. *Drug Discov. Des.* **1998**, *12*, 25–39. (d) Maddalena, D. J., *Expert. Opin. Ther. Pat.* **1998**, *8*, 249–258. (e) Chakraborty, A.; Pan, S.; Chattaraj, P. K., *Struct. Bond.* **2013**, *150*, 143–180.
11. a) Winkler, D. A., *Brief. Bioinform.* **2002**, *3*, 73–86. (b) Didziapetris, R.; Reynolds, D. P.; Japertas, P.; Zmuidinavicius, D.; Petrauskas, A., *Curr. Comput. Aided Drug Des.* **2006**, *2*, 95–103.
12. Ajay; Walters, W. P.; Murcko, M. A., *J. Med. Chem.* **1998**, *41*, 3314–3324.
13. Wiese, M.; Pajeva, I. K., *Curr. Med. Chem.* **2001**, *8*, 685–713.
14. a) Schultz, T. W.; Seward, J., *Sci. Total Environ.* **2000**, *249*, 73–84. (b) Benigni, R.; Giuliani, A.; Franke, R.; Gruska, A., *Chem. Rev.* **2000**, *100*, 3697–3714.
15. Gombar, V. K.; Enslein, K., *J. Chem. Inf. Comp. Sci.* **1996**, *36*, 1127–1134.
16. Agatonovic-Kustrin, S.; Beresford, R.; Yusof, A. P. M., *J. Pharm. Biomed Anal.* **2001**, *25*, 227–237.
17. Brusic, V.; Bucci, K.; Schönbach, C.; Petrovsky, N.; Zeleznikow, J.; Kazura, J. W., *J. Mol. Graphics Modell.* **2001**, *19*, 405–411.
18. Burden, F. R.; Winkler, D. A., *J. Chem. Inf. Comp. Sci.* **1999**, *39*, 236–242.
19. Lewis, D. F., *Toxicology* **2000**, *144*, 197–203.
20. Vedani, A.; Dobler, M., Multi-dimensional QSAR in drug research. In Progress in Drug Research, Springer: **2000**; pp 105–135.
21. a) Leo, A. J.; Hansch, C., Perspect. Drug Discov. Des. **1999**, 17, 1–25. (b) Klebe, G., *J. Mol. Med.* **2000**, *78*, 269–281. (c) Podlogar, B. L.; Ferguson, D. M., *Drug Des. Discov.* **2000**, *17*, 4. (d) Kurup, A.; Garg, R.; Hansch, C., *Chem. Rev.* **2000**, *100*, 909–924.

22. Winkler, D. A.; Burden, F. R., Application of Neural Networks to Large Dataset QSAR, Virtual Screening, and Library Design. In Combinatorial Library, Springer: 2002; pp 325–367.

23. a) Schultz, T. W.; Carlson, R.; Cronin, M.; Hermens, J.; Johnson, R.; O'Brien, P.; Roberts, D.; Siraki, A.; Wallace, K.; Veith, G., *SAR QSAR Environ. Res.* **2006**, *17*, 413–428. (b) Gerberick, F.; Aleksic, M.; Basketter, D.; Casati, S.; Karlberg, A.; Kern, P.; Kimber, I.; Lepoittevin, J. P.; Natsch, A.; Ovigne, J. M., *ATLA-NOTTINGHAM* **2008**, *36*, 215.

24. Schwöbel, J. A.; Koleva, Y. K.; Enoch, S. J.; Bajot, F.; Hewitt, M.; Madden, J. C.; Roberts, D. W.; Schultz, T. W.; Cronin, M. T. D., *Chem. Rev.* **2011**, *111*, 2562–2596.

25. a) Abraham, M. H.; Chadha, H. S.; Dixon, J. P.; Rafols, C.; Treiner, C., *J. Chem. Soc. Perkin Trans.* **1995**,*2*, 887–894. (b) Katritzky, A. R.; Lobanov, V. S.; Karelson, M., *Chem. Soc. Rev.* **1995**, *24*, 279–287. (c) Estrada, E. *Chem. Phys. Lett.* **2000**, *319*, 713–718. (d) Balaban, A. T., *J. Chem. Inf. Comput. Sci.* **1997**, *37*, 645–650.

26. a) Gupta, S.; Babu, M.; Sowmya, S., *Bioorg. Med. Chem.* **1998**, *6*, 2185–2192. (b) Chen, K.-x.; Xie, H.-y.; Li, Z.-g.; Gao, J.-r., *Bioorg. Med. Chem. Lett.* **2008**, *18*, 5381–5386. (c) Liu, Q.; Zhou, H.; Liu, L.; Chen, X.; Zhu, R.; Cao, Z., *BMC Bioinf.***2011**, *12*, 294. (d) Leonard, J.; Roy, K., *Drug Des. Discov.* 2003, *18*, 165–180. (e) Roy, K.; Leonard, J. T., *Bioorg. Med. Chem.* **2004**, *12*, 745–754.

27. Jalali-Heravi, M.; Asadollahi-Baboli, M.; Shahbazikhah, P., *Eur. J. Med. Chem.* **2008**, *43*, 548–556.

28. Shi, L. M.; Fan, Y.; Myers, T. G.; O'Connor, P. M.; Paull, K. D.; Friend, S. H.; Weinstein, J. N., *J. Chem. Inf. Comp. Sci.* **1998**, *38*, 189–199.

29. a) Tan, S. J.; Yan, Y. K.; Lee, P. P. F.; Lim, K. H., *Future Med. Chem.* **2010**, *2*, 1591–1608. (b) Boyles, J. R.; Baird, M. C.; Campling, B. G.; Jain, N., *J. Inorg. Biochem.* **2001**, *84*, 159–162. (c) Wang, D.; Lippard, S. J., *Nat. Rev. Drug Discov.* **2005**, *4*, 307–320. (d) Centerwall, C. R.; Goodisman, J.; Kerwood, D. J.; Dabrowiak, J. C., *J. Am. Chem. Soc.* **2005**, *127*, 12768–12769.

30. Shadnia, H.; Wright, J. S., *Chem. Res. Toxicol.* **2008**, *21*, 1197–1204.

31. Turabekova, M. A.; Rasulev, B. F., *Molecules* **2004**, *9*, 1194–1207.

32. Vlaia, V.; Olariu, T.; Vlaia, L.; Butur, M.; Ciubotariu, C.; Medeleanu, M.; Ciubotariu, D., *Farmacia* **2009**, *57*, 549–561.

33. a) Saquib, M.; Gupta, M. K.; Sagar, R.; Prabhakar, Y. S.; Shaw, A. K.; Kumar, R.; Maulik, P. R.; Gaikwad, A. N.; Sinha, S.; Srivastava, A. K., *J. Med. Chem.* **2007**, *50*, 2942-2950. (b) Ventura, C.; Martins, F., *J. Med. Chem.* **2008**, *51*, 612–624.

34. a) Katritzky, A. R.; Gordeeva, E. V., *J. Chem. Inf. Comp. Sci.* **1993**, *33*, 835–857. (b) Hawkins, D. M.; Basak, S. C.; Kraker, J.; Geiss, K. T.; Witzmann, F. A., *J. Chem. Inf. Model.* **2006**, *46*, 9–16.

35. a) Könemann, H., *Toxicology* **1981**, *19*, 209–221. (b) Schüürmann, G., *Environ. Toxicol. Chem.***1990**, *9*, 417–428. (c) Cronin, M. T.; Dearden, J. C., *Quant. Struct.-Act. Rel.* **1995**, *14*, 1–7. (d) Robert, D.; Carbó-Dorca, R., *SAR QSAR Environ. Res.* **1999**, *10*, 401–422. (e) Katritzky, A. R.; Tatham, D. B.; Maran, U., *J. Chem. Inf. Comp. Sci.* **2001**, *41*, 1162–1176.

36. Katritzky, A. R.; Maran, U.; Lobanov, V. S.; Karelson, M., *J. Chem. Inf. Comp. Sci.* **2000**, *40*, 1–18.

37. Katritzky, A. R.; Fara, D. C.; Petrukhin, R. O.; Tatham, D. B.; Maran, U.; Lomaka, A.; Karelson, M., *Curr. Top. Med. Chem.* **2002**, *2*, 1333–1356.

38. a) Grover, M.; Singh, B.; Bakshi, M.; Singh, S., *Pharm. Sci. Technol. To.* **2000**, *3*, 28–35. (b) Grover, M.; Singh, B.; Bakshi, M.; Singh, S., *Pharm. Sci. Technol. To.* **2000**, *3*, 50–57.

39. a) Cramer, R. D.; Patterson, D. E.; Bunce, J. D., *J. Am. Chem. Soc.* **1988**, *110*, 5959–5967. (b) Jayatilleke, P. R.; Nair, A. C.; Zauhar, R.; Welsh, W. J., *J. Med. Chem.* **2000**, *43*, 4446–4451. (c) Sippl, W.; Höltje, H.-D., *J. Mol. Struct.* **2000**, *503*, 31–50. (d) Hannongbua, S.; Nivesanond, K.; Lawtrakul, L.; Pungpo, P.; Wolschann, P., *J. Chem. Inf. Comp. Sci.* **2001**, *41*,

848–855. (e) Avery, M. A.; Alvim-Gaston, M.; Rodrigues, C. R.; Barreiro, E. J.; Cohen, F. E.; Sabnis, Y. A.; Woolfrey, J. R., *J. Med. Chem.* **2002**, *45*, 292–303. (f) Kubinyi, H., Drug Discov. Today **1997**, 2, 457–467. (g) Kubinyi, H., *Drug Discov. Today* **1997**, *2*, 538–546.

40. a) Roy, K.; Roy, P. P., *Chem. Biol. Drug des.* **2008**, *72*, 370–382. (b) Brito, M. A. j. d.; Rodrigues, C. R.; Cirino, J. J. V.; de Alencastro, R. B.; Castro, H. C.; Albuquerque, M. G., *J. Chem. Inf. Model.***2008**, *48*, 1706–1715. (c) Erickson, J. A.; Jalaie, M.; Robertson, D. H.; Lewis, R. A.; Vieth, M., *J. Med. Chem.* **2004**, *47*, 45–55. (d) Lei, B.; Li, J.; Lu, J.; Du, J.; Liu, H.; Yao, X., *J. Agric. Food Chem.* **2009**, *57*, 9593–9598. (e) Durdagi, S.; Mavromoustakos, T.; Chronakis, N.; Papadopoulos, M. G., *Bioorg. Med. Chem.* **2008**, *16*, 9957–9974. (f) Liu, H.; Huang, X.; Shen, J.; Luo, X.; Li, M.; Xiong, B.; Chen, G.; Shen, J.; Yang, Y.; Jiang, H., *J. Med. Chem.* **2002**, *45*, 4816–4827.

41. a) Hirokawa, S.; Imasaka, T.; Imasaka, T., *Chem. Res. Toxicol.* **2005**, *18*, 232–238. (b) Jäntschi, L.; Bolboacă, S. D.; Sestraş, R. E., *J. Mol. Model.* **2010**, *16*, 377–386.

42. Friesner, R. A.; Beachy, M. D., *Curr. Opin. Struct. Biol.* **1998**, *8*, 257–262.

43. Cartier, A.; Rivail, J.-L., *Chemom. Intell. Lab. Syst.* **1987**, *1*, 335–347.

44. a) Gupta, S. P.; Singh, P.; Bindal, M. C., *Chem. Rev.* **1983**, *83*, 633–649. (b) Gupta, S., *Chem. Rev.* **1987**, *87*, 1183–1253. (c) Gupta, S., *Chem. Rev.* **1991**, *91*, 1109–1119.

45. a) Brown, R. E.; Simas, A. M., *Theor. Chim. Acta.* **1982**, *62*, 1–16. (b) Buydens, L.; Massart, D. L.; Geerlings, P., *Anal. Chem.* **1983**, *55*, 738–744. c) Grüber, C.; Buss, V., *Chemosphere* **1989**, *19*, 1595–1609.

46. Karelson, M.; Lobanov, V. S.; Katritzky, A. R., *Chem. Rev.* **1996**, *96*, 1027–1044.

47. Asatryan, R. S.; Mailyan, N. S.; Khachatryan, L.; Dellinger, B., *Chemosphere* **2002**, *48*, 227–236.

48. Friesner, R. A.; Dunietz, B. D., *Acc. Chem. Res.* **2001**, *34*, 351–358.

49. a) Carloni, P.; Rothlisberger, U.; Parrinello, M., *Acc. Chem. Res.* **2002**, *35*, 455–464. (b) Andreoni, W.; Curioni, A.; Mordasini, T., *IBM J. Res. Dev.* **2001**, *45*, 397–407.

50. a) Raugei, S.; Gervasio, F. L.; Carloni, P., *phys. Status Solidi B* **2006**, *243*, 2500–2515. (b) Segall, M. D., *J. Phys. Condens. Matter* **2002**, *14*, 2957. (c) Shaik, S.; Cohen, S.; Wang, Y.; Chen, H.; Kumar, D.; Thiel, W., *Chem. Rev.* **2009**, *110*, 949–1017.

51. Sulpizi, M.; Folkers, G.; Rothlisberger, U.; Carloni, P.; Scapozza, L., *Quant. Struct. Act. Relat.* **2002**, *21*, 173–181.

52. Bayat, Z.; Vahdani, S., *J. Chem. Pharm. Res.* **2011**, *3*, 93–102.

53. a)   Chojnacki, H.; Kuduk-Jaworska, J.; Jaroszewicz, I.; Jański, J. J., *J. Mol. Model.* **2009**, *15*, 659–664. (b)   Sarmah, P.; Deka, R. C., *J. Comput. Aided Mol. Des.***2009**, *23*, 343–354.

54. Sarmah, P.; Deka, R. C., *J. Mol. Model.* **2010**, *16*, 411–418.

55. a) Arulmozhiraja, S.; Fujii, T.; Sato, G., *Mol. Phys.* **2002**, *100*, 423–431. (b) Arulmozhiraja, S.; Fujii, T.; Morita, M., *J. Phys. Chem. A* **2002**, *106*, 10590–10595. (c) Wan, J.; Zhang, L.; Yang, G., *J. Comp. Chem.* **2004**, *25*, 1827–1832. (d) Arulmozhiraja, S.; Morita, M., *J. Phys. Chem. A* **2004**, *108*, 3499–3508. (e) Arulmozhiraja, S.; Morita, M., *Chem. Res. Toxicol.* **2004**, *17*, 348–356. (f) Wan, J.; Zhang, L.; Yang, G.; Zhan, C.-G., *J. Chem. Inf. Comp. Sci.* **2004**, *44*, 2099–2105. g) Xiu–Fen, Y.; He–Ming, X.; Xue–Hai, J.; Xue–Dong, G., *Chin. J. Chem.* **2005**, *23*, 947–952. (h) Pasha, F.; Srivastava, H.; Singh, P., *Bioorg. Med. Chem.* **2005**, *13*, 6823–6829.

56. a) Elstner, M.; Frauenheim, T.; Suhai, S., *J. Mol. Struct.* **2003**, *632*, 29–41. (b) Elstner, M., *Theor. Chem. Acc.* **2006**, *116*, 316–325.

57. a) Putz, M. V.; Lacrămă, A.-M., *Int. J. Mol. Sci.* **2007**, *8*, 363–391. (b) Putz, M. V.; Lacrămă, A.-M., *Int. J. Mol. Sci.* **2007**, *8*, 363–391. c) Putz, M. V.; Duda-Seiman, C.; Duda-Seiman, D. M.; Putz, A.-M., *Int. J. Chem. Model.* **2008**, *1*, 45–62. (d) Putz, M. V.; Putz, A.-M.; Lazea, M.;

Ienciu, L.; Chiriac, A., *Int. J. Mol. Sci.* **2009**, 10, 1193–1214. (e) Chicu, S. A.; Putz, M. V., *Int. J. Mol. Sci.* **2009**, *10*, 4474–4497.

58. Duda-Seiman, C.; Duda-Seiman, D.; Dragos, D.; Medeleanu, M.; Careja, V.; Putz, M. V.; Lacrama, A.-M.; Chiriac, A.; Nutiu, R.; Ciubotariu, D., *Int. J. Mol. Sci.* **2006**, *7*, 537–555.

59. Duda-Seiman, C.; Duda-Seiman, D.; Putz, M.; Ciubotariu, D., *Digest J. Nanomat. Biostruct.* **2007**, *2*, 207–219.

60. Ciubotariu, D.; Deretey, E.; Oprea, T.; Sulea, T.; Simon, Z.; Kurunczi, L.; Chiriac, A., *Quant. Struct.–Act. Relat.* **1993**, *12*, 367–372.

61. Avram, S.; Buiu, C.; Duda-Seiman, D. M.; Duda-Seiman, C.; Mihailescu, D., *Sci. Pharm.* **2010**, *78*, 233.

62. Latosińska, J., *J. Pharm. Biomed. Anal.* **2005**, *38*, 577–587.

63. a) Holzgrabe, U.; Diehl, B. W.; Wawer, I., *J. Pharm. Biomed. Anal.* **1998**, *17*, 557–616. (b) Kalinkova, G., *Vib. Spectrosc.* **1999**, 19, 307.

64. Liu, S.-S.; Liu, H.-L.; Yin, C.-S.; Wang, L.-S., *J. Chem. Inf. Comp. Sci.* **2003**, *43*, 964–969.

65. Kaliszan, R., *Chem. Rev.* **2007**, *107*, 3212–3246.

66. Lobato, M.; Amat, L.; Besalú, E.; Carbó–Dorca, R., *Quant. Struct.–Act. Relat.* **1997**, *16*, 465–472.

67. Roy, K.; Popelier, P. L., *QSAR Comb. Sci.* **2008**, *27*, 1006–1012.

68. a) Mekenyan, O.; Veith, G., *SAR QSAR Environ. Res.* **1993**, *1*, 335–344. (b) Cronin, M.; Dearden, J.; Duffy, J.; Edwards, R.; Manga, N.; Worth, A.; Worgan, A., *SAR QSAR Environ. Res.* **2002**, *13*, 167–176.

69. a) Parr, R. G.; Yang, W., Density-Functional Theory of Atoms and Molecules. Oxford University Press: **1989**; Vol. 16. b) Geerlings, P.; De Proft, F.; Langenaeker, W., *Chem. Rev.* **2003**, *103*, 1793–1874.

70. a) Parr, R. G.; Donnelly, R. A.; Levy, M.; Palke, W. E., *J. Chem. Phys.* **1978**, *68*, 3801. (b) Chattaraj, P. K., *J. Ind. Chem. Soc.* **1992**, *69*, 173–183.

71. a) Parr, R. G.; Pearson, R. G., *J. Am. Chem. Soc.* **1983**, *105*, 7512–7516. (b) Pearson, R., Chemical hardness–Applications from molecules to solids, VCH. Wiley, Weinheim: **1997**.

72. a) Parr, R. G.; Szentpály, L. V.; Liu, S., *J. Am. Chem. Soc.* **1999**, *121*, 1922–1924. (b) Chattaraj, P. K.; Sarkar, U.; Roy, D. R., *Chem. Rev.* **2006**, *106*, 2065–2091. (c) Chattaraj, P. K.; Roy, D. R., *Chem. Rev.* **2007**, 107, PR46–PR74. (d) Chattaraj, P. K.; Giri, S.; Duley, S., *Chem. Rev.* **2011**, *111*, PR43–75.

73. Mulliken, R. S., *J. Chem. Phys.* **1955**, *23*, 1833.

74. Parr, R. G.; Yang, W., *J. Am. Chem. Soc.* **1984**, *106*, 4049–4050.

75. Yang, W.; Mortier, W. J., *J. Am. Chem. Soc.* **1986**, *108*, 5708–5711.

76. Mulliken, R. S., *J. Chem. Phys.* **1934**, *2*, 782.

77. Gyftopoulos, E. P.; Hatsopoulos, G. N., *Proc. Natl. Acad. Sci. U.S.A.* **1968**, *60*, 786.

78. a) Pearson, R. G., *J. Am. Chem. Soc.* **1963**, *85*, 3533–3539. (b) Pearson, R. G., *Science* **1966**, *151*, 172–177.

79. Pearson, R. G., *J. Chem. Edu.* **1987**, *64*, 561.

80. Gazquez, J. L.; Cedillo, A.; Vela, A., *J. Phys. Chem. A* **2007**, *111*, 1966–1970.

81. Chattaraj, P. K.; Chakraborty, A.; Giri, S., *J. Phys. Chem. A* **2009**, *113*, 10068–10074.

82. Ayers, P. W.; Levy, M., *Theor. Chem. Acc.* **2000**, *103*, 353–360.

83. a) Parr, R. G.; Chattaraj, P. K., *J. Am. Chem. Soc.* **1991**, *113*, 1854–1855. (b) Pearson, R. G., *Acc. Chem. Res.* **1993**, *26*, 250–255. (c) Pan. S.; Solà, M.; Chattaraj, P. K., *J. Phys. Chem. A* **2013**, *117*, 1843–1852. (d) Pan. S.; Chattaraj, P. K., *J. Mex. Chem. Soc.* **2013**, *57*, 23–24.

84. a) Chattaraj, P. K.; Sengupta, S., *J. Phys. Chem.* **1996**, *100*, 16126–16130. (b) Chattaraj, P. K.; Sengupta, S., *J. Phys. Chem. A* **1997**, *101*, 7893–7900. (c) Chattaraj, P. K.; Fuentealba, P.; Jaque, P.; Toro-Labbe, A., *J. Phys. Chem. A* **1999**, *103*, 9307–9312.

85. a) Chamorro, E.; Chattaraj, P. K.; Fuentealba, P., *J. Phys. Chem. A* **2003**, *107*, 7068–7072. (b) Parthasarathi, R.; Elango, M.; Subramanian, V.; Chattaraj, P. K., *Theor. Chem. Acc.* **2005**, *113*, 257–266.
86. Tanwar, A.; Pal, S.; Roy, D. R.; Chattaraj, P. K., *J. Chem. Phys.* **2006**, *125*, 056101–056102.
87. Vijayaraj, R.; Subramanian, V.; Chattaraj, P. K., *J. Chem. Theory. Comput.* **2009**, *5*, 2744–2753.
88. a) Frisch, M. J. *et al.,* Gaussian 98, Revision A. 6. Gaussian. Inc., Pittsburgh, PA, **1998**. (b) Frisch, M. J. *et al.,* Gaussian 03, revision B. 03. Gaussian Inc., Pittsburgh, PA **2003**. (c) Frisch, M. J. *et al.,* Gaussian09, Revision A.1.
89. Koopmans, T., *Physica* **1934**, *1*, 104–113.
90. Hirshfeld, F., *Theor. Chim. Acta* **1977**, *44*, 129–138.
91. DMOL3 User Guide, V., 4.2. 1 May 8 **2001**, Density Functional Theory Electronic Structure Program, Accelrys Inc.
92. Parthasarathi, R.; Subramanian, V.; Roy, D. R.; Chattaraj, P. K., *Bioorg. Med. Chem.* **2004**, *12*, 5533–5543.
93. Sarkar, U.; Roy, D. R.; Chattaraj, P. K.; Parthasarathi, R.; Padmanabhan, J.; Subramanian, V., *J. Chem. Sci.* **2005**, *117*, 599–612.
94. Roy, D. R.; Parthasarathi, R.; Maiti, B.; Subramanian, V.; Chattaraj, P. K. *Bioorg. Med. Chem.* **2005**, *13*, 3405–3412.
95. Padmanabhan, J.; Parthasarathi, R.; Subramanian, V.; Chattaraj, P. K., *Bioorg. Med. Chem.* **2006**, *14*, 1021–1028.
96. a) Sarkar, U.; Padmanabhan, J.; Parthasarathi, R.; Subramanian, V.; Chattaraj, P. K., *J. Mol. Struct.***2006**, *758*, 119–125. (b) Roy, D. R.; Sarkar, U.; Chattaraj, P. K.; Mitra, A.; Padmanabhan, J.; Parthasarathi, R.; Subramanian, V.; Damme, S. V.; Bultinck, P. *Mol. Div.* **2006**, *10*, 119–131.
97. Padmanabhan, J.; Parthasarathi, R.; Subramanian, V.; Chattaraj, P. K., *Chem. Res. Toxicol.* **2006**, *19*, 356–364.
98. Padmanabhan, J.; Parthasarathi, R.; Subramanian, V.; Chattaraj, P. K. *J. Mol. Struct.* **2006**, *774*, 49–57.
99. Padmanabhan, J.; Parthasarathi, R.; Subramanian, V.; Chattaraj, P. K., *J. Phys. Chem. A* **2006**, *110*, 2739–2745.
100. Roy, D. R.; Pal, N.; Mitra, A.; Bultinck, P.; Parthasarathi, R.; Subramanian, V.; Chattaraj, P. K., *Eur. J. Med. Chem.* **2007**, *42*, 1365–1369.
101. Chattaraj, P. K.; Roy, D. R.; Giri, S.; Mukherjee, S.; Subramanian, V.; Parthasarathi, R.; Bultinck, P.; Damme, S. v., *J. Chem. Sci.* **2007**, *119*, 475–488.
102. Giri, S.; Roy, D. R.; Damme, S. V.; Bultinck, P.; Subramanian, V.; Chattaraj, P. K., *QSAR Comb. Sci.* **2008**, *27*, 208–230.
103. Roy, D. R.; Giri, S.; Chattaraj, P. K., *Mol. Divers* **2009**, *13*, 551–556.
104. Pandith, A. H.; Giri, S.; Chattaraj, P. K., *Org. Chem. Int.* **2010**, *2010*, Article ID 545087.
105. Gupta, A. K.; Chakraborty, A.; Giri, S.; Subramanian, V.; Chattaraj, P. K., *Int. J. Chemoinformatics Chem. Eng.* **2011**, *1*, 61–74.
106. Giri, S.; Chakraborty, A.; Gupta, A.; Vijayaraj, D. R. R. R.; Parthasarathi, R.; Subramanian, V.; Chattaraj, P. K., Modeling ecotoxicity as applied to some selected aromatic compounds: a conceptual DFT Based Quantitative-Structure-Toxicity-Relationship (QSTR) Analysis. In Advanced Methods and Applications in Chemoinformatics: Research Progress and New Applications **2011**, Chapter 1.
107. Padmanabhan, J.; Parthasarathi, R.; Subramanian, V.; Chattaraj, P. K., *QSAR Comb. Sci.***2007**, *26*, 227–237.
108. Kyoto Encyclopedia of Genes and Genomes, Kanehisa Laboratories, Reaction: R01461.

109. Krause, B. R.; Black, A.; Bousley, R.; Essenburg, A.; Cornicelli, J.; Holmes, A.; Homan, R.; Kieft, K.; Sekerke, C.; Shaw-Hes, M. K.; Stanfield, R.; Trivedi, B.; Woolf, T., *J. Pharmacol. Exp. Ther.* **1993**, *267*, 734–743.

110. a) Patankar, S. J.; Jurs, P. C., *J. Chem. Inf. Comput. Sci.* **2000**, *40*, 706–723. (b) Chhabria, M. T.; Mahajan, B. M.; Brahmkshatriya, P. S., *Med. Chem. Res.* **2011**, *20*, 1573.

111. Peyrat-Maillard, M. N.; Cuvelier, M. E.; Berset, C. J. Am. Oil Chem. Soc. **2003**, 80, 1007–1012.

112. Brede, O.; Ganapathi, M. R.; Naumov, S.; Naumann, W.; Hermann, R. *J. Phys. Chem. A* **2001**, *105*, 3757–3764.

113. Meo, F. D.; Lemaur, V.; Cornil, J.; Lazzaroni, R.; Duroux, J.-L.; Olivier, Y.; Trouillas, P., *J. Phys. Chem. A* **2013**, *117*, 2082–2092.

CHAPTER 7

SYNOPSIS OF CHEMOMETRIC APPLICATIONS TO MODEL PPAR AGONISM

THEODOSIA VALLIANATOU, GEORGE LAMBRINIDIS, and
ANNA TSANTILI-KAKOULIDOU*

Department of Pharmaceutical Chemistry, Faculty of Pharmacy, University of Athens, Panepistimiopolis, Zografou 157 71, Athens, Greece

*Correspondence: Tel.: +30 210 7274530; fax: +30 210 7274747
e-mail: tsantili@pharm.uoa.gr

CONTENTS

ABSTRACT

The peroxisome proliferator-activated receptor (PPAR) family, consisting of three isoforms α, γ, and β/δ, attracts considerable research interest, offering drug targets primarily for dyslipidemia and hyperglycemia. In the present review the use of chemometrics in PPAR research is discussed highlighting its substantial contribution in identifying essential structural characteristics and understanding the mechanism of action. Although PPARs exert pleiotropic actions and may be involved in more pathophysiological conditions, currently quantitative structure–activity relationship studies aim to the design of novel antidiabeting agents. Achievements in biochemical research have influenced the focus of the chemometric techniques, which shifted from the search for PPAR-γ agonists to PPAR-α/γ dual agonists or PPAR-$\alpha/\gamma/\delta$ panagonists, as well as to partial PPAR-γ agonists, to reduce side effects. The different structural- and ligand-based models are analyzed in the light of both selectivity and multiple targeting.

7.1 INTRODUCTION

Chemoinformatics is an area of very active development and has great potential across the pharmaceutical research. In pharmaceutical industry *in silico* approaches have become increasingly important in reducing attrition rate and accelerating drug discovery and development (Cramer, 2012; Kortagere, 2013; Puzyn *et al.,*, 2010). Applications of chemoinformatics to chemical space navigation, virtual screening, and (quantitative) structure–activity relationship (Q) SAR analysis for affinity predictions toward a given therapeutic target have been extended to the consideration of multiple targets and antitargets and to multiobjective drug optimization with the aim to balance potency with physicochemical, absorption, distribution, metabolism, and excretion (ADME), and safety endpoints (Cronin, 2000; Glesson *et al.,*, 2011; Moroy *et al.,*, 2012). In fact, the evolution of QSAR methodology has progressed in parallel with an increasing appreciation and understanding of biological complexity and disease etiology and an enormous growth in size, complexity, and noise level of data that need to be analyzed (Searls, 2005; Tsantili-Kakoulidou and Agrafiotis, 2011). Public accessible databases with information on drugs, targets, and drug–target interactions are nowadays available and new ones are created. This evolution permits effective integration of data and knowledge management from many disparate sources, providing substantial aid to the development of *in silico* approaches (Searls, 2005; Wishart *et al.,*, 2006).

In principle the different methodologies in the QSAR field may be classified in structure- and in ligand-based strategies and can be used independently or in combination depending on the problem to be solved and the relevant information available. The first strategy, forming the area of molecular modeling, provides detailed information on protein–ligand interactions considering the three-dimensional (3D) conformation and taking advantage of crystal structures, if available (Bohacek et al.,, 1996; Klebe, 2000). The second strategy applies chemometric techniques to establish 3D or 2D QSAR prediction models from molecular structure representation. Further, 3D QSAR models are based on the GRID technique and the most popular methods are comparative molecular field analysis (CoMFA) and comparative molecular similarity indices analysis (CoMSIA) (Cramer et al.,, 1988; Cramer, 2011; Klebe, 1998). After construction of a hypermolecule through proper alignment of the compounds and the use of suitable probe atoms, placed at the various intersections of a regular 3D lattice, interactions energies are calculated, which are treated by partial least squares (PLS) analysis. CoMFA considers electrostatic and steric fields while in CoMSIA hydrophobic and hydrogen-bond donor and acceptor interactions are further included. Moreover, 3D QSAR models although very informative, especially through their graphical representations, suffer from certain limitations concerning ambiguity of the bioactive conformation and the difficulties associated with superposition in the alignment step. Alternatively, 2D-QSAR methods are not affected by alignment rules and/or assumptions on conformations and can therefore easily be applied to large compound libraries. In such a case, careful selection of biological data to guarantee analogous experimental protocols and data curation are crucial prerequisites (Cherkasov et al.,, 2014). Considerable progress has been achieved both in structure representation through molecular descriptors, which form the core of 2D QSAR models, as well as with regard to statistical techniques and model validation. Nowadays, a large arsenal of more than 4,000 descriptors encoding the molecular structure can be calculated by various software, Dragon (http://www.disat.unimib.it/chm/Dragon.htm) and Codessa (http://www.codessa-pro.com/descriptors/index.htm) being the most popular. An atlas of the available molecular descriptors has been compiled by Todeschini and Consonni (2009), along with their definitions, mathematical formulas, examples, and references. They reflect various levels of chemical structure representation ranging from molecular formula (the so-called 1D) to 2D structural formula to 3D conformation dependent. Higher dimension receptor dependent descriptors can also be calculated creating a bridge between ligand- and structure-based design (Polanski, 2009). Additional dimensions offer the possibility to represent each ligand molecule as an ensemble of conformations, orientations, tautomeric forms, and protonation states (Ekins et al.,, 1999; Hopfinger et al.,, 1997; Vedani et al.,, 2000, 2005). Using enhanced molecular dynamic simulations, the overall conformational change of the receptor upon ligand binding can be simulated, producing more vital structural descriptors (Sohn et al.,, 2013). Consequently, pharmacophore approaches being structurally focused but ligand-based can be considered as a very promising link between the two strategies (Caporuscio and Tafi, 2011). Some success stories of this approach are discussed in the following sections.

The large pool of descriptors in ligand-based drug design can be exploited by various statistical techniques to select the important variables from noise or irrelevant information and generate prediction models. Multiple linear regression (MLR) analysis, often combined with genetic algorithms for variable selection, and PLS are more frequently used to derive linear models. Other chemometric approaches like artificial neural networks (ANN), regression trees (RT), or support vector machines (SVM) allow for nonlinearity to be included in the models (Sakiyama, 2009).

The next crucial issue is to validate the models for their predictive performance applying different statistical techniques such as internal and external cross-validation and data scrambling. Internal cross-validation is performed by the leave-one-out (LOO) or leave-many-out (LMO) procedure. The omitted data are then considered as test set and the sum of squared differences between the measured response y_i and the predicted value y_i^{pred}, defined as PREdictive residuals sum of squares (PRESS), is used to calculate cross-validated correlation coefficient Q^2: Q^2=1–PRESS/SS, SS representing the sum of squared differences between the measured y_i and the mean value y_{mean}. External validation may be performed by splitting the data set into several training and test sets and comparing the resulting models. In addition, data scrambling through randomization of the response variable should lead to models with significantly lower R^2 and Q^2 than the original model to support its robustness.

However, it is still doubtful if these statistical tools guarantee the predictivity of the model and validation by an external blind test set is always recommended (Chirico and Gramatica, 2012; Tropsha et al.,, 2003; Roy et al.,, 2012). In addition, assessment of the applicability domain is very important in evaluating the reliability of predictions (Minovski et al.,, 2013; Stanforth et al.,, 2007). A comprehensive review on "good chemometric practice" has been recently published by Cherkasov et al., (2014).

The present review focuses on the application of chemometrics in the field of peroxisome proliferator-activated receptor (PPAR) research. PPARs, are considered as challenging molecular targets for the treatment of chronic diseases, such as type 2 diabetes mellitus (Lenhard, 2001; Staels and Fruchart, 2005), obesity (Vidal-Puig et al.,, 1996), atherosclerosis (Blaschke et al.,, 2006) , and cancer (Murphy and Holder, 2000), which constitute major health problems in developed societies, and the most frequent cause of death. The implication of

PPARs in central nervous system (CNS) disorders, like in neurodegenerated diseases or in brain trauma injury, is currently being investigated by several research groups and relevant reports are available in the literature (Gurley *et al.,*, 2008; Kapadia *et al.,*, 2009; Neher *et al.,*, 2012).

In silico techniques have considerably contributed to the designing of PPAR ligands, to the understanding of their mechanism of action on the different PPAR subtypes as well as to the identification of the essential pharmacophoric features. It is important to outline that PPARs represent a paradigm where biochemistry, synthesis of new chemotypes, X-ray crystallography, and QSAR studies advance in parallel and interactively.

7.2   THE PPAR FAMILY: A SHORT OVERVIEW

PPARs belong to the nuclear hormone receptor superfamily. They are transcription factors that bind DNA and regulate transcription in a ligand-dependent manner. PPARs were first identified in *Xenopus* frogs as receptors that induce the proliferation of peroxisomes in cells, a procedure related to carcinogenesis (Dreyer *et al.,*, 1992). To date, three major types of PPARs—encoded by separate genes—have been recognized: PPAR-α—encoded in NR1C1—PPAR-β/δ—NR1C2, and PPAR-γ—NR1C3 (Braissant *et al.,*, 1996; Desvergne and Wahli, 1999; Willson *et al.,*, 2000). In fact, the PPAR nomenclature is not strictly appropriate since activation of PPAR-β or PPAR-γ does not elicit peroxisome proliferation in rodents, while none of the PPAR subtypes has been associated with peroxisome proliferation in humans (Michalik *et al.,*, 2004).

Each of these subtypes appears to be differentiated in a distinct tissue-specific manner, playing a pivotal role in glucose and lipid homeostasis. PPAR-α is mostly expressed in tissues highly involved in metabolism, with increased rates of mitochondrial fatty acid oxidation, such as liver, kidneys, muscle, heart, and brown adipose (Escher *et al.,*, 2001). The classical biological activity of PPAR-α is the regulation of the rate of fatty acid uptake and their esterification into triglyceride or oxidation. Differently than PPAR-α, the expression of PPAR-γ is dramatically higher in fat, both in brown and white adipose tissues, than in liver and muscle. It is also, expressed in the large intestine and the spleen. In the CNS, PPAR-γ is mainly expressed in glia and astrocytes (Xu *et al.,*, 1999). PPAR-γ is classically involved in adipocyte differentiation, regulation of fat storage, and maintenance of glucose homeostasis. PPAR-δ (identical with PPAR-β) is present in all tissues at comparable levels and is the most highly expressed isoform, in neurons throughout the CNS. It is less investigated and its function is not completely understood. Its involvement in the regulation of myelination, glutamate-induced neurotoxicity, and signaling pathways of reactive oxygen species is being investigated (Aleshin *et al.,*, 2013; Braissant *et al.,*, 1996; Woods *et al.,*, 2003).

Unliganded PPARs exist as heterodimers with retinoid X receptor bound to DNA with corepressor molecules. The heterodimer binds to specific consensus DNA sequences, known as peroxisome proliferators responsive elements (PPREs) which are located in upstream of responsive genes. Upon ligand binding (small lipophilic ligands), conformational changes are triggered, the corepressors are dissociated and coactivators are recruited by the heterodimer, thus inducing an increase in gene transcription and exerting pleiotropic actions (Berger and Moller, 2002; Feige *et al.,*, 2006; Tugwood *et al.,*, 1992; Yu and Reddy, 2007). Natural ligands for all three subtypes are fatty acids, fatty acid derivatives, and prostaglandin derivatives (Ferry *et al.,*, 2001; Nosjean and Boutin, 2002). Well known PPAR-α synthetic ligands are the fibrates, already discovered in 1980, in fact before PPAR identification (Cabreroetal., 1999). For PPAR-γ several synthetic ligands have been and are currently being developed as drug candidates for type 2 diabetes mellitus. They belong mainly to thiazolidinediones, tyrosine analogues, indole analogues, propionic acid, and phenylacetic acid derivatives of nonsteroidal anti-inflammatory drugs (NSAIDs) (Willson *et al.,*, 2000). For PPAR-δ selective full agonist is a polyfluorinated arylo-oxo-acetic acid derivative, known as GW0742 (Sznaidman *et al.,*, 2003). Representative PPAR ligands are presented in **Figure 1**.

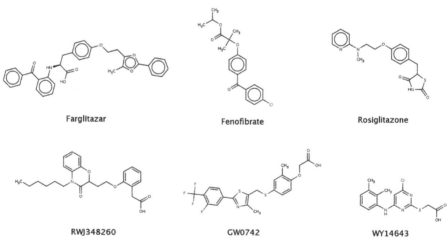

FIGURE 1   Representative structures of PPAR ligands: Fenofibrate, WY14643 (PPAR- α); Aleglitazar, Farglitazar (PPAR-α/γ); Rosiglitazone, RWJ348260 (PPAR-γ); GW0742 (PPAR-δ); Bezafibrate (PPAR panagonist).

7.3 PPARS AS DRUG TARGETS

The pleiotropic effects exerted by PPARs provide a challenging basis for drug development and novel experimental therapeutics, although specific attention should be paid in terms of drug safety. Considerable clinical progress has been made in the research of PPARs as molecular targets to prevent/inhibit various diseases, including dyslipidemias, diabetes, and metabolic syndrome. On the other hand, PPAR ligands are known to be associated with a variety of toxicities in a wide variety of species and cell types (Peraza et al.,, 2006).

According to the biological actions, described in Section 7.2, PPAR-α offers a target for the treatment dyslipidemia, with fibrates being well known approved drugs (Vidal-Puig et al.,, 1997). PPAR-α agonists are further associated with the prevention of the development of cardiac hypertrophy and left ventricular dysfunction (Duval et al.,, 2007), reduction of oxidative stress, apoptosis, and inflammation (Ichihara et al.,, 2006).

Most research is conducted in regard to PPAR-γ as a molecular target for the treatment of type 2 diabetes mellitus with rosiglitazone and piogliazone of the thiazolidinedione family being approved drugs in the market (Lenhard, 2001; Rieusset et al.,, 1999; Staels and Fruchart, 2005). More recently considerable interest has been oriented in combining the beneficial effects of dual PPAR-α and PPAR-γ activation, according to the concept of multitarget approach, with the aim to circumvent side effects including weight gain, fluid retention, and edema (Ebdrup et al.,, 2003; Henke, 2004; Lohray et al.,, 1999; Sauerberg et al.,, 2002; Wayman et al.,, 2002). The glitazar family, including PPAR-α/γ ligands, is considered to improve the lipid profile, while exerting antidiabetic action similar to a combination of a fibrate and a thiazolidinedione. However, failures in the dual agonism approach revealed that a critical requirement for safety is a balance of binding affinity such that the therapeutic dose range gives optimal biological effects of both PPAR-α-mediated and PPAR-γ-mediated actions (Balakumar et al.,, 2007). The latest shift from full agonists to partial PPAR-γ agonists seems to be another promising concept, since insulin sensitization is maintained, while side effects are reduced (Gandhi et al.,, 2013; Grether et al.,, 2010).

Given that insulin resistance, dyslipidemia, and obesity can be seen as components of a complex mixture of abnormalities known as "metabolic syndrome" or syndrome X, ongoing research efforts are focused on the investigation of pan-agonists, looking to combine the beneficial effects of PPAR-α, PPAR-γ, and PPAR-δ agonists (Nagasawa et al.,, 2006; Tenenbaum et al.,, 2005).

While no PPAR-δ agonists are yet approved for human use, ongoing studies have demonstrated their role in dyslipidemia, obesity, and wound healing (Barish et al.,, 2006; Kocalis et al.,, 2012), as well as in ameliorating cardiovascular complications through attenuating atherogenesis (Lee et al.,, 2003; Welch et *al.,*, 2003). The potential implications of both PPAR-γ and PPAR-δ in neurode-generative diseases (Parkinson, Alzheimer) and their beneficial effects in CNS and brain trauma injury are also under investigation (Carta, 2013; Iwashita *et al.,*, 2007; Paterniti *et al.,*, 2013).

7.4   THE PPARS TOPOLOGY–STRUCTURE-BASED DESIGN OF PPAR LIGANDS

The first PPAR-γ crystal structure was resolved in 1998 with rosiglitazone, a thiazolidinedione derivative, as the bound ligand (Uppenberg *et al.,*, 1998). This structure served to build a homology model for PPAR-α (Lewis *et al.,*, 2002) and to start considering the structural requirements of PPAR ligands. Nowadays more than 160 protein structures of the PPAR ligand binding domain (LBD), cocrystallized with ligands or in the apo-form, with or without coactivator, have been solved by X-ray crystallography and are available in the protein data bank (http://www.rcsb.org) (Berman *et al.,*, 2000, 2002; Gampe *et al.,*, 2000; Li *et al.,*, 2005; Xu *et al.,*, 2001). All three isotypes show a common overall LBD structure, which resembles the LBDs of other nuclear receptors (Bourguet *et al.,*, 1995; Renaud *et al.,*, 1995). The proteins fold into a single domain that contains a bundle of 13 helices and a small four-stranded β-sheet. Thus, in contrast to other nuclear receptors, the PPARs' LBD contains anextra helix, called H2¢, between the first β-strand and H3. A particular feature of LBD in PPARs is the very large Y-shaped cavity within the protein. Its total volume is 1,300–1,400 Å^3, substantially larger than in other nuclear receptors (Zoete *et al.,*, 2007). It includes a very flexible entrance allowing large ligands to enter the cavity and then branches into to two arms, each approximately 12 Å in length, as in **Figure 2** (Lu *et al.,*, 2006; Xu *et al.,*, 1999).

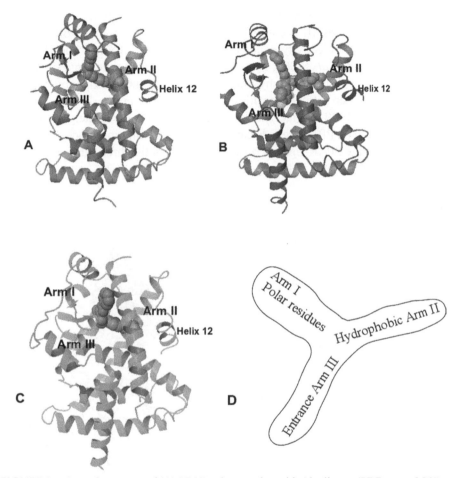

FIGURE 2   Crystal structure of (A) PPAR-α in complex with Aleglitazar (PDB entry 3G8I), (B) PPAR-β/δ in complex with GW2331 (PDB entry 1Y0S), and (C) PPAR-γ in complex with Aleglitazar (PDB entry 3G9E). Arms I, II, and III are depicted in each structure. Protein is presented with ribbons and ligands with CPK spheres. (D) Schematic representation of Y-shaped PPAR LBD.

Arm I, extending through helix H12, is the only region with substantially polar residues, which form part of a hydrogen-bond network involving the carboxylic group of fatty acids upon binding. It includes the AF-2 helix that contains the transcriptional activation domain. In PPAR-δ isoform the area next to AF2 is smaller than in the other two subtypes and cannot accommodate large hydrophobic groups linked to the acidic head. The hydrophobic arm II, situated between helix H3 and a β-sheet, and the interior of the entrance are mainly hydrophobic, occupied by the hydrophobic tail of the ligands. In contrast to the shape of arm II, the structure of arm III is conserved among the three receptor isoforms. Accordingly, subtype selectivity depends on the topology of arm I and II (Xu *et al.,*, 2001; Ebdrup *et al.,*, 2003; Fyffe *et al.,*, 2006). Due to the large size of the cavity and the flexibility in the hydrophobic entrance, the hydrophobic tail is in equilibrium between different positions (Burgermeister *et al.,*, 2006; Lu *et al.,*, 2006; Xu *et al.,*, 1999). In fact, none of the ligands fills completely the ligand-binding pocket, and PPAR ligands can adopt different binding modes.

Representative PPAR-ligand crystal structures for the three subtypes, reported in PDB are illustrated in **Figure 3.**

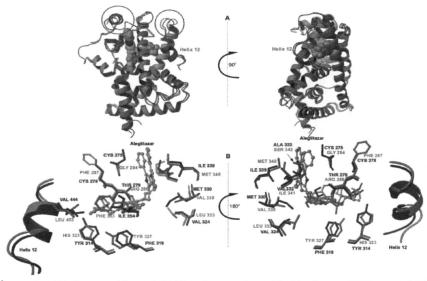

Figure 3   (A) Superposition of PPAR-α in complex with Aleglitazar (PDB entry 3G8I), PPAR-β/δ in complex with GW2331 (PDB entry 1Y0S), and PPAR-γ in complex with Aleglitazar (PDB entry 3G9E). Main differences in helices are marked in circle. (B) Detailed view of binding pocket of PPAR-α (black) and PPARγ (gray) in complex with Aleglitazar. Only aminoacids that differ are shown.

Docking studies in combination with 3D-QSAR methodologies, discussed in Section 7.5, have performed synergistically in defining pharmacophore units for PPAR ligand with crucial interactions. Typical PPAR-γ agonist molecules usually possess an acidic head involved in the hydrogen bond network, a central aromatic moiety, and a heteroaromatic hydrophobic tail as illustrated in **Figure 4**. This topology is maintained in a large number of synthetic PPAR-γ ligands, as representatively shown in **Figure 1**, which belong mainly to five chemical classes: thiazolidinediones (TZDs), tyrosine-based (TB), indole-based, propionic-acid and phenyl acetic acid derivatives (Haigh *et al.,*, 1999; Sohda *et al.,*, 1982; Liu et al 2001). In the case of chiral compounds, usually the S-enantiomers are the eutomers (Parks *et al.,*, 1998; Haigh *et al.,*, 1999). The same skeleton is essential for PPAR-α as well as for PPAR-δ ligands. In this aspect comparative (Q)SAR studies are of paramount importance in order to identify the particular features that are responsible for the affinity to different PPAR subtypes. The aforementioned increased interest for partial PPAR-γ agonists has prompted the investigation of their particular binding mode, which differs in regard to full PPAR-γ agonists. Full agonists occupy arm I and are involved in the hydrogen bond network with Ser 289, His323, His449, and Tyr473, stabilizing H12, as well as arm II through their hydrophobic tail. Stabilization of H12 is important for transactivation activity. In contrast, partial agonists occupy not only the mainly arm III forming a hydrogen bond with Ser 342 but also arm II, undergoing several hydrophobic interactions. Through this interaction a lesser degree of H12 and a higher degree of H3 stabilization is achieved, affecting the recruitment of coactivators and decreasing transactivation (Montanari *et al.,*, 2008; Pochetti *et al.,*, 2007). The orientation of Helix 12 plays a key role in agonism/antagonism/partial agonism to all nuclear receptors, and thus equilibrium has been proposed (Gangloff *et al.,*, 2001). A molecule acting as agonist pushes the equilibrium to the agonist conformation, a molecule acting as an antagonist pushes the equilibrium to the antagonist conformation while a molecule with partial agonist activity cannot stabilize H12 to the agonist conformation. The modulation of helix 12 and the surrounding key signaling residues by partial agonists with greatly reduced response has been further investigated by structural studies of indeglitazar, which is full PPAR-α agonist, but partial PPAR-γ and PPAR-δ agonist (Artis *et al.,*, 2009).

According to recent findings, Ser278 is another important receptor feature involved in transactivation, since at this residue PPAR-γ phosphorylation takes place. Inhibition of PPAR-γ phosphorylation may prevent the expression of genes associated with obesity and insulin sensitivity (Choi *et al.,*, 2010). This knowledge supports the understanding of the mechanism of action of partial agonists and is useful for the design of new candidates. Following these developments, Vidović *et al.,* (2011) created a virtual screening workflow combining rapid 3D ligand-shape-based screening with two stages of structure-based flexible docking of increasing accuracy. In addition, a prioritization protocol incorporating the docking scores, chemical diversity, and drug-like properties of the compounds was used to screen 341139 included in the National Institutes of Health (NIH) Molecular Libraries Small Molecule Repository (MLSMR) (http://mli.nih.gov/mli/compound-repository/mlsmr-compounds/). Further, Two hundred and thirty five compounds were selected for further experimental screening and the cell-based transactivation PPAR-γ assay confirmed 7 out of them as novel potent partial agonists.

Using available X-ray crystal structures from PDB, structure-based models were constructed for PPAR- α and PPAR- δ agonists, as well as for PPAR-γ agonists and partial agonists using 357 ligands (Markt et al.,, 2007). Because at the time no data were available for PPAR- α and PPAR- δ partial agonist no relevant models could be generated. Finally 47 PPAR models were constructed—7 for PPAR-α, 18 for PPAR-γ, 7 for PPAR-γ partial agonists, and 15 for PPAR-δ. Among them one PPAR-γ and one PPAR-δ were selected to represent the most selective models; however, one PPAR-α model proved highly selective to identify PPAR-α agonists, and one unselective PPAR-α model was useful to avoid a lot of negative false hits. Models were validated through parallel screening after integrating the 357 ligands and the 47 structure-based models into a database of 1,537 models for 181 different pharmacological targets. The results were promising since the PPAR target was prioritized by the ligands; thus, this approach may be used to identify ligands of the different PPAR subtypes.

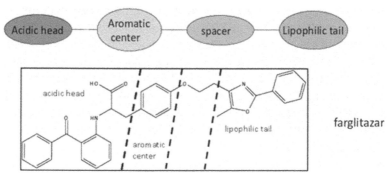

FIGURE 4   Structural characteristics of PPAR ligands.

7.5   LIGAND-BASED DESIGN OF PPAR AGONISTS

The research on drugs targeting PPARs is from its onset considerably supported by the use of chemometrics in parallel with the progress in the resolution of ligand–receptor crystal structures and structure-based design.

Thus, the first QSAR study concerning PPAR-γ ligands appeared in 1999, whereas the crystal structure of PPAR-γ complex with thiazolidinedione was reported in 1998 (Uppenberg et al.,, 1998). Kulkarni et al., (1999) used comparative molecular field analysis (CoMFA) to analyze in vivo hypoglycemic activity of 53 thiazolidinediones. Biological data were expressed as the negative logarithm of the effective molar dose required to reduce blood glucose by 25% pED_{25} in genetically obese and diabetic yellow KK mice. Alignment is a very critical step in CoMFA method, affecting the generation of molecular fields, which are subsequently treated by PLS to establish 3D QSAR models. The authors used atom-based and shape-based strategies for molecule alignment to obtain models with satisfactory statistics. Correlation coefficients R^2 range as observed was $0.689 < R^2 < 0.921$ and cross-validated Q^2 range as observed was $0.624 < Q^2 < 0.764$. Atom-based alignment gave the best results for the prediction of external test set ($R^2_{pred} = 0.750$). Steric and electrostatic fields were found to contribute almost to the same extent to the activity, while the introduction of calculated lipophilicity (c log P) as additional descriptor did not improve the models (Kulkarni et al.,, 1999). The CoMFA contour maps were used to propose a hypothetical receptor model, which was in agreement with the crystal structure of PPAR-γ thiazolidinedione complex, reported shortly before (Uppenberg et al.,, 1998). Thus, the aforementioned pharmacophoric features depicted in **Figure 4** have their origins in those early studies. At the same period a quite similar pharmacophore model for PPAR-α was proposed, combining homology modeling and QSAR equations for 12 fibrates (Lewis and Lake, 1998). Activity was expressed as potency relative to clofibric acid. A very good correlation was obtained between log relative potency and the calculated binding energy of the ligands to PPAR-α, including log D as an additional parameter ($r=0.988$). Further analysis of log relative potency with molecular descriptors led to two 2-parameter model equations of same quality ($r=0.86$), either with molecular mass and E_{LUMO} or with volume of the solvent-accessible surface and dipole moment. The latter equation was improved by introducing the distance between aromatic ring center and carboxylate (or isostere) group as an additional variable ($r=0.91$) (Lewis and Lake, 1998).

7.5.1 PPAR-γ FROM FULL TO PARTIAL AGONISTS

Beyond the aforementioned first attempts, application of QSAR analysis to PPAR research concerned mostly PPAR-γ ligands or ligands activating both PPAR-α and PPAR-γ and more recently PPAR-α and PPAR-δ, aiming either to find common features for dual agonists and pan-agonists or to explore selectivity. An important issue in these models turned out to be the measures for biological activity. As we discuss now, the initial preference from binding affinity data, K_i or IC_{50}, expressed as the negative logarithm (pK_i or pIC_{50}) was shifted toward transactivation data, EC_{50}, expressed as pEC_{50}. Although the latter constitute more complex quantities and is therefore more difficult to treat, they actually represent true biological activity indicating whether the compound is a full or partial agonist, an issue that is becoming very important for the design of new safer PPAR ligands, as already discussed.

Liao $et\ al.,$ (2004a) used both CoMFA and CoMSIA to derive QSAR models for a data set of PPAR-γ, including 74 tyrosine analogues and 5 thiazolidinediones. In CoMSIA five types of similarity indices—steric, electrostatic, hydrophobic, and hydrogen-bond donor and acceptor—were calculated using a distance-depended Guassian functional form and used as input variables in a PLS analysis, as in the CoMFA protocol. Activity was expressed as the negative logarithm of binding affinity constants (pK_i). While in the CoMFA model steric fields dominated, the CoMSIA model showed a considerable contribution of hydrophobicity indices next to a crucial hydrogen bond acceptor role of the oxygen atom, serving as a bridge between the aromatic central moiety and the heterocyclic tail (Liao $et\ al.,$ 2004a).

The authors applied eigenvalue analysis (EVA) for the same data set in order to further investigate the importance of hydrogen bonding network, associated with the acidic head (Liao $et\ al.,$ 2004b). To derive the EVA models, infrared-range vibrational frequencies were calculated after energy minimization, as conformational sensitive but superposition-free descriptors and were used as input in PLS analysis. Such descriptors characterized also as 2½ D descriptors, although do not intend to simulate experimental IR spectra, can be interpreted in an analogous way and may be useful to recognize the most important parts of the molecules, which contribute through their interactions to binding affinity (Ferguson $et\ al.,$ 1997; Turner $et\ al.,$ 1999). With EVA descriptors statistical data of the PLS models depend on the Hamiltonians used to calculate normal modes of vibrations as well as on the resolution factor (σ) and the distance between sampled frequencies (δ) . For the training set R^2 and Q^2 values up to 0.920 and 0.587 were obtained for the AM1 method and 0.863 and 0.586 for the PM3 method, respectively. The predictive ability of the models was validated by a test set. The best R^2_{pred} values were R^2_{pred} = 0.614 for the AM1 and R^2_{pred} = 0.822 for the PM3 method. According to the EVA models (Liao $et\ al.,$ 2004b), the two hydrogen bond donor sites in the tyrosine analogues, for example, the carboxylic OH group and the NH group with prominent peaks in the hydrogen bond stretching frequency region (at about 3,200 cm^1) showed important contribution to binding affinity. For the TZD analogues, with only one hydrogen bond donor, the corresponding peak was attenuated, thus leading to the assumption that the higher number of hydrogen bonds is responsible for the stronger activity of the tyrosine analogues compared to TZDs. In addition, bulk substituents on the tyrosine nitrogen atom proved favorable to the higher affinity, since they may be able to interact with an area of the ligand-binding domain of PPAR-γ that is not accessible to the TZDs. Such bulk structural elements cause the acidic head to appear located near the center of the molecule, while all other essential pharmacophoric features remain intact.

The bridge oxygen as spacer, the electron density clouds over this bridge oxygen as well as the carboxylic carbonyl group were confirmed as essential pharmacophore sites by another 3D QSAR study on 23 tyrosine analogues (Rathi *et al.,*, 2004). In that publication the logico-structural based approach, implemented in Apex-3D software was used to analyze binding affinities pK_i. According to this approach the molecular structures after energy minimization serve to derive certain physico-chemical properties which are used for the automated identification of pharmacophores (biophores), the superimposition of compounds, and the building of the QSAR model (Kashaw *et al.,*, 2003). Two models of comparable probability were selected with two and three variables and R^2 =0.66 and 0.69, respectively. The models included 18 and 19 compounds as training set, respectively, and were evaluated with the remaining compounds as test set. The three pharmacophore features differ slightly in the two models regarding their physico-chemical properties and their in between distance. These features consist of electron-rich sites capable of donating electrons and may be involved in electrostatic, ionic, and π–π interactions, while the electronic cloud on the oxygen atom may form hydrogen bonds with the receptor. Using these pharmacophore features as template for superimposition, two secondary pharmacophore sites were further suggested: S2 located on the carbon atom of the phenyl ring attached to the acidic head and S3 located on a carbon atom in the spacer region between the lipophilic tail and the aromatic center (sites can be identified in the template of **Figure 4**). The importance of the secondary sites in PPAR-γ agonism was further supported by two QSAR equations based on the two models.

BA = 0.004(±0.001) Total refractivity + 0.017 (±0:005) Steric refractivity at S2

–0.308

n=19, r=0.814

BA=0.004(±0.001) Total refractivity + 0.019 (±0.005) Steric refractivity at S2–0.010(±0.005) Steric refractivity at S3 + 0.252

n=18, r=0.83

(BA stands for biological activity)

The positive sign of steric refractivity at site S2 reflects the necessity of bulk groups at that position while small groups should be present at S3, as indicated by the negative sign of the relevant steric refractivity parameter. The equations were successfully validated using a test set (Rathi *et al.,*, 2004).

Vedani *et al.*, (2007) used a data set of 89 tyrosine analogues + 6 thiazoli-dinediones previously reported by Liao *et al.*, (2004a) to establish a 6D QSAR model, according to the *Quasar* concept. *Quasar* is a quasi-atomistic receptor—modeling concept offering a bridge between 3D QSAR and receptor modeling. It considers protonation state, solvation issues, and induced fit as additional dimensions, while performing flexible 3D docking to the receptor-binding pocket (Vedani and Zbinden, 1998). Using 75 compounds as the training set, a model family was generated, which converged to a cross-validated Q^2=0.832. A predictive R^2_{pred}=0.723 was obtained for the test set of the remaining 20 compounds. The robustness of the model was demonstrated by performing scramble tests, while the model was further challenged by three compounds of different chemical category, two with high activity and one with low activity, which were successfully predicted. The graphical representation of the models, showing the receptor properties instead of the ligand properties, demonstrated extended areas with hydrophobic properties, areas with H-bond donor functions, limited areas with H-bond acceptors, and a site positively charged to form a salt bridge. The model was included as a virtual test kit in the VirtualToxLab platform created by the same authors (Vedani *et al.,*, 2012), considering PPAR-γ as a target inducing toxicity potential upon activation rather than as a drug target.

It is evident that 3D and higher dimension QSAR provide highly informative graphical representations which are very useful to map the receptor-binding site and to identify the pharmacophore, complimentary to structure based drug design techniques. On the other hand 2D QSAR techniques remain very popular since they focus on the physico-chemical and structural characteristics of the ligands themselves and can guide further synthetic modifications for ligand optimization.

Using multiple linear regression and various physico-chemical descriptors—thermodynamic, topological, structural, electronic, and geometrical—calculated according to TATA BioSuite 1.0 software, 2D QSAR models were generated for the 23 tyrosine analogues previously analyzed by Rathi *et al.*, (2004). The relative negative charge was the most important factor to PPAR-γ binding, as well as molar refractivity, total hydrophobic surface area, and hydrogen bond acceptor sites. These descriptors were implemented in five different QSAR equations which were validated by an external test set of five compounds (Dixit and Saxena, 2008).

Rücker *et al.*, (2006) developed 2D QSAR models using a carefully compiled data set of 177 PPAR-γ ligands. The data set comprised structural diverse compounds, the majority of which were tyrosine analogues. Some thiazolidine-diones, indole derivatives, amino-propoxyphenoxy acetic acid derivatives, isopropoxy-phenylpropanoic acid derivatives as well as some natural fatty acids and thiazolidinedione-fatty acids hybrids were included. The authors used a large number of descriptors including atom and bond counts, connectivity indices, partial charge descriptors, pharmacophore feature descriptors, physico-chemical descriptors, like lipophilicity, and the MACCS keys. The latter represent bit string representations of structures, where each bit refers to the presence or absence of a unique substructural pattern (Durant et al.,, 2002). The descriptors were calculated considering the protonation state of the compounds. After variable selection by means of genetic algorithm, multiple linear regression analysis was applied to derive 2D QSAR models for both binding affinity, expressed as pK_i and for gene transactivation, expressed as pEC_{50}. With respect to binding affinity, two models were derived, one for the whole data set and one after partitioning the data into a training and a test set. Considering the structural diversity, correlation coefficients were satisfactory with $R^2=0.79$ and $Q^2=0.76$ and $R^2=0.79$ and $Q^2=0.75$ for the complete data set and for the training set, respectively. In the latter case for the test set $R^2_{pred} = 0.70$. However, the two models contained different variables sharing only three MACCS descriptors in common, one of them referring to the formal charge on carboxylate. Lipophilicity of the neutral species (log P) was included with a positive sign in the model for the training set but not in the overall model. A positive effect of lipophilicity was demonstrated in the model generated for pEC_{50} values, which, however, had inferior statistics, $R^2 = 0.65$ and $Q^2 = 0.57$. The difficulties encountered in building up QSAR models for transactivation were attributed to the lower quality of experimental data, which are measured in cellular level and to the higher complexity of the biological processes involved. Therefore the authors suggested that pEC_{50} values may be better predicted from the pK_i values, if available, by means of an activity–activity model, which they constructed by introducing three additional descriptors in the pEC_{50}/pK_i relationship. The additional descriptors were the sum of negative charge and two MACCS keys related to the number of O in rings and the number of rings at a certain position. To this point, it should be noted that the described models, although characterized by the authors as portable and easy to use for predictions, contain descriptors, some of which are not straightforwardly understood. A concern, noticed also by the authors, is that the good correlation found for observed versus predicted pK_i for the entire set of the heterogeneous compounds, becomes obscure or diminishes if the data set is broken down to subgroups. A rather poor pattern was observed for the indole-based derivatives, the tyrosine-based derivatives with lower molecular weight and the TZD-fatty acid hybrids. This is an indication that the leverage of the tyrosine analogues, which form the majority in the data set, drives the model toward its direction; the 6 TZDs are well accommodated within the model, whereas for the remaining subgroups other factors, not incorporated in the model, may be important.

These results elucidate the importance of the applicability domain of a QSAR model, which often is restricted within a given chemical class. Considering that tyrosine analogues and indole-based derivatives constitute highly populated, interesting chemical categories of PPAR-γ ligands, Giaginis *et al.,* (2008a, 2009) focused their research on the development of relevant separate 2D QSAR models to investigate the effect of chemical scaffold to the binding affinity and to identify potential common or specific features. For this purpose they applied multivariate data analysis based on physico-chemical and structural descriptors, which are easily interpretable for the medicinal chemist and can be further evaluated in respect to the drug-likeness concept (Lipinski *et al.,,* 1997; Veber *et al.,,* 2002). Models were derived for both binding affinity and transactivation data. For 106 tyrosine analogues a 2-component PLS model for pK_i with $R^2=0.82$ and $Q^2=0.78$ was generated (Giaginis *et al.,,* 2008a). Molecular size and surface parameters were found to exert considerable positive influence in binding affinity. Lipophilicity of the neutral form and flexibility (expressed as the number of rotatable bonds) contributed positively but at a lesser extent to the model. A number of substructural descriptors were also included in the model. For pEC_{50} data, less statistically inferior models were obtained. However, a highly satisfactory 2-component PLS model was reported for the 22 highly active compounds with $R^2 = 0.89$, $Q^2 = 0.78$, and very low $RMSEE = 0.17$ (pEC_{50} range: 8.5 to 10, pKi range 8.4 to 9.1). The descriptors included in the pEC_{50} model for the highly active compounds were different from those which proved important for the global pK_i model. Specific structural descriptors were found to be most important, whereas lipophilicity had a strong positive impact, (variable influence to projection, VIP >1), if expressed by the distribution coefficient at pH 7.4, log $D_{7.4}$, instead of the log P of the neutral form. This finding was attributed to the requirements of the cell-based experimental protocol. It should be noted that for that limited subset, a poor correlation between pK_i and pEC_{50} was observed. For the entire data, there was a better activity–activity interrelation with $R^2 = 0.58$. Correlation coefficient and cross-validated correlation coefficient raised to $R^2=0.76$, $Q^2=0.67$ in a 4-component PLS model with 12 additional descriptors, next to pK_i. Among the most important descriptors, hydrogen bond basicity, polarizability, and presence of acidic and basic groups exerted a negative effect, while molecular volume parameters showed an excessive positive contribution.

Using the pK_i values of 109 indole-based PPAR-γ ligands, a 3-component PLS model with comparable statistics was obtained with $R^2=0.82$ and $Q^2=0.80$ (Giaginis *et al.,,* 2009). Differently from the case of tyrosine analogues, the lipophilicity proved to be the most important factor, followed by the molecular weight, both with a positive influence. Flexibility and surface parameters exerted a negative effect, an indication that indole-based PPAR-γ agonists should be more rigid and compact molecules, compared to the tyrosine analogues, where these properties showed a positive contribution (Giaginis *et al.,*, 2008a). Moreover, electrophilicity—expressed by E_{LUMO}—was found to be another important factor for the PPAR-γ binding affinity of indole derivatives, while not included in the tyrosine model (Giaginis *et al.,*, 2008a). These findings explain the difficulties associated with the establishment of a general model for the prediction of PPAR-γ agonism, as already observed by Rücker *et al.,* (2006). Such difficulties may be related to the large flexible cavity, which has the ability to accommodate ligands in different modes according to the chemical type, as already commented. Analysis of pEC_{50} transactivation data of the indole derivatives led to a 3-component model with inferior statistics (R^2=0.69 and Q^2=0.64.) that also differed from the pK_i model as well as from the corresponding model for the tyrosine analogues. The number of ionizable groups, the dipole moments, as well as two volume parameters (van der Waals volume and molar refractivity) were found to have an additional positive contribution to the activity. Differently from the tyrosine model, lipophilicity was expressed as log P of the neutral form. The moderate of pK_i/pEC_{50} interrelation (r^2=0.77) was improved to r^2=0.84 if the molecular weight, the nonpolar surface area, and E_{LUMO} were introduced to establish an MLR activity–activity model.

The high demands for both lipophilicity and molecular weight in the case of indole derivatives should be carefully considered in further design, since they could lead to a violation score of 2 concerning the widely accepted "rule-of-five" for oral bioavailability (Lipinski *et al.,*, 1997). In fact, a survey on drug-like characteristics of a large number of PPAR-γ ligands demonstrated that 40% of active compounds (pEC50>7) violate the "rule-of-five" in respect to lipophilicity and molecular weight (Giaginis *et al.,*, 2008b). Analogous study concerning mainly tyrosine and TZD analogues has shown, however, that high activity can be achieved with moderate lipophilicity (Giaginis *et al.,*, 2007). To this point it should be noted that the indole analogues analyzed by Giaginis *et al.,* (2009) possess affinity also for PPAR-α, being in fact dual agonists. As demonstrated recently by the same authors and discussed hereunder, according to a QSAR study for dual PPAR α/γ activity, high lipophilicity is an essential demand for PPAR-α, while high molecular weight is more critical for PPAR-γ (Vallianatou *et al.,*, 2013).

The above QSAR studies bring into light two major problems associated with PPAR-γ ligands: the difficulties to establish a global QSAR model for PPAR-γ ligands belonging to different chemical categories and the not straightforward correlation between binding and transactivation.

Al-Najjar *et al.*, (2011) attempted to face the first problem by combining pharmacophore modeling and classical QSAR. They used a data set of 88 compounds with adequate diversity, collected from different sources. The chemical features considered to construct the phramacophores were hydrogen bond donors and acceptors, aliphatic and aromatic hydrophobes, positive and negative ionizable groups, and aromatic planes. The models were ranked according to their "total cost", for example, the error cost, weight cost, and configuration cost as well as the cost of the null hypothesis and they were validated through scrambling of the biological data. The fact that many pharmacophore models were optimal and statistically comparable further supports the ability of the large, flexible binding pocket of PPAR-γ to accommodate ligands according to multiple pharmacophoric binding modes. The authors consequently employed genetic function approximation and multiple linear regression (GFA–MLR) to identify the best combination of pharmacophore(s) as well as the most essential 2D descriptors, capable to explain bioactivity variation. They derived a QSAR equation, using 71 compounds as the training set and 17 as the external test set, with satisfactory statistics (training set: R^2=0.80, cross-validated R^2 (LOO)=0.73, test set: R^2_{pred}=0.67). The model contains three orthogonal pharmacophoric models and additionaly the molecular fractional polar surface area, FPSA (the ratio of the polar surface area divided by the total surface area) with positive sign and the number of hydrogen bond donors, the number of rotatable bonds and E_{LUMO} with negative signs. The emergence of three orthogonal pharmacophoric models in the QSAR equation suggests that there are three complementary binding modes accessible to ligands within the binding pocket of PPAR-γ, meaning that one of the pharmacophores can optimally explain the activity of some ligands, while the others explain the activity of the remaining ligands. The QSAR equation and the associated pharmacophoric models were further validated experimentally by the identification of three nanomolar to micromolar PPAR-γ activators retrieved via *in silico* screening.

The moderate or even poor correlation between PPAR-γ binding affinity and gene transctivation in many cases as well as the longstanding paradox (why PPAR-γ activation does not always correlate with the ligands' in vivo efficacy) cannot be explained simply by the complexity of the process and the consideration of cell and nucleus penetration issues, as suggested by Rücker *et al.*, (2006) and Giaginis at al. (2008a, 2009). The activity–activity models reported by these groups actually do not support this assumption, since many of the additional factors involved are structural specific and/or not directly related to permeability. The recently proposed new mechanism for the antidiabetic effect of some PPAR-γ ligands, relating the inhibition of phosphorylation of Ser278 with transactivation, promotes the disengagement between binding and transactivation (Choi *et al.,*, 2010). More to the point, since inhibition of PPAR-γ phosporylation prevents the unregulated expression of certain genes linked to obesity and insulin resistance, targeting PPAR-γ becomes more rationalized toward the design of partial agonists with high binding affinity but with low or moderate transactivation (Houtkooper and Auwerx, 2010). This rationale can be guided by tracking the different binding modes of full and partial agonists, already discussed in **Section 7.4**. In this aspect, Guasch *et al.,* (2011) conducted a study to define which ligand interactions in the PPAR-γ LBD ligand increase their binding affinity without increasing their transactivation activity. They used a data set of 205 ligands with available binding affinities and/or transactivation data expressed as percentage to maximal activation to discriminate partial agonists. After classifying the compounds in five clusters according to their Tanimoto similarities, an energetically optimized pharmacophores for each cluster was constructed. The pharmacophores were compared between the different clusters as well as with the pharmacophore constructed for a full agonist. Although the latter showed similar binding sites, their locations were very different highlighting the binding differences between full and partial agonists. The results were in agreement with those of the crystal structures previously reported (Montanari *et al.,*, 2008; Pochetti *et al.,*, 2007) according to which full agonists interact prudentially with arms I and II, and partial agonists with arms II and III, the main differentiation concerning the hydrogen bond interaction network. Slight differences in the binding mode were observed also between the clusters of partial agonists. These findings were further supported by the construction of a pair of atom-based 3D QSAR models, one for binding affinity and one for percentage of maximal activation. For this purpose 82 indole-based ligands with available both binding and maximal activation data (measured under the same conditions) were used, with 80% of them randomly selected as training set. Based on the selected ligand conformations, the basic characteristics of the chemical structures were defined according to six categories concerning hydrogen bond donors (hydrogens attached to polar atoms), hydrophobic/non polar atoms (carbons, halogens, C-H), explicit negative ionic charge, explicit positive ionic charge, electron-withdrawing atoms (nonionic nitrogen and oxygen atoms), and miscellaneous (all other atom types) and used as inputs in PLS. Considering statistical data for both the training and test sets 2-component PLS models were chosen. Statistical data for the binding affinity model were R^2=0.67 and Q^2=0.55 for the training set and Pearson r=0.77 for the test set. Slightly inferior statistics in terms of predictions was obtained for percentage maximal activation, with R^2=0.71, Q^2=0.40, and Pearson r=0.72, respectively. Graphical representation of the models revealed that hydrophobic and electron-withdrawing atoms are most important for binding affinity, the latter contributing in arm I interactions. The compound with lowest percentage maximal activation occupies arm II and III, while it makes hardly any of the favorable interactions in arm I. The compound with highest percentage maximal activation occupies all favorable regions at arms I, II, and III. The authors suggest that despite the fact that interactions with arm I increase binding affinity, this region should be avoided in order to decease the transactivation activity of potential PPAR-γ agonists. On the other hand, differences in the binding mode may be observed also between full agonists due to the large cavity of the LBD. This fact constitutes an additional factor, affecting the binding affinity/transactivation interrelationship. Thus, the same authors extended their study to investigate the structural differences between the features of PPAR-γ full agonists used for binding and those needed for transactivation. For this purpose they applied the above described procedure to develop 3D-atom-based QSAR models, one for the binding affinity and another for the transactivation activity, for 49 tyrosine-based full PPAR-γ agonists (Guasch et al.,, 2012). Despite the common molecular scaffold of the ligands the correlation between binding affinity (pIC_{50}) and transactivation (pEC_{50}) was moderate ($R^2=0.645$) with certain compounds lying far from the fit line. The aim of the study was therefore to investigate the structural features required for binding and those needed for transactivation; 2-component PLS models were chosen, which showed satisfactory and comparable statistics (for IC_{50}, $R^2=0.90$, $Q^2=0.70$, and Pearson $r=0.86$; for EC_{50}, $R^2=0.92$, $Q^2=0.64$, Pearson $r=0.90$). Graphical representation of the models with respect to the receptor–ligand binding domain showed the importance of arm II as the favorable region for transactivation mainly through hydrophobic interactions and to a lesser extent through electron withdrawal. This region corresponds to the effector part of PPAR-γ full agonists and may be responsible for the differences in affinity and potency. For binding affinity arm II was also characterized as the favorable region with predominance of hydrophobic interactions, while unfavorable regions were found to be located in arm I and beginning of arm II.

The techniques mentioned so far can facilitate rational drug design using the appropriate in silico screening algorithms. Petersen et al., (2011) recently build pharmacophore model based on crystal structure of PPAR-γ in order to screen the Chinese Natural Product Database (CNPD). They successfully identified oleanonic acid (found in Chios mastic gum) as a new partial PPAR-γ agonist. At the same time, Sohn et al., (2013) introduced multiconformation dynamic pharmacophore modeling (MCDPM) for novel PPAR-γ agonist discovery. Highly populated structures derived from MD simulations were used as template for pharmacophore model build. Those models were utilized in virtual screening of NCI (http://cactus.nci.nih.gov/download/nci/) and Maybridge (http://www.maybridge.com/) libraries to identify novel scaffolds.

7.5.2   DUAL PPAR-α/γ AGONISTS

The preference for partial agonists in the development of safer drugs for the treatment of T2DM was only recently well documented. Before this knowledge, the concept of dual PPAR-α/γ agonists attracted and continues to attract considerable interest in the aim to achieve synergistic action, while reducing side effects. Faced with the frequent coexistence of dyslipidemia and hyperglycemia, the hypolipidemic and cardioprotective effect of PPAR-α agonists may counterbalance obesity and cardiotoxicity often caused by PPAR-γ. Glitazars emerged as a compound family of dual PPAR-α/γ agonists with promising results; however, they were finally discontinued because of toxicity problems (Fagerberg *et al.,*, 2005; Kendall *et al.,*, 2006; Rosenson *et al.,*, 2012). As already commented a critical issue to achieve optimal results in terms of risk and efficacy is the proper balance in binding affinity toward each PPAR subtype (Balakumar *et al.,*, 2007). In this aspect the challenge of chemometric approaches is to scrutinize interactions of ligands with the two PPAR subtypes simultaneously and to suggest models with the desired degree of selectivity.

The first 3D QSAR studies for α/γdual activity were based on the sum of activities, which implies "additivity" of fields in a CoMFA model. In this sense biological activities for the individual receptors are added to get the combined activity for both receptors on which CoMFA is performed. This strategy was used for a set of thiazolidinedione and oxazolidinedione derivatives with PPAR-α/γdual binding affinity (Khanna *et al.,*, 2005). The dual model was compared to independent CoMFA models derived for the PPAR-α and PPAR-γ activity of the compounds. It was clearly shown that the electrostatic fields contribute relatively more in the α-model, while the steric fields play an important role in the γ-model with large molecular regions, including the acidic head, favorable for bulkier groups. In the dual model a proper balance between these field contributions was observed, confirming that the resulting fields represent indeed "additivity fields" which incorporate features of both receptors.

Considering the advantages of 2D QSAR as simpler and easier interpretable models while maintaining receptor information, Lather *et al.,* (2009) developed receptor dependent volume descriptors suitable to be to be used for the design of multitarget ligands. These quantitative descriptors, labelled V_{site}, measure the volume occupied by a ligand within the common and/or specific regions defined by the superimposed binding sites of the targets under consideration, assuming that receptors targeted by the same ligand should share some common features in their binding sites. In the case of PPARs, V_α and V_γ correspond to the volume occupied by the ligands in the region specific for PPARα and PPARγ binding sites, respectively. These volume parameters in combination with other descriptors were used for the investigation of dual PPAR-α/γ activity of the thiazolidinedione and oxazolidinedione derivatives used by Khana et al., (2005) in the "sum model". Adapting the summation of pIC_{50} values for PPAR-α and PPAR-γ to express dual activity, three independent 2D QSAR models were established (for PPAR-α, PPAR-γ, and dual PPAR- α/γ ligands) with 27 compounds as training set and 7 as test set. In the PPAR-α model, with R^2=0.90, Q^2=0.85, and test set R^2_{pred}=0.62, volume $V_α$ was the main descriptor with a positive sign. Since this region at PPAR-α binding site is lined with hydrophobic residues this result outlines the importance of hydrophobic interactions in binding to this subtype. The second most important descriptor is a topographic electronic index reflecting electrostatic interactions, followed by two geometrical descriptors and a hydrogen bond related descriptor. In the PPAR-γ model, with R^2=0.89, Q^2=0.85, and R^2_{pred}=0.50 the main descriptor was related to hydrogen bonding, followed by the relative number of N atoms with positive sign. A gravitation index related to molecular mass and the number of double bonds contributed with a negative sign. The corresponding $V_γ$ descriptor, accounting for the small hydrophilic pocket which is specific of the PPAR-γ subtype, showed a lower negative contribution. The dual model with R^2=0.85, Q^2=0.77, and R^2_{pred}=0.69 showed molecular size, expressed as the number of atoms, as the most important descriptor with a negative sign; followed by a valence connectivity index, depicting different aspects of atom connectivity within a molecule, such as branching, flexibility, or the steric crowding around an atom and/bond. The number of oxygen atoms showed a negative contribution, while strong contribution of electrostatic interactions was reflected by other relevant descriptors. These models were used to design three new molecules, a dual agonist and two PPAR-α and PPAR-γ specific agonists according to docking results.

The key role of electronic properties of the substituents in the phenyl ring of the hydrophobic tail play was demonstrated in another 2D QSAR on dual PPAR-α/γ agonism of a series of 2-alkoxydihydrocinnamates, while the bulky substituents in the acidic head were found not to confer selectivity toward the PPAR activity (Kumar et al.,, 2008).

In order to circumvent the "sum of activity" assumption Vallianatou et al., (2013) established consensus 2D-QSAR models using PLS to analyze transactivation of a larger data set of 71 diverse dual PPAR-α/γ agonists compiled from different sources. PLS permits the simultaneous analysis of more than one interrelated response variables, providing overall global statistics, as well as separate statistics for each individual response variable. The authors used two pools of descriptors, one including a large number of physico-chemical, constitutional, and topological descriptors and a second including a limited number of easily interpretable drug-like and constitutional descriptors. The activity was expressed as pEC_{50}-α and pEC_{50}-γ values which were analyzed separately and concurrently. The size of the descriptor pool was found to have minor influence in the quality of the PLS models; thus, the authors chose the simpler model for further interpretation. Statistics for PPAR-α model were $R^2=0.791/Q^2=0.754$ and for PPAR-γ $R^2=0.782/Q^2=0.742$. The total statistics of the consensus dual activity model were $R^2=0.755$, $Q^2=0.713$, while individual statistics for each subtype were $R^2=0.757$, $Q^2=0.728$ and $R^2=0.752$, $Q^2=0.698$ for PPAR-α and PPAR-γ, respectively. The differentiation of important descriptors in the separate models is reflected in the higher impact of lipophilicity in PPAR-α, while bulk descriptors are more crucial for PPAR-γ activity and in certain specific structural descriptors, like the number of sulfur atoms in rings (Sr), which is important for PPAR-γ but is not included in the PPAR-α model, and the number of double bonds, which contribute considerably to PPAR-α, but less to PPAR-γ activity. The acidity (expressed as pka_{acid}) constitutes another important difference between the two receptor subtypes: pka_{acid} shows positive contribution to PPAR-γ activity, indicating that compounds with lower acidity are preferable, while this descriptor was not included in PPAR-α. The consensus PPAR-α/γ model displayed the same molecular features as the separate models, in a balanced "combination". The differentiations in receptor requirements for PPAR-α and γ subtypes as revealed by the separate models were supported by detailed inspection of the relevant crystal structures and molecular simulation studies. A blind test set was used to evaluate the performance of all models. A very good fit of the blind test set was obtained in the PPAR-α model, while pEC_{50}-γ values were in most cases considerably underestimated by the corresponding model. An explanation provided by the authors concerned the presence of oxadiazole in the test set, a structural feature not included in the training set. The presence of this feature seems to be essential in PPAR-γ activity while it did not affect PPAR-α. For the consensus PPAR-α/γ model acceptable predictions were obtained for both PPAR subtypes.

Dual PPAR-α/γ agonists have attracted interest in respect to other therapeutic areas such as ultraviolet B (UVB)-Induced skin inflammation (Park *et al.,*, 2013). Using molecular docking simulations, a synthetic compound MHY966 designed to treat UVB-induced skin inflammation proved to exhibit affinity for both PPARα/γ, being more selective for PPARα; however, this activity was validated in animal models.

7.5.3 Pan-AGONISTS, THE δ-RECEPTOR

PPAR-δ is the less investigated PPAR subtype. Its higher distribution in brain tissue renders it a possible drug target for neurodegenerative diseases, as already mentioned in Section 7.1. Nevertheless, the selective PPAR-δ agonist GW501516 has been shown to be associated with improved insulin sensitivity, elevated high density lipoproteins, and prevention of weight gain (Luquet $et\ al.$,, 2005). Following the problems associated with dual PPAR-α/γ agonists, many pharmaceutical companies have initiated efforts toward the design of compounds that activate all three PPAR subtypes (Adams $et\ al.$,, 2003; Mahindroo $et\ al.$,, 2006; Rudolph $et\ al.$,, 2007) Pan-agonists may offer a better pharmacological profile for drugs related to diabetes, obesity, and metabolic disorders, as validated also by animal studies.

The "sum of activities" approach was applied to analyze by the CoMFA methodology compounds with affinity toward the three PPAR subtypes (Shah $et\ al.$,, 2008); the training set included 23 oxadiazole-substituted a-isopropoxy phenylpropanoic acids with activities mainly not only on PPAR-α and PPAR-γ but also on PPAR-δ. The activity was expressed as transactivation pEC_{50} data. Three individual CoMFA models were first generated with satisfactory PLS statistics, followed by dual and multiple models; however, all models were validated using an external testset. A dual 5-component PPAR-α/γ CoMFA model was successfully developed with $R^2=0.998$ and $R^2_{cv}=0.756$. However, dual PPAR-γ/δ, dual PPAR-α/δ and multiple PPAR-α/γ/δ CoMFA models although with equally good correlation coefficients R^2 showed poor cross-validated R^2_{cv} (R^2_{cv}: 0.233, 0.267, and 0.430 respectively). This failure was attributed to the rather poor activity of the compounds toward PPAR-δ.

The same methodology was used for a different training set of 28 indanyl-acetic acid derivatives, carrying 4-thiazloyl-phenoxy tail groups; 9 more compounds were used as test set (Sundriyal and Bharatam, 2009). In this case, the activity was more pronounced for PPAR-δ relative to the two other subtypes. All generated models were found to be statistically significant with satisfactory statistics. The 5-component sum-model showed $R^2 = 0.981$, $R^2_{cv} = 0.757$; the corresponding values for the separate models were $R^2 = 0.969$, $R^2_{cv} = 0.670$ for the 5-component PPAR-α model, $R^2 = 0.969$, $R^2_{cv} = 0.555$ for the 6-component PPAR-δ model, and $R^2 = 0.941$, $R^2_{cv} = 0.549$ for the 5-component PPAR-γ model. Standard error of estimation (SEE) values ranged from 0.097 to 0.160. In the PPAR-δ model steric and electrostatic fields contribution was quasi-equal, whereas for PPAR-α and PPAR-γ subtypes steric fields had a considerably stronger contribution, their ratio in regard to electrostatic fields being larger for PPAR-α. This large ratio was maintained in the pan-agonist "sum model".

Dual PPAR-δ/α selectivity was studied for a larger data set of 70 compounds with α- and δ- activity and three PLS models were created, which in combination with molecular docking studies were used to understand the main reasons for PPAR-δ selectivity. The obtained results showed that some molecular descriptors such as log P, hydration energy, steric, and polar properties are related to the main interactions that can direct ligands to a particular PPAR subtype (Maltarollo and Honório, 2012).

Molecular modeling with a core hopping approach was used to screen multiple   scaffolds to generate a series of novel compounds with affinity toward all three PPAR subtypes (Zhang et al, 2012). After flexible docking procedures and molecular dynamics simulations, seven novel compounds were found using LY465608, a typical PPAR pan-agonist, as a guiding structure. The compounds not only showed a similar function in activating PPAR-α, PPAR-γ, and PPAR-δ but also assumed a conformation more favorable in binding to PPAR receptors. Prediction of drug-like properties according to QickProp showed that none of the compounds violated Lipinski's rule of 5 (Lipinski *et al.,*, 1997), with molecular weight and log P values lower than the typical PPAR-α and PPAR-γ ligands (Giaginis 2008b). Such lower values may be the result of structure compromise so that the compounds can fit PPAR-δ binding pocket as well. In any case this study shows that PPAR activity can be achieved also with smaller and less lipophilic compounds.

The above models consider PPAR-δ in conjunction to the other PPAR subtypes. Recently QSAR models have been developed for PPAR-δ agonists per se in order to better highlight the factors influencing binding to this PPAR subtype. The role of physico-chemical properties in the activation of PPAR-δ, expressed as pEC_{50}, was investigated for 35 structurally diverse compounds using PLS. A 4-component model was obtained with $R^2 = 0.90$, $Q^2 = 0.80$ and was successfully validated with an external test set of 10 compounds (Maltarollo *et al.,*, 2011). The authors identified important physico-chemical properties such as E_{LUMO} dipole moment, log P, which have been previously reported to contribute to the PPAR-γ activation by indole-based ligands (Giaginis *et al.,*, 2009). This fact was attributed to the high similarity of amino acid residues in the LBD of all PPAR isoforms. However, although not commented by the authors, log P as well as the volume descriptor appears with a negative sign, which may be explained by the smaller size of arm I in PPAR-δ LBD. Further to these properties, atomic charge at the phenyl carbon atom attached to an oxygen bridge, a topological descriptor related to atomic polarizabilty and aromaticity index were statistically significant with positive contribution (Maltarollo *et al.,*, 2011).

The negative contribution of lipophilicity was demonstrated also in a recent QSAR study of a large data set including 86 compounds with PPAR-δ as training set and 19 compounds as test set (Garcia *et al.,*, 2013). A PLS model was established with good statistics ($R^2=0.87$, $Q^2=0.83$). Next to lipophilicity (log P), electronegativity, expressed as the half sum of $E_{LUMO} + E_{HOMO}$, partial charge at the nitrogen atom of the heteroaromatic ring, as well as the number of oxygen and sulfur atoms contributed in a negative way, while positive sign was assigned to the partial charge at the carbonyl oxygen of the carboxylate and to molecular volume. Hologram QSAR (HQSAR) and CoMFA performed in the same study (Garcia *et al.*,, 2013) also resulted in good models with R^2=0.90, Q^2=0.73 and R^2=0.94, Q^2=0.88, respectively. HQSAR is a highly predictive technique and is used to estimate the biological activity of unknown compounds according to molecular fragment information (Honorio *et al.*,, 2007). Graphical representation of the HQSAR model pinpointing the positive and negative fragment contributions and the CoMFA contour maps indicated possible interactions between the PPAR-δ receptor and its agonists and led to suggestions for molecular modifications to design new compounds with improved biological properties (Garcia *et al.*,, 2013).

7.6 CONCLUSIONS

In PPAR research, structure- and ligand-based modeling advanced in parallel with both the resolution of X-ray crystal structures and the progress in biochemical investigation. Such studies have substantially contributed to the understanding of the mechanism of action and the identification of the essential structural requirements. A common skeleton is suggested for ligands activating all three subtypes; however, there is still considerable structural variation which may contribute to selectivity or to multiple targeting. Such subtle details in molecular structures are still being investigated through QSAR modeling. For this purpose structure- and ligand-based approaches or a combination of both are employed by means of different chemometric techniques. The difficulties associated with the establishment of global models, due to the large LBD cavity of PPARs, often lead to contradictory results in terms of the importance of molecular descriptors and differences in pharmacophoric models, corresponding to various chemical classes. It should be noted that although PPARs exert pleiotropic actions and may be involved in more pathophysiological conditions, currently QSAR studies aim to the design of novel antidiabeting agents. Achievements in biochemical research have influenced the focus of the chemometric techniques, to shift from the search of PPAR-γ agonists to PPAR-α/γ dual agonists or PPAR-α/γ/δ panagonists, as well as to partial PPAR-γ agonists, with the aim to reduce side effects. The critical balance of activities toward the different PPAR subtypes offers a challenge for a consensus between QSAR models. More to the point, ongoing investigations on the implication of PPARs in inflammation as well as in CNS may guide QSAR modeling under a new perspective.

KEYWORDS

- **Chemoinformatics**
- **Chemometrics**
- **Dual PPAR agonists**
- **Ligand based drug design**
- **PPAR agonists**
- **PPAR pan-agonists**
- **Structure based drug design**

REFERENCES

Adams, A. D.; Yuen, W.; Hu, Z.; Santini, C.; Jones, A. B.; MacNaul, K. L.; Berger, J. P.; Doebber, T. W.; Moller, D. E. Amphipathic 3-Phenyl-7-Propylbenzisoxazoles; Human PPAR gamma, delta and alpha Agonists. *Bioorg. Med. Chem. Lett.* **2003**, *13*, 931–935.

Aleshin, S.; Strokin, M.; Sergeeva, M.; Reiser, G. Peroxisome Proliferator-Activated Receptor (PPAR) β/δ, a Possible Nexus of PPARα- and PPARγ-Dependent Molecular Pathways in eurodegenerative Diseases: Review and Novel Hypotheses. *Neurochem. Int.* **2013**, *63*, 322–330.

Al-Najjar, B. O.; Wahab, H. A.; Tengku Muhammad, T. S.; Shu-Chien A. C.; Ahmad Noruddin, N. A.; Taha M. O. Discovery of New Nanomolar Peroxisome Proliferator-Activated Receptor γ Activators via Elaborate Ligand-Based Modeling. *Eur. J. Med. Chem.* **2011**, *46*, 2513–2529.

Artis, D. R..; Lin, J. J.; Zhang, C.; Wang, W.; Mehra, U.; Perreault, M.; Erbe, D.; Krupka, H. I.; England, B. P.; Arnold, J.; Plotnikov, A. N.; Marimuthu, A.; Nguyen, H.; Wil,l S.; Signaevsky, M.; Kral, J.; Cantwell. J.; Settachatgull, C.; Yan, D. S.; Fong, D.; Oh, A.; Shi, S.; Womack, P.; Powell, B.; Habets, G.; West, B. L.; Zhang, K. Y. J.; Milburn, M. V.; Vlasuk, G. P.; Hirth, K. P.; Nolop, K.; Bollag, G.; Ibrahim, P. N.; Tobin, J. F.; Scaffold-based discovery of indeglitazar, a PPAR pan-active anti-diabetic agent. *Proc Natl Acad Sci U S A* **2009**; *106*, 262–267.

Balakumar, P.; Rose, M.; Ganti, S. S.; Krishan, P.; Singh, M. PPAR dual agonists: Are they opening pandora's box? *Pharmacol. Res.* **2007**, *56*, 91–98.

Barish, G. D.; Narkar, V. A.; Evans, R.M. PPAR delta: A Dagger in the Heart of the Metabolic Syndrome. *J. Clin. Invest.* **2006**, *116*, 590–597.

Berger, J.; Moller, D. E. The Mechanisms of Action of PPARs. *Ann. Rev. Med.* **2002**, 53, 409–435.

Berman, H. M.; Westbrook, J.; Feng, Z.; Gilliland, G.; Bhat, N.; Weissig, H.; Shindyalov, I. N.; Bourne, P. E. The Protein Data Bank. *Nucleic Acids Res.* **2000**, *28*, 235–242.

Berman, H. M.; Battistuz, T.; Bhat, T. N.; Bluhm, W. F.; Bourne, P. E.; Burkhardt, K.; Feng, Z.; Gilliland, G. L.; Iype, L.; Jain, S.; Fagan, P.; Marvin, J.; Padilla, D.; Ravichandran, V.; Schneider, B.; Thanki, N.; Weissig, H.; Westbrook, J. D.; Zardecki, C. The Protein Data Bank. *Acta Crystallogr. D* **2002**, *58*, 899–907.

Blaschke, F.; Takata, Y.; Caglayan, E.; Law, R.E.; Hsueh, W.A. Obesity, Peroxisome Proliferator-Activated Receptor, and Atherosclerosis in Type 2 Diabetes. *Arterioscler. Thromb. Vasc. Biol.* **2006**, *26*, 28–40.

Bohacek, R. S.; McMartin, C.; Guida, W. C. The Art and Practice of Structure-Based Drug Design: A Molecular Modeling Perspective. *Med. Res. Rev.* **1996**, *16*, 3–50.

Bourguet, W.; Ruff, M.; Chambon, P.; Gronemeyer, H.; Moras, D. Crystal Structure of the Ligand-Binding Domain of the Human Nuclear Receptor RXR-alpha. *Nature* **1995**, *375*, 377–382.

Braissant, O.; Foufelle, F.; Scotto, C.; Dauça, M.; Wahli, W. Differential Expression of Peroxisome Proliferator-Activated Receptors (PPARs): Tissue distribution of PPAR-α, β- and –γ in the Adult Rat. *Endocrinology* 1996, *137*, 354–366.

Burgermeister, E.; Schnoebelen, A.; Flament, A.; Benz, J.; Stihle, M.; Gsell, B.; Rufer, A.; Ruf, A.; Kuhn, B.; Marki, H.P.; Mizrahi, J.; Sebokova, E.; Niesor, E.; Meyer, M. A Novel Partial Agonist of Peroxisome Proliferators Activated Receptor-gamma (PPAR gamma) Recruits PPAR gamma-Coactivator-1alpha, Prevents Triglyceride Accumulation, and Potentiates Insulin Signaling in Vitro. *Mol. Endocrinol.* 2006, *20*, 809–830.

Cabrero, A.; Llaverias, G.; Roglans, N.; Alegret, M.; Sanchez, R.; Adzet, T.; Laguna, J. C.; Vázquez, M. Uncoupling Protein-3 mRNA Levels Are Increased in White Adipose Tissue and Skeletal Muscle of Bezafibrate-Treated Rats. *Biochem. Biophys. Res. Commun.* 1999, *260*, 547–556.

Caporuscio, F.; Tafi, A. Pharmacophore Modelling: A Forty Year Old Approach and Its Modern Synergies. *Curr. Med. Chem.* 2011, *18*, 2543–2553.

Carta, A. R. PPAR-γ: Therapeutic Prospects in Parkinson's Disease. *Curr. Drug Targets* 2013, *14*, 743–751

Cherkasov, A.; Muratov, E. N.; Fourches, D.; Varnek, A.; Baskin, I.I.; Cronin, M.; Dearden, J.; Gramatica, P.; Martin, Y. C.; Todeschini, R.; Consonni, V.; Kuz'min, V. E.; Cramer, R.; Benigni, R.; Yang, C.; Rathman, J.; Terfloth, L.; Gasteiger, J.; Richard, A.; Tropsha, A. QSAR Modeling: Where Have You Been? Where Are You Going To? *J. Med. Chem.* 2014 [Epub ahead of print].

Chirico, N.; Gramatica, P. Real External Predictivity of QSAR Models. Part 2. New Intercomparable Thresholds for Different Validation Criteria and the Need for Scatter Plot Inspection. *J. Chem. Inf. Model.* 2012, *52*, 2044–2058.

Choi, J. H.; Banks, A. S.; Estall, J. L.; Kajimura, S.; Boström, P.; Laznik, D.; Ruas, J.L.; Chalmers, M. J.; Kameneck, T. M.; Blüher, M.; Griffin, P. R.; Spiegelman, B. M. Anti-Diabetic Drugs Inhibit Obesity-Linked Phosphorylation of PPARγ 3 by Cdk5. *Nature* 2010, *466*, 451–456.

Cramer, R. D., III; Patterson, D. E.; Bunce, J. D. Comparative Molecular Field Analysis (CoMFA). 1. Effect of Shape on Binding of Steroids to Carrier Proteins. *J. Am. Chem. Soc.* 1988, *110*, 5959–5967

Cramer R. D., III. The Inevitable QSAR Renaissance. *J. Comput. Aided Mol. Des.* 2012, *26*, 35–38.

Cramer R. D., III. Rethinking 3D-QSAR. *J. Comput. Aided Mol. Des.* 2011, *25*, 197–201.

Cronin, M.T. Computational Methods for the Prediction of Drug Toxicity. *Curr. Opin. Drug Disc. Develop.* 2000, *3*, 292–297

Desvergne, B.; Wahli, W. Peroxisome Proliferator-Activated Receptors: Nuclear Control of Metabolism. *Endocr. Rev.* 1999, *20*, 649–688.

Dixit, A.; Saxena, A.K. QSAR Analysis of PPAR-gamma Agonists as Anti-Diabetic Agents. *Eur. J. Med. Chem.* 2008, *43*, 73–80.

Dreyer, C.; Krey, G.; Keller, H.; Givel, F.; Helftenbein, G.; Wahli, W. Control of the Peroxisomal b-Oxidation Pathway by a Novel Family of Nuclear Hormone Receptors. *Cell* 1992, *68*, 879–887.

Durant, J. L.; Leland, B. A.; Henry, D. R.; Nourse, J. G. Reoptimization of MDL Keys for Use in Drug Discovery. *J. Chem. Inf. Comput. Sci.* 2002, *42*, 1273–1280.

Duval, C.; Müller, M.; Kersten, S. PPARα and Dyslipidemia. *Biochim. Biophys. Acta* 2007, *1771*, 961–971.

Ebdrup, S.; Pettersson, I.; Rasmussen, H. B.; Deussen, H.; Jensen, A. F.; Mortensen, S. B.; Fleckner, J.; Pridal, L.; Nygaard, L.; Sauerberg, P. Synthesis and Biological and Structural Characterzation of the Dual-Acting Peroxisome Proliferator- Activated Receptor α/γ Agonist Ragaglitazar. *J. Med. Chem.* 2003, *46*, 1306–1317.

Ekins, S.; Bravi, G.; Binkley, S.; Gillespie, J. S.; Ring, B. J.; Wikel, J. H.; Wrighton, S. A. Three-and Four-Dimensional Quantitative Structure–Activity Relationship Analyses of Cytochrome P450 3A4 Inhibitors. *J. Pharmacol. Exp. Ther.*1999, *290*, 429–438.

Escher, P.; Braissant, O.; Basu-Modak, S.; Michalik, L.; Wahli, W.; Desvergne, B. Rat PPARs: Quantitative Analysis in Adult Rat Tissues and Regulation in Fasting and Refeeding. *Endocrinology* 2001, *142*, 4195–4202.

Fagerberg, B.; Edwards, S.; Halmos, T.; Lopatynski, J.; Schuster, H.; Stender, S.; Stoa-Birketvedt, G.; Tonstad, S.; Halldórsdóttir, S.; Gause-Nilsson, I. Tesaglitazar, a Novel Dual Peroxisome Proliferators-Ativated Receptor α/γ Agonist, Dose-Dependently Improves the Metabolic Abnormalities Associated with Insuln Resistance in a Non-Diabetic Population. *Diabetologia* 2005, 48, 1716–1725.

Fajas, L.; Auboeuf, D.; Raspé, E.; Schoonjans, K.; Lefebvre, A.M.; Saladin, R.; Najib, J.; Laville, M.; Fruchart, J.C.; Deeb, S.; Vidal-Puig, A.; Flier, J.; Briggs, M.R.; Staels, B.; Vidal, H.; Auwerx, J. The Organization, Promoter Analysis, and Expression of the Human PPARγ Gene. *J. Biol. Chem.* 1997, 272, 18779–18789.

Feige, J. N.; Gelman, L.; Michalik, L.; Desvergne, B.; Wahli, W. From Molecular Action to Physiological Outputs: Peroxisome Proliferator-Activated Receptors Are Nuclear Receptors at the Crossroads of Key Cellular Functions. *Progr. Lipid Res.* 2006, 45, 120–159.

Ferguson, A. M.; Heritage, T.; Jonathon, P.; Pack, S. E.; Philips, L.; Rogan, J.; Snaith, P. J. EVA: A New Theoretically Based Molecular Descriptor for Use in QSAR/QSPR Analysis. *J. Comput. Aided Mol. Des.* 1997, *11*, 143–152.

Ferry, G.; Bruneau, V.; Beauverger, P.; Goussard, M.; Rodriguez, M.; Lamamy, V.; Dromaint, S.; Canet, E.; Galizzi, J.-P.; Boutin, J. A. Binding of Prostaglandins to Human PPAR-γ: Tool Assessment and New Natural Ligands. *Eur. J. Pharmacol.*2001, *77*, 417–489.

Fyffe, S. A.; Alphey, M. S.; Buetow, L.; Smith, T. K.; Ferguson, M. A.; Sørensen, M. D.; Björkling, F.; Hunter, W. N. Recombinant Human PPAR-β/δ Ligand-binding Domain is Locked in an Activated Conformation by Endogenous Fatty Acids. *J. Mol. Biol.*2006, *356*, 1005–1013.

Gandhi, G. R.; Stalin, A.; Balakrishna, K.; Ignacimuthu, S.; Paulraj, M. G.; Vishal, R. Insulin Sensitization via Partial Agonism of PPARγ and Glucose Uptake through Translocation and Activation of GLUT4 in PI3K/p-Akt Signaling Pathway by Embelin in Type 2 Diabetic Rats. *Biochim. Biophys. Acta* 2013, *1830*, 2243–2255.

Gampe, R. T., Jr.; Montana, V. G.; Lambert, M. H.; Miller, A. B.; Bledsoe, R. K.; Milburn, M. V.; Kliewer, S. A.; Willson, T. M.; Xu, H. E. Asymmetry in the PPARγ/RXRR Crystal Structure Reveals the Molecular Basis of Heterodimerization Among Nuclear Receptors. *Mol. Cell* 2000, *5*, 545–555.

Gangloff, M.; Ruff, M.; Eiler, S.; Duclaud, S.; Wurtz, J. M.; Moras, D. Crystal Structure of a Mutant hERalpha Ligand-Binding Domain Reveals Key Structural Features for the Mechanism of Partial Agonism. *J. Biol. Chem.*2001, *276*, 15059–15065.

Garcia , T. S.; Silva , D. C.; Gertrudes, J. C.; Maltarollo, V. G.; Honorio, K. M. Molecular Features Related to the Binding Mode of PPARδ Agonists from QSAR and Docking Analyses. *SAR QSAR Environ. Res.* 2013, *24*, 157–173.

Giaginis, C.; Theocharis, S.; Tsantili-Kakoulidou, A. A Consideration of PPAR-γ Ligands in respect to Lipophilicity: Current Trends and Perspectives. *Expert Opin. Investig. Drugs* 2007, *16*, 413–417.

Giaginis, C.; Theocharis, S.; Tsantili-Kakoulidou, A. Application of Multivariate Data Analysis For Modeling Receptor Binding and Gene Transactivation of Tyrosine-Based PPAR-γ Ligands, *Chem. Biol. Drug Des.*2008a, *72*, 257–264.

Giaginis, C.; Zira, A.; Theocharis, S.; Tsantili-Kakoulidou, A. Property Distribution in the Chemical Space of PPAR-γ Agonists: Evaluation of Drug-like Characteristics. *Rev. Clin. Pharmacol. Pharmacokin. Intern. Ed.*2008b, *22*, 366–368.

Giaginis, C.; Theocharis, S.; Tsantili-Kakoulidou,A. A QSAR Study on Indole-based PPAR-γ Agonists with respect to Receptor Binding and Transactivation Data. *QSAR Comb. Sci.* **2009**, *28*, 802–805.

Glesson, P.; Hersey, A.; Hannongbua, S. *In Silico* ADME Models: A General Assessment of their Utility in Drug Discovery Applications. *Curr. Top. Med. Chem.* **2011**, *11*, 358–381.

Grether, U.; Klaus, W.; Kuhn, B.; Maerki, H. P.; Mohr, P.; Wright, M. B. New Insights on the Mechanism of PPAR-targeted Drugs, *ChemMedChem* **2010**, *5*, 1973–1976.

Guasch, L.; Sala, E.; Valls, C.; Blay, M.; Mulero, M.; Arola, L.; Pujadas, G.; Garcia-Vallvé, S. Structural Insights for the Design of New PPARgamma Partial Agonists with High Binding Affinity and Low Transactivation Activity. *J. Comput. Aided Mol. Des.* **2011**, *25*, 717–728.

Guasch, L.; Sala, E.; Valls, C.; Mulero, M.; Pujadas, G.;Garcia-Vallvea, S. Development of Docking-based 3D-QSAR Models for PPARgamma Full Agonists. *J. Mol. Graph. Model.***2012**, *36*, 1–9.

Gurley, C.; Nichols, J.; Liu, S.; Phulwani, N. K.; Esen, N.; Kielian, T. Microglia and Astrocyte Activation by Toll-Like Receptor Ligands: Modulation by PPAR-γ Agonists. *PPAR Research* **2008**, 1–15.

Haigh, D.; Allen, G.; Birrell, H. C.; Buckle, D. R.; Cantello, B. C. C.; Eggleston, D. S.; Halti-wanger, R. C.; Holder, J. C.; Lister, C. A.; Pinto, I. L.; Rami, H. K.; Sime, J. T.; Smith, S. A.; Sweeney, J. D. Non-Thiazolidinedione Antihyperglycaemic Agents. Part 3: The Effects of Stereochemistry on the Potency of α-methoxy-β-Phenylpropanoic Acids. *Bioorg. Med. Chem.***1999**, *7*, 821–830.

Henke, B. R. Peroxisome Proliferator-Activated Receptor α/γDual Agonists for the Treatment of Type 2 Diabetes. *J. Med. Chem.***2004**, *47*, 4118–4127.

Honorio, K. M.; Montanari, C. A.; Andricopulo, A. D. Two-Dimensional Quantitative Structure Activity Relationships: Hologram QSAR. In *Current Methods in Medicinal Chemistry and Biological Physics*; Taft, C. A., Silva, C. H. T. P., Eds, Research Signpost: India, **2007**; Vol. 1, pp. 49–60.

Hopfinger, A. J.; Wang, S.; Tokarski, J. S.; Jin, B.; Albuquerque, M.; Madhav, P.J.; Duraiswami, C. Construction of 3D-QSAR Models Using 4D-QSAR Analysis Formalism. *J. Am. Chem. Soc.***1997**, *119*, 10509–10524.

Houtkooper, R. H.; Auwerx, J. Obesity, New Life for Anti-Diabetic Drugs. *Nature* **2010**, *466*, 443 444.

Ichihara, S.; Obata, K.; Yamada, Y.; Nagata, K.; Noda, A.; Ichihara, G.; Yamada, A.; Kato, T.; Izawa, H.; Murohara, T.; Yokota, M. Attenuation of Cardiac Dysfunction by a PPAR-α Agonist is Associated with Down-Regulation of Redox-regulated Transcription Factors. *J. Mol. Cell. Cardiol.***2006**, *41*, 318–329.

Iwashita, A.; Muramatsu, Y.; Yamazaki, T.; Muramoto, M.; Kita, Y.; Yamazaki, S.; Mihara, K.; Moriguchi, A.; Matsuoka, N. Neuroprotective Efficacy of the Peroxisome Proliferator-Acti-vated Receptor δ-Selective Agonists in Vitro and in Vivo. *J. Pharmacol. Exp. Ther.***2007**, *320*, 1087–1096.

Kapadia, R.; Yi, J -H.; Vemuganti, R. Mechanisms of Anti-Inflammatory and Neuroprotective Actions of PPAR-gamma Agonists. *Front. Biosci.***2009**, *13*, 1813–1826.

Kashaw, S. K.; Rathi, L. G.; Mishra, P.; Saxena, A. K. Development of 3D-QSAR Models in Cy-clic Ureidobenzenesulfonamides: Human beta3-Adrenergic Receptor Agonist. *Bioorg. Med. Chem. Lett.* **2003**, *13*, 2481–2484.

Kendall, D. M.; Rubin, C. J.; Mohideen, P.; Ledeine, J. M.; Belder, R.; Gross, J.; Norwood, P.; O'Mahony, M.; Sall, K.; Sloan, G.; Roberts, A.; Fiedorek, F. T.; DeFronzo, R. A. Improve-ment of Glycemic Control, Triglycerides, and HDL Cholesterol Levels with Muraglitazar, a Dual (α/γ) Peroxisome Proliferator-Activated Receptor Activator, in Patients with Type 2 Diabetes Inadequately Controlled with Metformin Monotherapy: A Double-blind, Randomized, Pioglitazone-Comparative Study. *Diabetes Care* **2006**, *29*, 1016–1023.

Khanna, S.; Sobhia, M. E.; BharatamP. V. Additivity of Molecular Fields: CoMFA Study on Dual Activators of PPARα and PPARγ. *J. Med. Chem.* **2005**, *48*, 3015–3025.

Klebe, G. Recent Developments in Structure-Based Drug Design. *J. Mol. Med.* **2000**, *78*, 269–281.

Klebe, G. Comparative Molecular Similarity Indices Analysis: CoMSIA. *Perspect. Drug Discov. Des.* **1998**, *12*, 87–104.

Kocalis, H. E.; Turney, M. K.; Printz, R. L.; Laryea, G. N.; Muglia, L. J.; Davies, S. S.; Stanwood, G. D.; McGuinness, O. P.; Niswender, K. D. Neuron-Specific Deletion of Peroxisome Proliferator-Activated Receptor Delta (PPARδ) in Mice Leads to Increased Susceptibility to Diet-Induced Obesity. *PLoS One* **2012**, *7*, art. no. e42981.

Kortagere, S. (ed). *In Silico* Models for Drug Discovery. In Methods in Molecular Biology. Vol 993 Springer; New York **2013**.

Kulkarni, S. S.; Gediya, L. K.; Kulkarni, V. M. Three-dimensional Quantitative Structure Activity Relationships (3-D-QSAR) of Antihyperglycemic Agents. *Bioorg. Med. Chem.* **1999**, *7*, 1475–1485.

Kumar, P. M.; Hemalatha, R.; Mahajan, S. C.; Karthikeyan, C.; Moorthy, N. S.; Trivedi, P. Quantitative Structure-Activity Analysis of 2-Alkoxydihydrocinnamates as PPARα /γ Dual Agonist. *Med. Chem.* **2008**, *4*, 273–277.

Lather, V.; Kairys, V.; Fernandes, M. X. Quantitative Structure Activity Relationship Model with Receptor-dependent Descriptors for Predicting Peroxisome Proliferator Activated Receptor Affinities of Thiazolidinedione and Oxazolidinedione Derivatives. *Chem. Biol. Drug Des.* **2009**, *73*, 428–441.

Lee, C. H.; Chawla, A.; Urbiztondo, N.; Liao, D.; Boisvert, W. A.; Evans, R. M.; Curtiss, L. K. Transcriptional Repression of Atherogenic Inflammation: Modulation by PPAR delta. *Science* **2003**, *302*, 453–457.

Lenhard, J. M. PPAR Gamma/RXR as a Molecular Target for Diabetes. *Receptors Channels* **2001**, *7*, 249–258.

Lewis, D. F. V.; Lake B. G. Molecular Modelling of the Rat Peroxisome Proliferator-activated Receptor -α (rPPARα) by Homology with the Human Retinoic Acid X Receptor a (hRXRa) and Investigation of Ligand Binding Interactions I: QSARs. *Toxicol. In Vitro* **1998**, *12*, 619–632.

Lewis, D. F. V.; Jacobs, M. N.; Dickins, M.; Lake, B. G. Molecular Modelling of the Peroxisome Proliferator-Activated Receptor α (PPARα) from Human, Rat and Mouse, Based on Homology with the Human PPARγ Crystal Structure. *Toxicol. In Vitro* **2002**, *16*, 275–280.

Li, Y.; Choi, M.; Suino, K.; Kovach, A.; Daugherty, J.; Kliewer, S.A.; Xu, H. E. Structural and Biochemical Basis for Selective Repression of the Orphan Nuclear Receptor Liver Receptor Homolog 1 by Small Heterodimer Partner. *Proc. Natl. Acad. Sci. U. S. A.* **2005**, *102*, 9505–9510.

Liao, C. Z.; Xie, A. H.; Shi, L. M.; Zhou, J. J.; Lu, X. P. 3D QSAR Studies on Peroxisome Proliferator-Activated Receptor gammaAgonists using CoMFA and CoMSIA. *J. Mol. Model.* **2004**, *10*, 165–177.

Liao, C. Z.; Xie, A. H.; Shi, L. M.; Zhou, J. J.; Lu, X. P. Eigen value Analysis of Peroxisome Proliferator-Activated Receptor-γAgonists, *J. Chem. Inf. Comput. Sci.* **2004**, *44*, 230–238.

Lipinski, C. A.; Lombardo, F.; Dominy, B. W.; Feeney, P. J. Experimental and Computational Approaches to Estimate Solubility and Permeability in DrugDiscovery and Development Settings. *Adv. Drug. Deliv. Rev.* **1997**, *23*, 3–25.

Liu, K.; Black, R. M.; Acton, J. J. 3rd; Mosley, R.; Debenham, S.; Abola, R.; Yang, M.; Tschirret-Guth, R.; Colwell, L.; Liu, C.; Wu, M.; Wang, C. F.; MacNaul, K. L.; McCann, M. E.; Moller, D. E.; Berger, J. P.; Meinke, P. T.; Jones, A. B.; Wood, H. B. Selective PPARγ Modulators with Improved Pharmacological Profiles. *Bioorg. Med. Chem. Lett.* **2005**, *15*, 2437–2440.

Lohray, B. B.; Bhushan, V.; Bajji, A. C.; Kalchar, S.; Poondra, R. R.; Padakanti, S.; Chakra-barti, R.; Vikramadityan, R. K.; Mishra, P.; Juluri, S.; Mamidi, N. V. S. R.; Rajagopalan, R. (-)3-[4-[2-(Phenoxazin-10-yl) ethoxy]phenyl]-2-ethoxypropanoic Acid [(-)DRF 2725]: A Dual PPAR Agonist with Potent Antihyperglycemic and Lipid Modulating Acitivity. *J. Med. Chem.* **1999**, *42*, 2569–2581.

Lu, I.-L.; Huang, C.-F.; Peng, Y.-H.; Lin, Y.-T.; Hsieh, H.-P.; Chen, C.-T.; Lien, T.-W.; Lee, H.-J.; Mahindroo, N.; Prakash, E.; Yueh, A.; Chen, H.-Y.; Goparaju, C.M.V.; Chen, X.; Liao, C.-C.; Chao, Y.-S.; Hsu, J.-T.A.; Wu, S.-Y. Structure-based Drug Design of a Novel Family of PPAR Partial Agonists: Virtual Screening, X-ray Crystallography, and in Vitro/in Vivo Biological Activities. *J. Med. Chem.* **2006**, *49*, 2703–2712.

Luquet, S.; Gaudel, C.; Holst, D.; Lopez-Soriano, J.; Jehl-Pietri, C.; Fredenrich, A.; Grimaldi, P. A. Roles of PPAR Delta in Lipid Absorption and Metabolism: A New Target for the Treatment of Type 2 Diabetes. *Biochim. Biophys. Acta* **2005**, *1740*, 313–317.

Mahindroo, N.; Wang, C. C.; Liao, C.C.; Huang, C. F.; Lu, I. L.; Lien, T. W.; Peng, Y. H.; Huang, W. J.; Lin, Y. T.; Hsu, M. C.; Lin, C. H.; Tsai, C. H.; Hsu, J. T.; Chen, X.; Lyu, P. C.; Chao, Y. S.; Wu, S. Y.; Hsieh, H. P. Indol-1-yl Acetic Acids as Peroxisome Proliferator-Activated Receptor Agonists: Design, Synthesis, Structural Biology, and Molecular Docking Studies. *J. Med. Chem.* **2006**, *49*, 1212–1216.

Maltarollo, V. G.; Homem-de-Mello, P.; Honorio, K. M. Role of Physicochemical Properties in the Activation of Peroxisome Proliferator-Activated Receptor δ. *J. Mol. Model.* **2011**, *17*, 2549–2558.

Maltarollo, V. G.; Honório, K. M. Ligand- and Structure-based Drug Design Strategies and PPARδ/α Selectivity. *Chem. Biol. Drug Des.* **2012**, *80*, 533–544.

Markt, P.; Schuster, D.; Kirchmair, J.; Laggner, C.; Langer, T. Pharmacophore Modeling and Parallel Screening for PPAR Ligands. *J. Comput. Aided Mol. Des.* **2007**, *21*, 575–590.

Michalik, L.; Desvergne, B.; Wahli, W. Peroxisome-Proliferator-Activated Receptors and Cancers: Complex Stories. *Nat. Rev. Cancer* **2004**, *4*, 61–70.

Minovski, N.; Zuperl, S.; Drgan, V.; Novic, M. Assessment of Applicability Domain for Multi-variate Counter-Propagation Artificial Neural Network Predictive Models by Minimum Euclidean Distance Space Analysis: A Case Study. *Anal. Chim. Acta* **2013**, *759*, 28–42.

Montanari, R.; Saccoccia, F.; Scotti, E.; Crestani, M.; Godio, C.; Gilardi, F.; Loiodice, F.; Frac-chiolla, G.; Laghezza, A.; Tortorella, P.; Lavecchia, A.; Novellino, E.; Mazza, F.; Aschi, M.; Pochetti, G.Crystal Structure of the Peroxisome Proliferator-Activated Receptor γ (PPARγ) Ligand Binding Domain Complexed with a Novel Partial Agonist: A New Region of the Hydrophobic Pocket Could Be Exploited for Drug Design. *J. Med. Chem.* **2008**, *51*, 7768–7776.

Moroy, G.; Martiny, V. Y.; Vayer, P.; Villoutreix, B. O.; Miteva, M. A. Towards *in Silico* Structure-Based ADMET Prediction in Drug Discovery. *Drug Discov. Today* **2012**, *17*, 44–55.

Murphy, G.J.; Holder, J.C. PPAR-gamma Agonists: Therapeutic Role in Diabetes, Inflammation and Cancer. *Trends Pharmacol. Sci.* **2000**, *21*, 469–474.

Nagasawa, T.; Inada, Y.; Nakano, S.; Tamura, T.; Takahashi, T.; Maruyama, K.; Yamazaki, Y.; Kuroda, J.; Shibata, N. Effects of Bezafibrate, PPAR Pan-agonist, and GW501516, PPARdelta Agonist, on Development of Steatohepatitis in Mice Fed a Methionine- and Choline-Deficient Diet. *Eur. J. Pharmacol.* **2006**, *536*, 182–191.

Neher, M. D.; Weckbach, S.; Huber-Lang, M. S.; Stahel, P. F. New Insights into the Role of Peroxisome Proliferator-Activated Receptors in Regulating the Inflammatory Response after Tissue Injury. *PPAR Research* **2012**, *2012*, 1–13.

Nosjean, O.; Boutin, J.A. Natural Ligands of PPARγ: Are Prostaglandin J(2) Derivatives Really Playing the Part? *Cell Signal.* **2002**, *14*, 573–583.

Park, M. H.; Park, J. Y.; Lee, H. J.; Kim, D. H.; Chung, K. W.; Park, D.; Jeong, H. O.; Kim, H. R.; Park, C. H.; Kim, S. R.; Chun, P.; Byun, Y.; Moon, H. R.; Chung, H. Y. The Novel PPAR α/γ Dual Agonist MHY 966 Modulates UVB-induced Skin Inflammation by Inhibiting NF-κB Activity. *PLoS One* **2013**, *8*, art. no. e76820.

Parks, D. J.; Tomkinson, N. C. O.; Villeneuve, M. S.; Blanchard, S. G.; Willson, T. M. Differential Activity of Rosiglitazone Enantiomers at PPARγ. *Bioorg. Med. Chem. Lett.***1998**, *8*, 3657–3658.

Paterniti, I.; Impellizzeri, D.; Crupi, R.; Morabito, R.; Campolo, M.; Esposito, E.; Cuzzocrea, S. Molecular Evidence for the Involvement of PPAR-δ and PPAR-γ in Anti-Inflammatory and Neuroprotective Activities of Palmitoylethanolamide after Spinal Cord Trauma. *J. Neuroinflammation***2013**, *10*.

Peraza, M. A.; Burdick, A. D.; Marin, H. E.; Gonzalez, F. J.; Peters, J. M. The Toxicology of Ligands for Peroxisome Proliferator-Activated Receptors (PPAR). *Toxicol. Sci.***2006**, *90*, 269–295.

Petersen, R. K.; Christensen, K. B.; Assimopoulou, A. N.; Fretté, X.; Papageorgiou, V. P.; Kristiansen, K.; Kouskoumvekaki, I. Pharmacophore-driven Identification of PPARγ Agonists from Natural Sources. *J Comput. Aided Mol Des.***2011**, *25*, 107–116.

Pochetti, G.; Godio, C.; Mitro, N.; Caruso, D.; Galmozzi, A.; Scurati, S.; Loiodice, F.; Fracchiolla, G.; Tortorella, P.; Laghezza, A.; Lavecchia, A.; Novellino, E.; Mazza, F.; Crestani, M. Insights into the Mechanism of Partial Agonism: Crystal Structures of the Peroxisome Proliferator-Activated Receptor γ Ligand-binding Domain in the Complex with two Enantiomeric Ligands. *J. Biol. Chem.***2007**, *282*, 17314–17324.

Polanski, J. Receptor Dependent Multidimensional QSAR for Modeling Drug–Receptor Interactions. *Curr. Med. Chem.* **2009**, *16*, 3243–3257.

Puzyn, T.; Leszczynski, J.; Cronin, M. T. Recent Advances in QSAR Studies: Methods and Applications. In *Challenges and Advances in Computational Chemistry and Physics;* Leszczynski, J., Ed.; Springer: Vol 8, **2010**.

Rathi, L.; Kashaw, S. K.; Dixit, A.; Pandey, G.; Saxena, A. K. Pharmacophore Identification and 3D-QSAR Studies in N-(2-benzoyl phenyl)-L-tyrosines as PPARγ Agonists. *Bioorg. Med. Chem.***2004**, *12*, 63–69.

Renaud, J.; Rochel, N.; Ruff, M.; Vivat, V.; Chambon, P., Gronemeyer, H.; Moras, D. Crystal Structure of the RAR-[gamma] Ligand-binding Domain Bound to all-trans Retinoic Acid. *Nature* **1995**, *378*, 681–689.

Rieusset, J.; Andreelli, F.; Auboeuf, D.; Roques, M.; Vallier, P.; Riou, J. P.; Auwerx, J.; Laville, M.; Vidal, H. Insulin Acutely Regulates the Expression of the Peroxisome Proliferator-Activated Receptor-γ in Human Adipocytes. *Diabetes* **1999**, *48*, 699–705.

Rosenson, R. S.; Wright, R. S.; Farkouh, M.; Plutzky, J. Modulating Peroxisome Proliferator-Activated Receptors for Therapeutic Benefit? Biology, Clinical Experience, and Future Prospects. *Am. Heart J.***2012**, *164*, 672–680.

Roy, K.; Mitra, L.; Kar, S.; Ojha, P. K.; Das, R. N.; Kabir, H. Comparative Studies on Some Metrics for External Validation of QSPR Models. *J. Chem. Inf. Model.***2012**, *52*, 396–408.

Rücker, C.; Scarsi, M.; Meringer, M. 2D QSAR of PPARγ Agonist Binding and Transactivation. *Bioorg. Med. Chem.* **2006**, *14*, 5178–5195.

Rudolph, J.; Chen, L.; Majumdar, D.; Bullock, W. H.; Burns, M.; Claus, T.; Dela Cruz, F. E.; Daly, M.; Ehrgott, F. J.; Johnson, J. S.; Livingston, J. N.; Schoenleber, R. W.; Shapiro, J.; Yang, L.; Tsutsumi, M.; Ma, X. Indanylacetic Acid Derivatives Carrying 4-Thiazolyl-phenoxy Tail Groups, a New Class of Potent PPAR α/γ/δ Pan Agonists: Synthesis, Structure-Activity Relationship, and Iin Vivo Efficacy. *J. Med. Chem.***2007**, *50*, 984–1000.

Sakiyama, Y. The Use of Machine Learning and Nonlinear Statistical Tools for ADME Prediction. *Expert Opin. Drug Metab. Toxicol.***2009**, *5*, 149–169.

Sauerberg, P.; Pettersson, I.; Jeppesen, L.; Bury, P. S.; Mogensen, J. P.; Wassermann, K.; Brand, C. L.; Sturis, J.; Woldike, H. F.; Fleckner, J.; Andersen, A. T.; Mortensen, S. B.; Svensson, L.

A.; Rasmussen, H. B.; Lehmann, S. V.; Polivka, Z.; Sindelar, K.; Panajotova, V.; Ynddal, L.; Wulff, E. M. Novel Tricyclic-Ralkoxyphenylpropionic Acids: Dual PPARα/γAgonists with Hypolipidemic and Antidiabetic Activity. *J. Med. Chem.* **2002**, *45,* 789–804.

Searls, D. B. Data Integration: Challenges for Drug Discovery. *Nature Rev. Drug Disc.***2005**, *4,* 45–58.

Shah, P.; Mittal, A.; Bharatam, P. V. CoMFA Analysis of Dual/Multiple PPAR Activators. *Eur. J. Med. Chem.* **2008**, *43,* 2784–2791.

Sohda, T.; K., M.; Imamiya, E.; Sugiyama, Y.; Fujita, T.; Kawamatsu, Y. Studies on Antidiabetic Agents. II. Synthesis of 5-[4-(1-Methylcyclohexyl methoxybenzyl] thiazolidine-2,4-dione (ADD-3878) and Its Derivatives. *Chem. Pharm. Bull.***1982**, *30,* 3580–3600.

Sohn, Y. S.; Park, C.; Lee, Y.; Kim, S.; Thangapandian, S.; Kim, Y.; Kim, H. H.; Suh, J. K.; Lee, K. W. Multi-conformation Dynamic Pharmacophore Modeling of the Peroxisome Proliferator-Activated Receptor γ for the Discovery of Novel Agonists. *J. Mol. Graph. Model.***2013**, *46,* 1–9.

Staels, B.; Fruchart, J. C. Therapeutic Roles of Peroxisome Proliferators Activated Receptor Agonists. *Diabetes* **2005**, *54,* 2460–2470.

Stanforth, R. W.; Kolossov, E.; Mirkin, B. A Measure of Domain of Applicability for QSAR Modelling Based on Intelligent K-means Clustering. *QSAR Comb. Sci.***2007**, *26,* 837–844.

Sundriyal, S.; Bharatam, P.V. 'Sum of Activities' as Dependent Parameter: A New CoMFA-based Approach for the Design of Pan PPAR Agonists. *Eur. J. Med. Chem.* **2009**, *44,* 42–53.

Sznaidman, M. L.; Haffner, C. D.; Maloney, P. R.; Fivush, A.; Chao, E.; Goreham, D.; Sierra, M, L.; LeGrumelec, C.; Xu, H. E.; Montana, V. G.; Lambert, M. H.; Willson, T. M.; Oliver, W. R., Jr; Sternbach, D. D. Novel selective Small Molecule Agonists for Peroxisome Proliferator-Activated Receptor δ (PPARδ)–Synthesis and Biological Activity. *Bioorg. Med. Chem. Lett.***2003**, 13, 1517–1521.

Tenenbaum, A.; Motro, M.; Fisman, E. Z. Dual and Pan-Peroxisome Proliferator-Activated Receptors (PPAR) Co-Agonism: the Bezafibrate Lessons. *Cardiovasc. Diabetol.* **2005**, *4,* 1–5.

Todeschini, R.; Consonni, V. Molecular Descriptors for Chemoinformatics. In *Methods and Principles in Medicinal Chemistry*; Mannhold, R., Kubinyi, H., Folkers, G., Eds.; Wiley; Weinheim, **2009**.

Tropsha, A.; Gramatica, P.; Gombar, V. K. The Importance of Being Earnest: Validation is the Absolute Essential for Successful Application and Interpretation of QSPR Models. *QSAR Comb. Sci.* **2003**, *22,* 69–77.

Tsantili-Kakoulidou, A.; Agrafiotis, D. 18th EuroQSAR: Perspectives on QSAR, Molecular Informatics and Drug Design. *Mol. Inf.***2011**, *30,* 87–88.

Tugwood, J. D.; Issemann, I.; Anderson, R. G.; Bundell, K. R.; McPheat, W. L.; Green, S. The Mouse Peroxisome Proliferator Activated Receptor Recognizes a Response Element in the 5' Flanking Sequence of the Rat Acyl CoA Oxidase Gene. *EMBO J.*, **1992**, *11,* 433–439.

Turner, D. B.; Willett P., Ferguson, A. M.; Heritage, T. W. Evaluation of a Novel Molecular Vibration-based Descriptor (EVA) forQSAR Studies: 2. Model Validation Using a Benchmark Steroid Dataset. *J. Comput. Aided Mol. Des.***1999**, *13,* 271–296.

Uppenberg, J.; Svensson, C.; Jaki, M.; Bertilsson, G.; Jendeberg, L.; Berkenstam, A. Crystal Structure of the Ligand Binding Domain of the Human Nuclear Receptor PPAR Gamma. *J. Biol. Chem.***1998**, *273,* 31108–31112.

Vallianatou, T.; Lambrinidis, G. ; Giaginis, C.; Mikros, E.; Tsantili- Kakoulidou, A. Analysis of PPAR-α/γ Activity by Combining 2-D QSAR and Molecular Simulation. *Mol. Inf.***2013**, *32,* 431–445.

Veber, D. F.; Johnson, S. R.; Cheng, H. Y.; Smith, B. R.; Ward, K. W.; Kopple, K. D. PropertiesthatInfluencetheOralBioavailabilityofDrugCandidates. *J. Med. Chem.***2002**, *45,* 2615–2623.

Vedani, A.; Briem, H.; Dobler, M.; Dollinger, H.; McMasters, D. M. Multiple Conformation and Protonation-State Representation in 4D-QSAR: The Neurokinin-1 Receptor System. *J. Med. Chem.* **2000**, *43*, 4416–4427.

Vedani, A.; Dobler, M.; Lill, M.A. Combining Protein Modelling and 6D-QSAR—Simulating the Binding of Structurally Diverse Ligands to the Estrogen Receptor. *J. Med. Chem.* **2005**, *48*, 3700–3703.

Vedani, A.; Descloux, A. V.; Spreafico, M.; Ernst, B. Predicting the Toxic Potential of Drugs and Chemicals *in Silico*: A Model for the Peroxisome Proliferator-Activated Receptor gamma (PPAR gamma). *Toxicol Lett.* **2007**, *173*, 17–23.

Vedani, A.; Zbinden, P. Quasi-atomistic Receptor Modeling. A Bridge Between 3D QSAR and Receptor Fitting. *Pharm. Acta Helv.* **1998**, *73*, 11–18.

Vedani, A.; Dobler, M.; Smieško, M. VirtualToxLab - a Platform for Estimating the Toxic Potential of Drugs, Chemicals and Natural Products. *Toxicol. Appl. Pharmacol.* **2012**, *261*, 142–153.

Vidal-Puig, A.; Jimenez-Liñan, M.; Lowell, B. B.; Hamann, A.; Hu, E.; Spiegelman, B.; Flier, J. S.; Moller, D.E. Regulation of PPAR gamma Gene Expression by Nutrition and Obesity in Rodents. *J. Clin. Invest.* **1996**, *97*, 2553–2561.

Vidal-Puig, A. J.; Considine, R. V.; Jimenez-Liñan, M.; Werman, A.; Pories, W. J.; Caro, J. F.; Flier, J. S. Peroxisome Proliferator-Activated Receptor Gene Expression in Human Tissues. Effects of Obesity, Weight Loss, and Regulation by Insulin and Glucocorticoids. J. *Clin. Invest.* **1997**, *99*, 2416–2422.

Vidović, D.; Busby, S. A.; Griffin, P. R.; Schürer, S. C.; A combined ligand- and structure-based virtual screening protocol identifies submicromolar PPARγ Partial agonists. *ChemMedChem* **2011**; *6*, 94–103.

Wayman, N.S.; Hattori, Y.; McDonald, M.C.; Mota-Filipe, H.; Cuzzocrea, S.; Pisano, B.; Chatterjee, P.K.; Thiemermann, C. Ligands of the Peroxisome Proliferator-Activated Receptors (PPAR-γ and PPAR-α) Reduce Myocardial Infarct Size. *FASEB J.* **2002**, *16*, 1027–1040.

Welch, J. S.; Ricote, M.; Akiyama, T. E.; Gonzalez, F. J.; Glass, C. K. PPARγ and PPARδ Negatively Regulate Specific Subsets of Lipopolysaccharide and IFN-γ Target Genes in Macrophages. *Proc. Natl. Acad. Sci.* **2003**, *100*, 6712–6717.

Willson, T. M.; Brown, P. J.; Sternbach, D. D.; Henke, B. R. The PPARs: From Orphan Receptors to Drug Discovery. *J. Med. Chem.* **2000**, *43*, 527–550.

Wishart, D. S.; Knox, C.; Guo, A. C.; Shrivastava, S.; Hassanali, M.; Stothard, P.; Chang, Z.; Woolsey J. DrugBank: A Comprehensive Resource for *in Silico* Drug Discovery and Exploration. *Nucleic Acids Res.* **2006**, *34*, D668–D672.

Woods, J. W.; Tanen, M.; Figueroa, D. J.; Biswas, C.; Zycband, E.; Moller, D. E.; Austin, C. P.; Berger, J. P. Localization of PPARδ in Murine Central Nervous System: Expression in Oligodendrocytes and Neurons. *Brain Res.* **2003**, *975*, 10–21.

Xu, H. E.; Lambert, M. H.; Montana, V. G.; Parks, D. J.; Blanchard, S. G.; Brown, P. J.; Sternbach, D. D.; Lehmann, J. M.; Wisely, W. G.; Willson, T. M.; Kliewer, S. A.; Milburn, M. V. Molecular Recognition of Fatty Acids By Peroxisome Proliferator-Activated Receptors. *Mol. Cell* **1999**, *3*, 397–403.

Xu, H. E.; Lambert, M. H.; Montana, V. G.; Plunket, K. D.; Moore, L. B.; Collins, J. L.; Oplinger, J. A.; Kliewer, S. A.; Gampe, R. T. Jr.; McKee, D. D.; Moore, J. T.; Willson, T. M. Structural Determinants of Ligand Binding Selectivity Between the Peroxisome Proliferator-Activated Receptors, *Proc. Natl. Acad. Sci.* **2001**, *98*, 13919–13924.

Yu, S.; Reddy, J. K. Transcription Coactivators for Peroxisome Proliferator-Activated Receptors. *Biochim. Biophys. Acta* **2007**, *1771*, 936–951.

Zhang, L.; Wang S.; Xu, W.; Wang, R.; Wang, J. Scaffold-Based Pan-Agonist Design for the PPARα, PPARβ and PPARγ Receptors. *PLoS ONE* **2012**, *7*(10), art. no. e48453

Zoete, V.; Grosdidier, A.; Michielin, O. Peroxisome Proliferator-Activated Receptor Structures: Ligand Specificity, Molecular Switch and Interactions with Regulators. *Biochim. Biophys. Acta* **2007**, *1771*, 915–925.

CHAPTER 8

ANTIMICROBIAL AND IMMUNOSUPPRESSIVE ACTIVITITES OF CYCLOPEPTIDES AS TARGETS FOR MEDICINAL CHEMISTRY

ALICIA B. POMILIO, STELLA M. BATTISTA, and ARTURO A. VITALE

Instituto de Bioquímica y Medicina Molecular (IBIMOL) (UBA-CONICET), Facultad de Farmacia y Bioquímica, Universidad de Buenos Aires, Junín 956, C1113AAD Buenos Aires, Argentina. Phone/Fax: +54 11 4814 3952;
e-mail: battistasm@yahoo.com.ar; e-mail: pomilio@ffyb.uba.ar; e-mail: avitale@ffyb.uba.ar

CONTENTS

ABSTRACT

Cyclopeptides are natural products that show a range of structures from cyclic dipeptides to circular proteins and cyclotides with 30 amino acids. Synthetic analogues have also been developed. These compounds display distinct biological activities. In this chapter, we focus on the structure and quantitative structure–activity relationships (QSARs) of antimicrobial and immunosuppressive cyclopeptides. However, few QSAR studies have been performed on cyclopeptides compared to small organic molecules. The balance of antimicrobial and hemolytic activities is discussed for designing novel antimicrobial cyclic peptides. Furthermore, we stress the importance of developing P-glycoprotein inhibition *in silico* predictive models in the process of drug discovery and development.

8.1 INTRODUCTION

Cyclic peptides are a particular group of bioactive peptides, containing cycles generated by the formation of either an amide, ester, or a disulfide bond, or by a new carbon–carbon, carbon–nitrogen, nitrogen–oxygen, or carbon–sulfur bond (neither esters nor amides) linking both terminal residues of acyclic peptides. These new connections are indicated with the prefix *anhydro*, *cyclo* or *epoxy*, or a combination thereof.[1] However, these cyclic peptides are usually called cyclopeptides.

Cyclopeptides can be formed by proteinogenic L-α-amino acids, and also by D-isomers, and nonprotein amino acids. The 20 proteinogenic L-α-amino acids may be all obtained from protein hydrolysates. The D-isomers and nonprotein amino acids are usually not available from natural sources, and must be obtained through chemical synthesis. Interest in unnatural synthetic amino acids is increasing because of their potential use in therapeutic and biological applications.[2]

Cyclopeptides show a variety of structures, from cyclodipeptides *via* cyclo-hepta- and octapeptides to the so-called circular proteins, and cyclotides with 30 amino acids, which can be found in bacteria, insects, higher plants, fungi, animals, and humans.[3] The most important structural features are that cyclopeptides not only show the primary structure, but also secondary and tertiary ones, perhaps quaternary, which give them properties and a behavior similar to those of large proteins. Bioactivity can be explained accordingly.

The electronic structures and conformations of the cyclopeptides, *O*-methyl-α-amanitin, phalloidin, and antamanide have been obtained from molecular parameters on the basis of semiempiric and *ab initio* methods.[4] The electronic structures and conformational analysis of the toxic cyclopeptides, α-amanitin,

O-methyl-α-amanitin, *S*-deoxo-α-amanitin, α-amanitin-(*S*)-sulfoxide, and α-amanitin-sulfone were obtained from molecular parameters on the basis of AM1 and *ab initio* methods.[5] The planar indole moiety of α-amanitin showed to be located in front of the rest of the bean-shaped bicyclic structure (**Figure 1**). Therefore, the upper and lower sides of the π-heterocycle were able to interact with any π-compounds, forming stable π-complexes. This region was also so lipophilic as required for transport through membranes to enter into cells.[4,5]

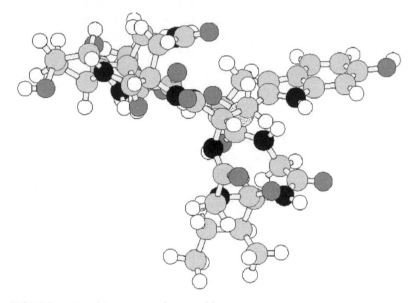

FIGURE 1   Spatial structure of α-amanitin.

The conformations of cyclopeptides from the fungus *Amanita phalloides*, and some derivatives have been related to its toxicity through total and point-charge dipole moments. Dipole moment's direction was nearly alike for α-amanitin, *O*-methyl-α-amanitin, *S*-deoxo-α-amanitin, and α-amanitin-sulfone; however, only α-amanitin-(*S*)-sulfoxide showed quite a distinct orientation. Therefore, on the basis of dipole moment calculations it was possible to explain the decrease in toxicity and binding of this molecule, and the results were in agreement with the inhibitory constant K_i of RNA polymerase II and lethal doses in mice.[3,5]

The most important cyclopeptides from higher plants and fungi have been reviewed, focusing on their structures, spectral and conformational studies, classification, occurrence, and bioactivity.[3] Recently, structure and quantitative structure–activity relationship (QSAR) studies on bioactive cyclopeptides have been analyzed and discussed.[6]

Peptides and particularly cyclopeptides are therapeutic targets that play an important role in medicinal chemistry, including drug design and QSARs. However, few QSAR studies have been conducted on cyclopeptides compared to small organic molecules. Some structural features, substructures, functional groups, and conformations contribute to their enhanced bioactivity.

Some physico-chemical properties, such as the partition coefficient (log P) and several molecular parameters are relevant to the activity. QSAR models including a number of descriptors have been applied to natural and synthetic cyclopeptides, and their analogues. The balance of antimicrobial and hemolytic properties is discussed herein for the design of antimicrobial cyclic peptides. The immunosuppressive activity is also analyzed in the present chapter. Such studies will also help to design selective drugs.

8.1.1 ABBREVIATIONS

ABC, ATP-binding cassette; ADME/Tox, absorption, distribution, metabolism, excretion, and toxicity; ADRs, adverse drug reactions; CYP_3A_4, cytochrome P_{450} $_3A_4$; 2D, two-dimensional; 3D, three-dimensional; DOE, design of experiments; ED_{50}, 50% effective dose; ESI-MS, electrospray ionization mass spectrometry; HBA, hydrogen bond acceptor; HBD, hydrogen bond donor; hERG, human ether-a-go-go-related gene; IC_{50}, 50% inhibitory concentration; IL-2, interleukin 2; LA, lipid A; LPS, lipopolysaccharide; MD, molecular dynamics; MDR, multidrug resistance; MHC, minimal hemolytic concentration; MIC, minimum inhibitory concentration; MIF, molecular interaction field; MM, molecular mechanics; MS, mass spectrometry; MS/MS, tandem mass spectrometry; NMR, nuclear magnetic resonance; PA, peptide association; PC, phosphatidylcholine; PE, phosphatidylethanolamine; PG-1, protegrin-1; P-gp, P-glycoprotein, also known as ABCB1; PhE/SVM, pharmacophore ensemble/support vector machine; PLCγ1, phospholipase $Cgamma1$; PPIase, peptidyl-propyl *cis–trans* isomerase; 3D-QSAR, three-dimensional quantitative structure–activity relationship; QSAR, quantitative structure–activity relationship; RP-HPLC, reversed-phase high-performance liquid chromatography; SAR, structure–activity relationship.

Amino acids: Ala, alanine; Asn, asparagine; Asp, aspartic acid; Cys, cysteine; Glu, glutamic acid; Phe, phenylalanine; Gly, glycine; Ile, isoleucine; HOIle, δ-hydroxyl isoleucine; Leu, leucine; OMet, *S*-oxomethionine; Pro, proline; Ser, serine; Thr, threonine; Trp, tryptophan; Tyr, tyrosine; Val, valine.

A, alanine; C, cysteine; D, aspartic acid; E, glutamic acid; F, phenylalanine; G, glycine; H, hystidine; I, isoleucine; K, lysine; L, leucine; M, methionine; N, asparagine; P, proline; Q, glutamine; R, arginine; S, serine; T, threonine; V, valine; W, tryptophan; Y, tyrosine.

8.2 ANTIMICROBIAL ACTIVITY OF PEPTIDES

8.2.1 STRUCTURES OF ANTIMICROBIAL PEPTIDES

The extensive clinical use of the classical antibiotics has led to resistant bacterial strains, in particular those responsible for infectious diseases such as Gram-negative bacteria.[7,8] Therefore, there is a search for new effective antibiotics,[9] such as cationic antimicrobial peptides.[10,11]

The endotoxin of the Gram-negative bacteria is a lipopolysaccharide (LPS), which is a component of the outer membrane, and the endotoxic membrane anchor moiety is a lipid A (LA).[12] LPS is spread out during Gram-negative bacterial infection and antimicrobial therapy and/or bacteria lysis, and may result in a lethal endotoxemia.[13]

Therefore, the target of any novel class of antimicrobial peptides is the neutralization of LPS and/or LA.[14] Endotoxin-binding host defence proteins showed that an LPS- and LA-binding substructure was formed by amphipathic sequences, for example, hydrophilic and hydrophobic moieties into opposite faces of the molecule,[15,16] rich in cationic residues with a β-sheet conformation.[17] To understand how these cationic molecules overcome the free energy barrier to insert into the lipid membrane, solid-state NMR spectroscopy was recently used to determine the membrane-bound topology of these peptides.[18]

Cytoplasmic membrane is the main target of some antimicrobial peptides,[19] in particular all cationic amphipathic peptides interact with membranes.[20] Recently, the molecular basis for the differences in activity of cyclic and linear antimicrobial peptides have been reported.[21] Molecular dynamics (MD) simulations and biophysical measurements were used to probe the interaction of a cyclic antimicrobial peptide and its inactive linear analogue with model membranes.[21] The cyclopeptide bound stronger than the linear one to negatively charged membranes. Moreover, the cyclopeptide folded at the membrane interface, and adopted a β-sheet structure characterized by two turns. Subsequently, the cyclopeptide penetrated deeper into the bilayer, while the linear peptide remained essentially at the surface. Finally, a model was proposed to characterize the mode of action of antimicrobial cyclopeptides, and can be used as a guideline for designing novel antimicrobial peptides.[21]

Although extremely variable in length, amino acid composition and secondary structure, all antimicrobial peptides can adopt a distinct membrane-bound amphipathic conformation.[22] Recent studies demonstrated that the compounds achieved their antimicrobial activity by disrupting various key cellular processes. Some peptides can even use multiple mechanisms. Moreover, several intact proteins or protein fragments are now being shown to have inherent antimicrobial activity. A better understanding of the structure–activity relationships (SARs) of antimicrobial peptides is required to facilitate the rational design of novel antimicrobials.[22]

The amphipathicity of antimicrobial peptides is necessary for their mechanism of action, because the positively charged polar face would reach the biomembrane through electrostatic interaction with the negatively charged head groups of phospholipids (negatively charged LPS or LA of Gram-negative bacteria[23,24]); then, the peptide molecules permeate the membrane by different mechanisms, such as hydrophobic interactions, causing increased permeability and loss of the barrier function of target cells.[17,25] Therefore, cationic peptides have got an increasing attention as broad spectrum antimicrobial agents, especially against Gram-negative bacteria.[11,26] Even though antimicrobial peptides show a different mode of action compared to traditional antibiotics, problems in application such as toxicity, susceptibility to proteolysis, manufacturing cost, and molecular size have delayed their clinical development. Nevertheless, antimicrobial peptides can be a new hope in developing novel, effective, and safe therapeutics without antibiotic resistance.[27] Therefore, it is necessary to study their structures and physico-chemical properties more in depth. Recent advances in the areas of screening and *in silico* modeling have been reviewed.[26] The ability to accurately predict peptide activity *in silico* and in a high-throughput manner should benefit all classes of cationic antimicrobial peptides and provide candidate structures for clinical evaluation.

Since the target of the antimicrobial peptides is the cytoplasmic membrane, resistance development is not expected because this would imply severe changes in the lipid composition of microorganism's cell membranes.[27] Therefore, an obvious approach against multidrug-resistant bacterial strains involves antimicrobial peptides and mimics thereof. The impact of α- and β-peptoid as well as β(3)-amino acid modifications on the activity profile against β-lactamase-producing *Escherichia coli* was recently assessed by testing different types of cationic peptidomimetics obtained by a monomer-based solid-phase synthesis.[28] Most of the peptidomimetics showed high-to-moderate activity toward multidrug-resistant *E. coli*. Differences in hemolytic activities indicated that a careful choice of backbone design is a significant parameter in the search for effective cationic antimicrobial peptidomimetics targeting specific bacteria.[28]

Another strategy against resistant bacteria consists of combining antibiotics with nanoparticles. Genuine synergy against bacterial resistance is raised when using nanoparticles with antimicrobial peptides, together with essential oils.[29,30]

The mechanisms of the antimicrobial peptides for permeabilizing cell membranes in order to induce bacterial death have been extensively discussed in the literature, and have been recently reported.[31,32] After the adhesion of the peptides on the external face of the membrane parallel to the bacterial lipid bilayer, the peptide would insert into the membrane according to either a "barrel-stave", "toroidal-pore", or "carpet mechanisms" as a result of their amino acid composition, amphipathicity, and cationic charge. However, neither of these mechanisms alone can fully explain the experimental data.

The mechanism of action depends on the difference in membrane composition between prokaryotic and eukaryotic cells.[33] If the peptides formed pores/channels in the hydrophobic core of the eukaryotic bilayer, they would cause hemolysis of human erythrocytes. On the contrary, for prokaryotic cells the peptides lysed cells in a detergent-like mechanism as described in the carpet mechanism.

The extent of interaction between peptide and biomembrane depends on the composition of the lipid bilayer. Liu et al.,[34,35] used a polyleucine-based α-helical transmembrane peptide to demonstrate that the peptide reduced the phase transition temperature to a higher extent in phosphatidylethanolamine (PE) bilayers than in phosphatidylcholine (PC) or phosphatidylglycerol bilayers, indicating a higher disruption of PE organization. The zwitterionic PE is the main lipid component in prokaryotic cell membranes, and PC is the main lipid component in eukaryotic cell membranes.[36]

According to results, the carpet mechanism is essential for strong antimicrobial activity, and if there were a preference by the peptide for penetration into the hydrophobic core of the bilayer, the antimicrobial activity would actually decrease.[33]

Membrane interactions of designed cationic antimicrobial peptides have been reported.[37]

Antimicrobial peptides take part in the innate immune response by providing a rapid first-line defence against infection.[38,39] Examples of antimicrobial peptides are magainins, cecropins, defensins, lactoferricins, tachyplesins, protegrins, thanatin, and others.[40] Antimicrobial peptide databases have been reported.[41,42] The design of new molecules has been achieved using combinatorial chemistry procedures coupled to high-throughput screening systems and data processing with design-of-experiments (DOE) methodology to obtain QSAR equation models and optimized compounds.

These compounds have been classified into three classes on the basis of secondary structures: (a) *linear peptides with propensity for amphiphilic α-helical structure*,[43,44] which are disordered structures in aqueous media and become amphipathic helices upon interaction with hydrophobic membranes,[45–47] for example, cecropins, magainins, and melittins; (b) *peptides with β or αβ structure stabilized by a different number of disulfide bridges*. The β-sheet class consists of cyclic peptides constrained in this conformation either by intramolecular disulfide bonds, for example, defensins[48] and protegrins,[49] or by an N-terminal to *C*-terminal covalent bond, for example, tyrocidins and gramicidin S (**Figure 2**);[50] and (c) *peptides with overrepresentation of certain amino acids or unusual structures*. This group has been reviewed;[51] it includes aromatic amino acid-rich peptides, (Pro-Arg)-rich peptides, unusual defensins and defensin-like molecules, unusual antimicrobial peptides from amphibians, bacteriocins with unusual structures, and anionic antimicrobial peptides.[51]

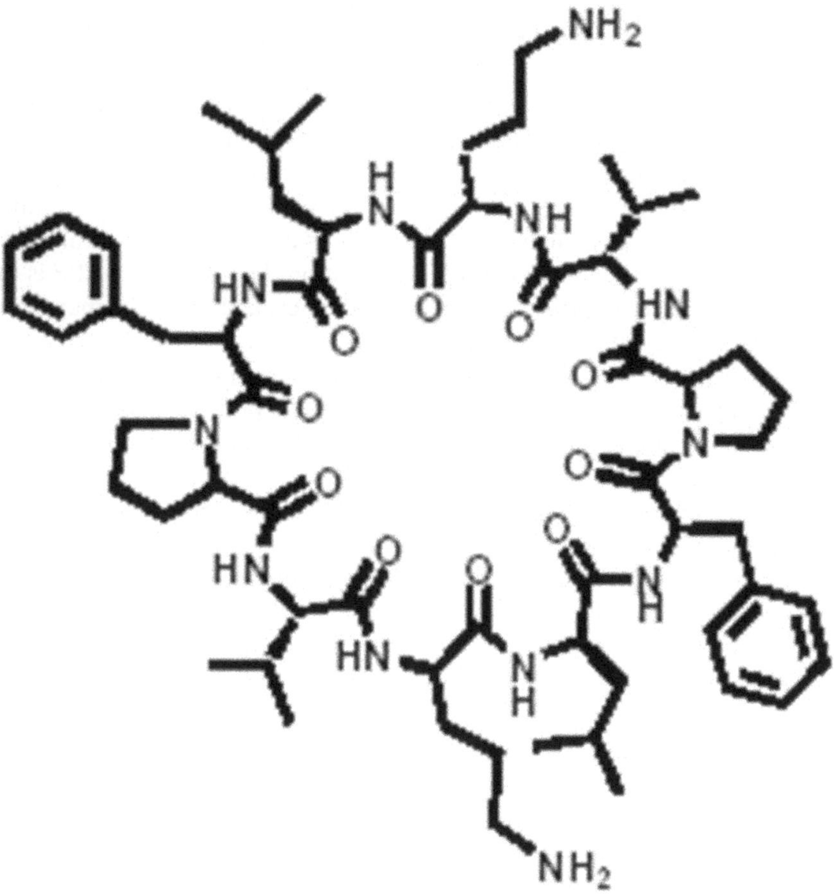

FIGURE 2　　Structure of gramicidin S.

Varieties of human proteins and peptides have antimicrobial activity and play important roles in innate immunity. There are three important groups of human antimicrobial peptides—defensins, histatins, and cathelicidins.[52] Defensins are cationic nonglycosylated peptides containing six cysteine residues that form three intramolecular disulfide bridges, resulting in a triple-stranded β-sheet structure, for example, α- and β-defensins in humans. The second group is the family of histatins, which are small, cationic, histidine-rich peptides present in human saliva. Histatins adopt a random coil conformation in aqueous solvents and form α-helices in nonaqueous solvents. The third group comprises only one antimicrobial peptide, cathelicidin LL-37. This peptide is derived proteolytically from the *C*-terminal end of the human CAP18 protein. Just like the histatins, it adopts a largely random coil conformation in a hydrophilic environment, and forms an α-helical structure in a hydrophobic environment.[52]

Cathelicidin and *defensin gene families* are multifunctional natural antibiotic peptides and signaling molecules that activate host cell processes involved in immune defence and repair.[53,54] In mammals, defensins have evolved to have a central function in the host defence properties of granulocytic leukocytes, mucosal surfaces, skin, and other epithelia. Three structural subgroups of mammalian defensins are involved as effectors of antimicrobial innate immunity.[55]

Furthermore, over 80 different α-defensin or β-defensin peptides are expressed by the leukocytes and epithelial cells of birds and mammals. Although these compounds may be candidates for therapeutic development due to the broad spectrum antimicrobial properties, there are technical limitations related to their size (30–45 residues) and complex structure. Therefore, minidefensins have been developed, which are antimicrobial peptides with 16–18 residues, approximately half the number found in α-defensins.[56] The θ-defensins are evolutionarily related to α- and β-defensins, but other minidefensins probably arose independently. Like α- or β-defensins, minidefensin molecules have a net positive charge and a largely β-sheet structure that is stabilized by intramolecular disulfide bonds. Whereas α-defensins are found only in mammals and θ-defensins only in nonhuman primates, the other minidefensins come from widely divergent species, including horseshoe crabs, spiders, and pigs. Several α-defensins and minidefensins are effective inhibitors of human immunodeficiency virus-1 (HIV-1) infection *in vitro*, and recent evidence implicates α-defensins in resistance to HIV-1 progression *in vivo*.[56]

8.2.2 QSAR MODELS FOR ANTIMICROBIAL CYCLOPEPTIDES

Cyclopeptides have been and are under study as potential antimicrobial therapeutic agents. Cyclopeptides usually exhibit broad-spectrum activity against Gram-positive and Gram-negative bacteria, yeasts, fungi, and enveloped viruses.[52] Combinatorial synthesis of cyclic peptides together with antimicrobial screening and other bioactivities can provide new lead identification, and construction of QSARs. Redman *et al.,*[57] reported a new sequencing protocol for rapid identification of the members of a *cyclic peptide library* based on automated computer analysis of mass spectra, new lead identification, and construction of QSARs. The utility of the new MS sequencing approach was demonstrated using sonic spray ionization ion trap MS and MS/MS spectrometry on a single compound per bead cyclic peptide library and validated with individually synthesized pure cyclic D, L-α-peptides.[57]

Also, complex libraries of glycosidated cyclopeptides, which are an important class of drug-like compounds, have been developed by incorporating glycosidated amino acids into linear peptides via solid-phase peptide synthesis followed by thioesterase-mediated peptide cyclization.[58]

The two major classes of cationic amphipathic antimicrobial peptides are α-helical and β-sheet peptides.[59,60] Potent antimicrobial cyclopeptides selective for Gram-negative bacteria have been successfully developed on the basis of the β-stranded framework mimicking the putative LPS-binding sites of the LPS-binding protein family.[61]

The disadvantage of antimicrobial peptides for clinical use as antibiotics is their toxicity or ability to lyse eukaryotic cells.[10] Therefore, it is necessary to dissociate antieukaryotic activity from antimicrobial activity in order to use them as broad spectrum antibiotics. SAR studies indicated that changes in the amphipathicity of these antibacterial peptides could be used to dissociate the antimicrobial activity from the hemolytic activity.[62,63] Furthermore, peptide cyclization increased the selectivity for bacteria because of substantially reducing the hemolytic activity.[64]

QSARs were obtained by associating the experimental biological potencies to physicochemical molecular properties obtained from the peptide sequences. A rational strategy was used to design cationic antimicrobial peptides via repeated sequences of alternating cationic and nonpolar residues. To achieve a high level of antimicrobial activity and selectivity toward bacteria instead of eukaryotic cells, systematic modifications of molecular properties were made by varying the amino acid residues of the amphipathic LPS- and LA-binding motifs,[17] while preserving the size, symmetry, and amphipathic character of the peptides. Therefore, antimicrobial and hemolytic activities of *de novo* designed cyclic β-sheet gramicidin S analogues have been successfully dissociated by systematic alterations in amphipathicity/hydrophobicity through D-amino acid substitutions.[65,66]

Frecer *et al.,*[67] reported the *de novo* design of a series of synthetic *amphipathic cationic cyclopeptides* for which a high affinity of binding to LA was predicted from molecular modeling. These V peptides were composed of two identical symmetric amphipathic LPS- and LA-binding motifs containing cationic residues, such as *HBHPHBH* and *HBHBHBH* (where *B* is a cationic residue, *H* is a hydrophobic residue, and *P* is a polar residue), that formed two strands of a β-hairpin joined by a $G_9S_{10}G_{11}$ turn on one side, and a Cys_1-Cys_{19} disulfide bond linking the *N*- and *C*-terminal residues on the other (**Figure 3**).

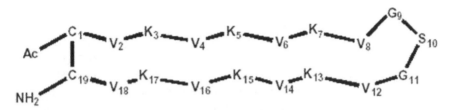

FIGURE 3   Chemical structure of the cationic cyclopeptide V1.

The V peptides exhibited strong effects against five Gram-negative bacteria (*E. coli*, *Klebsiella pneumoniae*, and *Pseudomonas aeruginosa*), with MICs in the nanomolar range, and low cytotoxic and hemolytic activities at concentrations significantly exceeding their MICs.

Each β-sheet conformation would bind to the bisphosphorylated glucosamine disaccharide head group of LA, primarily by ion-pair formation between anionic phosphates of LA and the cationic side chains.[17]

The two LPS- and LA-binding sites showed structural similarity to cyclic β-sheet defence peptides, such as protegrin 1, thanatin, and androctonin.[39] Peptides were further characterized by electrospray ionization mass spectrometry (ESI-MS) and amino acid analysis.

MD simulations showed that the backbone conformations of free V peptides evolved from the initial β-hairpin with defined patterns of secondary structure into flexible random conformations. The patterns of the molecular shape fluctuations and torsional flexibility indicated high degrees of flexibility of the free V peptides in solution.[67]

Antibacterial activity test, hemolytic activity assay, and cytotoxicity test were carried out. The therapeutic index of antimicrobial reagents is the ratio of the MHC (hemolytic activity) and MIC (antimicrobial activity); therefore, larger values in therapeutic index indicated higher antimicrobial specificity.[8,68]

High peptide hydrophobicity and amphipathicity also led to a higher peptide self-association in solution. Temperature profiling in RP-HPLC from 5 to 80°C was used to measure self-association of small amphipathic molecules, including cyclic β-sheet peptides.[69] However, a higher ability to self-associate in solution was correlated with weaker antimicrobial activity and stronger hemolytic activity of the peptides. In addition, self-associating ability was correlated with the secondary structure of peptides, that is, disrupting the secondary structure by replacing the L-amino acid with its D-amino acid counterpart decreased the peptide association (*PA*) parameter values,[67] thus leading to an enhanced average antimicrobial activity.

In peptides V1 to V7, the molecular charges, amphipathicities, and lipophilicities of the peptides were modulated by varying the cationic (polar) amino acid residues in the center of the binding motifs, where *B(P)* was Lys or Arg (Ser or Gln), and the hydrophobic residues, where *H* was Ala, Val, Phe, or Trp, which preserved the symmetries, sizes, and amphipathic characters of the peptides with alternating polar and nonpolar residues. Lysine residues were previously shown to contribute mostly to the high affinity to LA when placed at the flanking basic residue position of the *HBHB(P)HBH* motif with a β-sheet conformation.[17,67]

QSAR analysis revealed that the substitution of residues in the hydrophobic face of the amphipathic peptides with less lipophilic residues selectively decreased the hemolytic effect without significantly affecting the antimicrobial or cytotoxic activity. On the other hand, the antimicrobial effect was enhanced by substitutions in the polar face with more polar residues, which increased the amphipathicity of the peptide.[70]

Simple properties derived from the V-peptide sequences, such as the molecular charge (Q_M), amphypathicity index (*AI*), and lipophilicity index ($\Pi_{o/w}$), were correlated to the mean antimicrobial effect against Gram-negative bacteria by multivariate linear regression as shown in **Figure 4a**.[67] The *t*-test of the multivariate correlation (**Figure 4a**) revealed that the antimicrobial effect on bacteria was mainly determined by Q_M and *AI*, that is, by the number of cationic and polar residues forming the polar face of the V peptides and their distribution throughout the two symmetric amphipathic LPS- and LA-binding motifs.[67] A higher affinity to the outer bacterial membrane seemed to be a favorable prerequisite for the antimicrobial effects, since the V peptides displayed low micromolar K_d values and antimicrobial activities at concentrations in the nanomolar range. K_d accounted for the dissociation constant of the peptide-LA.

For antimicrobial effect:
ln (MIC) = 9.49 . Q_M + 10.17 . AI - 0.05 . $\Pi_{o/w}$ - 22.16   (a)

For haemolysis:
ln (EC$_{50}$) = - 5.34 . Q_M - 4.94 . AI - 0.23 . $\Pi_{o/w}$ + 31.87   (b)

For cytotoxicity:
ln (EC$_{50}$) = 8.98 . Q_M + 11.74 . AI - 0.04 . $\Pi_{o/w}$ - 8.70   (c)

FIGURE 4 Correlations obtained for antimicrobial effect (a), haemolysis (b), and cytotoxicity (c).

According to the antimicrobial effect correlation (**Figure 4a**), the QSAR model predicted rapid increases in the antimicrobial activity with an increase in Q_M over 4 è (in units of electron charge) when amphipathicity and hydrophobicity were kept constant at the levels of the most promising peptide, V4. The model analogues of V4 that shared the polar *HKHQHKH* motif and that differed only in the *H* residues (which retained the amphipathicity index of V4) were predicted to possess decreasing hemolytic activities with decreasing lipophilicities, while their predicted antimicrobial and cytotoxic activities remained unchanged. In other analogues of V4, the replacement of the two central Gln residues by more polar Asn residues was predicted to lead to significantly increased antimicrobial potencies due to the increased amphipathicity independent of the *H* residues (predicted MICs were lower than that of V4).[67]

Therefore, variations in the *H* residues forming the hydrophobic face of the analogues of V4 mainly affected the hemolytic activity, which was shown to depend strongly on $\Pi_{o/w}$, but did not affect the predicted antimicrobial activity of the analogues. Therefore, substitution of the *H* residues with less hydrophobic residues in the nonpolar face of the amphipathic analogues decreased the hemolytic activities of the V peptides.

Furthermore, directed substitutions of the *B* and *P* residues in the polar faces of the V peptides with more polar residues, which increased the amphipathic character (more negative *AI* values) of the peptide while keeping the net charge, the symmetry of the binding motifs, and the composition of the hydrophobic face, were predicted to bring about a significant increase in antimicrobial potencies.[8,67]

The positively charged antimicrobial peptide *cyclo*[VKLdKVdYPLKVKLdYP] (GS14dK4), which is a diastereomeric lysine ring-size analogue of the naturally occurring antimicrobial cyclopeptide gramicidin S (**Figure 1**), exhibited enhanced antimicrobial and markedly reduced hemolytic activities compared to gramicidin S itself.[71]

The hemolytic activity of the peptides against human erythrocytes was determined as a main measure of peptide toxicity to higher eukaryotic cells. Since both antimicrobial and hemolytic activities of the cationic peptides involved cell membrane lysis, and depended on the same physico-chemical properties[65,72] a similar correlation (**Figure 4b**) was obtained for the hemolytic activities of the V peptides.[67]

The correlation parameters and *t*-statistics showed that the hemolytic activity against eukaryotic cells (**Figure 4b**) was mainly influenced by the molecular lipophilicity, with the major contribution coming from the *H* residues, which formed the nonpolar face of the V peptides, which was predicted to acquire a β-hairpin-like structure in the peptide-LA complexes.[67]

The EC_{50} values of the V peptides for cytotoxicity ranged from 40 M to 5.7 mM, which exceeded their MICs by up to 3 orders of magnitude. For the cytotoxic effects of the V peptides, the correlation of **Figure 4c** was obtained.[67] The correlation parameters and t-statistics indicated that the cytotoxic activity was determined mainly by the peptide charge and amphipathicity. Hydrophobicity coefficients were determined by RP-HPLC at pH 7 (phosphate buffer).[67]

Since the antimicrobial activities of the V peptides strongly increased with the increasing amphipathicity of the molecules at constant Q_M and $\Pi_{o/w}$, then aggregates of V peptides rather than individual molecules would behave as strong antimicrobials.[67] The ability of cationic peptides to form aggregates has been related to their antimicrobial potencies, as previously reported for dermaseptin S4,[73,74] protegrin-1,[75] and human defensins.[8,76]

The validity of the QSAR model for the antimicrobial potencies of the V peptides against Gram-negative bacteria was verified with the set of *cationic amphipathic cyclopeptides* designed by Muhle and Tam,[61] which were similar to the V peptides, for example, sequences *cyclo*(PA*C*R*C*RAG-PA*R*C*R*CAG) constrained by two cross-linking disulfide bonds. These peptides displayed potent activities against Gram-negative bacteria (*E. coli* and *P. aeruginosa*). The MICs of these peptides were 20 nM for *E. coli*. New analogues have been proposed on the basis of QSARs, displaying strong antimicrobial effects without hemolytic activity.[67]

Protegrin-1 (PG-1) (**Figure 5**) is an 18-residue β-hairpin peptide containing two disulfide bridges (Cys_{6-15} and Cys_{8-13}), which belongs to the cathelicidin class of antimicrobial peptides. These disulfides constrained the peptide backbone into a β-hairpin conformation, with a β-turn formed by residues 9–12, as detected by NMR. SAR studies were carried out on over 100 single site substituted synthetic analogues, and the biological profiles were assessed. Some analogues showed slightly improved antimicrobial activities (2–4-fold lowering of MICs), while other substitutions caused large increases in hemolytic activity.[77]

SAR studies[78] led to the discovery of the analogue IB367 with Cys_{5-14} and Cys_{7-12} disulfide bridges, which has been clinically tested to treat ulcerative oral mucositis, ventilator-associated pneumonia, and respiratory infections associated with cystic fibrosis. An approach to PG-1 peptidomimetics has been earlier reported[79,80] based on the use of β-hairpin-stabilizing organic templates. The template D-Pro-Pro was chosen for its ability to promote a β-hairpin loop structure. This design was used to prepare β-hairpin peptidomimetics.[81–83]

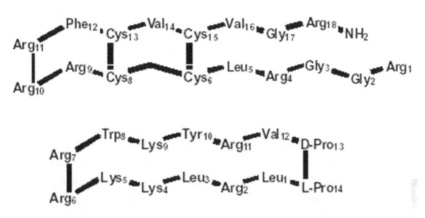

FIGURE 5 Structure of protegrin-1 (PG-1) and cyclic β-hairpin peptides-analogues of PG-1.

The lead compound, containing the sequence *cyclo*(Leu-Arg-Leu-Lys-Lys-Arg-Arg-Trp-Lys-Tyr-Arg-Val-*D*-Pro-Pro), showed antimicrobial activity against Gram-positive and Gram-negative bacteria, but a much lower hemolytic activity than PG-1.

Frecer[84] quantitatively analyzed antimicrobial and hemolytic activities of PG-1 mimetics-cationic cyclopeptides with β-hairpin fold synthesized by Robinson *et al.*,[77] (**Figure 5**).

The polar face of the lead cyclopeptide R1[77] was formed by the side chains of cationic residues 2, 4, 6, 7, 9, 11, and D-Pro$_{13}$ and Pro$_{14}$, while the nonpolar face consisted of residues 1, 3, 5, 8, 10, and 12 with predominant lipophilic/aromatic character.

For the QSAR models, the selected properties, which characterized peptide's charge, lipophilicity, amphipathicity, size, shape, and flexibility were used, including the following descriptors: charge (Q), overall lipophilicity (L), lipophilicity of polar and nonpolar faces (P and N), surface areas of polar and nonpolar faces (S_P and S_N), molecular mass of the polar and nonpolar faces (M_{wP} and M_{wN}), count of small lipophilic, highly lipophilic and aromatic residues forming the nonpolar face (C_{SL}, C_{HL} and C_{AR}), total number of hydrogen bond donor and acceptor centers (HB_{don} and HB_{acc}), total number of rotatable bonds (RotBon), and various amphipathicity descriptors (P/L, P/N, L/N, Q/L, Q/N, S_P/S_N, M_{wP}/M_{wN}, Q/C_{SL}, Q/C_{HL}, and Q/C_{AR}).[84] These simple additive molecular descriptors were easily derived from peptide sequences and tabulated amino acid properties.[85]

Frecer[84] assumed that the analogues adopted an amphipathic β-hairpin secondary structure, which was in agreement with the fact that protegrins and synthetic analogues with a constrained β-hairpin conformation displayed higher antimicrobial potencies than linear or nonconstrained counterparts.[18,86]

The best models obtained by application of genetic function approximation algorithm correlated antimicrobial potencies (log MIC_a) to peptide's charge and amphipathicity index, while hemolytic effect (log %Hem) correlated well with the lipophilicity of residues forming the nonpolar face of the β-hairpin.[84]

The lipophilicity of the nonpolar face N and the amphipathicity parameter Q/N showed some relation to the antimicrobial activity, while N and the inter-correlated count of highly lipophilic residues in the nonpolar face (C_{HL}) appeared to be related to the hemolytic activity. This finding was consistent with the above mentioned QSAR studies (**Figure 4 a, b, c**), which suggested that charge and amphipathicity correlated with MIC of cationic cyclopeptides and overall lipophilicity was very important for the hemolytic activity.[67]

A large set of QSAR models combining up to five descriptors in each correlation equation was prepared by the genetic function approximation (GFA) algorithm[87] of the Cerius2 package. The best performing QSAR model of the antimicrobial effect for the R1 analogues accounted for two descriptors, molecular charge Q and amphipathicity parameter Q/N, which are determined by the cationic residues forming mainly the polar face and the lipophilicity of the nonpolar face, N (**Figure 6a**).[84]

$$log\ MIC_a = 1.291 - 0.180 \cdot Q + 1.438 \cdot (Q/N) \quad \text{(a)}$$

$$log\ \%Hem = -2.551 + 0.431 \cdot N \quad \text{(b)}$$

FIGURE 6   QSAR models of the antimicrobial effect (a) and the haemolytic effect (b) for the R1 analogues.

The antimicrobial effect of cationic peptides related to molecular charge and amphipathicity has been previously reported.[67,88]

Based on this QSAR model, the best variants of R1 lead should have polar faces formed only by charged residues and nonpolar faces by highly lipophilic residues in order to display strong antimicrobial activity. Any analogue with the same charge as the lead peptide R1 ($Q = 7$ è) should show more potent antimicrobial activity than R1 when the lipophilicity of its nonpolar face $N \geq 6.84$ (value of N for R1).[84] MIC_a values were validated for the 97 peptides of Robinson et al.,[77] for their Q and N descriptors.[84]

The best QSAR model of the hemolytic effect for the R1 analogues related the lysis of human erythrocytes to the lipophilicity of the nonpolar face, N (**Figure 6b**).[84] Therefore, the hemolytic potency of R1 analogues depended mainly on the lipophilicity of the nonpolar face, thus being almost independent on the charge and composition of the polar face. Based on this QSAR model, any analogue with $N \leq 6.84$ should show lower levels of hemolytic activity than the lead peptide R1.[84] The %Hem values of the 97 peptides of Robinson *et al.*,[77] fitted this model.

The combination of the QSAR models with the cyclic backbone of the protegrin analogues, sequence amphipathicity (regular alternation of cationic and nonpolar residues) and peptide symmetry provided a sufficient strategy for peptide design. Circular dichroism experiments showed that cyclic protegrins containing one to three Cys bonds displayed some degree of β-strand structure in solution.[88] The occurrence of the β-hairpin fold was essential for membrane permeation/disruption by PG-1 analogues as previously reported.[88–90]

Bhonsle *et al.*,[91] used 3D-QSAR for identification of descriptors defining the bioactivity of antimicrobial peptides. The resulting 3D physico-chemical properties were controlled by the placement of amino acids with well-defined properties (hydrophobicity, charge density, electrostatic potential, and those mentioned above) at specific locations along the peptide backbone. These peptides exhibited different *in vitro* activity against *Staphylococcus aureus* and *Mycobacterium ranae*. Differences in bioactivity seem to be due to different physico-chemical interactions that occur between the peptides and bacteria cell membranes. 3D-QSAR analysis showed that specific physico-chemical properties were responsible for the antibacterial activity and selectivity. There were five physico-chemical properties specific to the *S. aureus* QSAR model, while five properties were specific to the *M. ranae* QSAR model.[91]

Naturally occurring antimicrobial peptides contain a large number of amino acid residues, which limit their clinical applicability. Recent studies indicated that it is possible to decrease the chain length of these peptides without loss of activity, and suggested that a minimum of two positive ionizable (hydrophilic) and two bulky groups (hydrophobic) are required for antimicrobial activity. By employing the HipHop module of the software package CATALYST, these experimental findings have been translated into 3D pharmacophore models by finding common features among active peptides.[92] Positively ionizable and hydrophobic features were the important characteristics of compounds used for pharmacophore model development. Based on the highest score and the presence of amphiphilic structure, two separate hypotheses, Ec-2 and Sa-6 for *E. coli* and *S. aureus*, respectively, were selected for mapping analysis of active and inactive peptides against these organisms.

The resulting models not only provided information on the minimum requirement of positively ionizable and hydrophobic features, but also indicated the importance of their relative arrangement in space. The minimum requirement for positively ionizable features was two in both cases, but the number of hydrophobic features required in the case of *E. coli* was four, while for *S. aureus* was three.[92]

A new screening assay was developed to characterize and optimize short antimicrobial peptides.[93] This assay is based on peptides synthesized on cellulose, combined with a bacterium, where a luminescence gene cassette was introduced. Tens of thousands of peptides can be screened per year. Information gained by this high-throughput screening can be used in QSAR analysis. QSAR modeling of antimicrobial peptides to date has been based on predicting differences between peptides that are highly similar. The studies have largely addressed differences in lactoferricin and protegrin derivatives or similar *de novo* peptides. "Inductive" QSAR in combination with more complex mathematical modeling algorithms such as artificial neural networks (ANNs) may yield powerful new methods for *in silico* identification of novel antimicrobial peptides.[93]

Fjell *et al.*,[94] reported the successful *in silico* screening for potent antibiotic peptides using a combination of QSAR and machine learning techniques. On the basis of initial high-throughput measurements of activity of over 1,400 random peptides, ANN models were built using QSAR descriptors and subsequently used to screen an *in silico* library of approximately 100,000 peptides. *In vitro* validation of the modeling showed 94% accuracy in identifying highly active peptides. The best peptides identified through screening were found to have activities comparable or superior to those of four conventional antibiotics and superior to the peptide most advanced in clinical development against a broad array of multiresistant human pathogens.[94]

Cruz-Monteagudo *et al.*,[95] recently reported chemoinformatics approaches for antimicrobial cyclopeptides with high selectivity and lower hemolytic activity, which consisted on a multicriteria virtual screening strategy based on the use of a desirability-based multicriteria classifier combined with similarity and chemometrics concepts. The authors proposed a new quantitative feature encoding information related to the desirability, the degree of credibility ascribed to this desirability and the similarity of a candidate to a highly desirable query, which can be used as ranking criterion in a virtual screening campaign, the desirability-credibility-similarity (DCS) score. The enrichment ability of a multicriteria virtual screening strategy based on the use of the DCS score was also assessed and compared to other virtual screening options. Specifically, by using the DCS score it was possible to rank a selective antibacterial peptidomimetic earlier than a biologically inactive or nonselective antibacterial peptidomimetic with a probability of *ca.* 0.9.[95] These results showed that promising chemoinformatics tools were obtained by considering both the multicriteria classification rule and the virtual screening strategy, which could, for instance, be used to aid the discovery and development of potent and nontoxic antimicrobial peptides.

8.3   IMMUNOSUPPRESSIVE ACTIVITY OF CYCLOPEPTIDES

8.3.1   STRUCTURES OF IMMUNOSUPPRESSIVE CYCLOPEPTIDES

A wide variety of natural products have immunosuppressive activity, but it is often difficult to distinguish this activity from the cytotoxicity associated with the compounds.

Mann[96] has recently reviewed the natural products that show immunosuppressive activity, for example, macrocyclic lactones, polyketides and fatty acid derivatives, prenylated glycosphingolipids, isoprenoids such as diterpenoids, triterpenoids, and withanolides, acridine alkaloids, β-carboline alkaloids, geranylphenols, *bis*-guanidines, cyclic carbamate cytoxazones, cyclic peptides, and polypeptides. The immunosuppressive cyclopeptides cyclosporin A (**Figure 7**) and astin C (**Figure 8**) are used in clinics, and in clinical trials, respectively, together with the antitumor cyclopeptides aplidine (**Figure 9A**), RA-V and RA-VII (**Figure 10**). The progress in these drug research studies has been recently reviewed. [97]

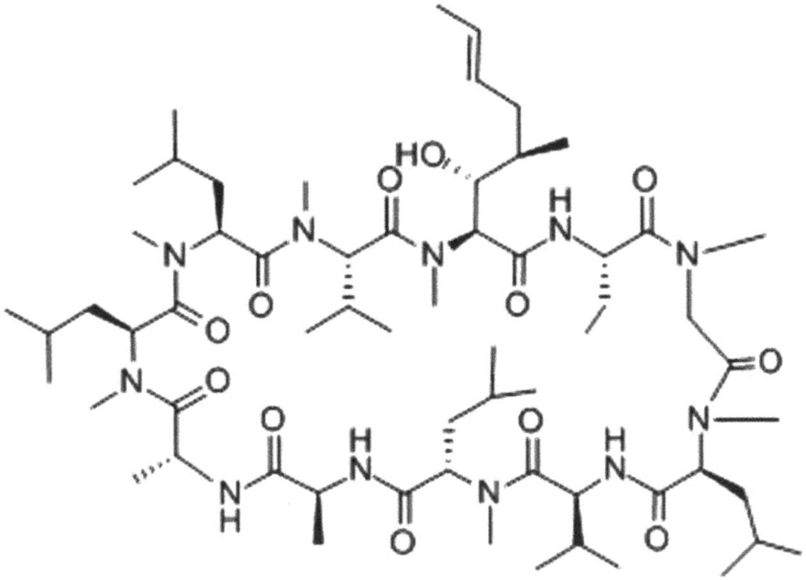

FIGURE 7   Structure of cyclosporin A.

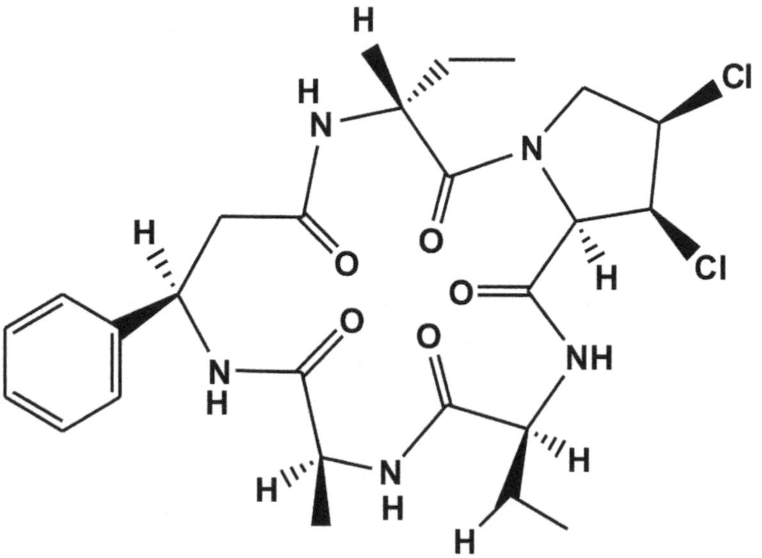

FIGURE 8 Structure of astin C, cyclic heptapeptide with a cis 3,4-dichlorinated proline residue.

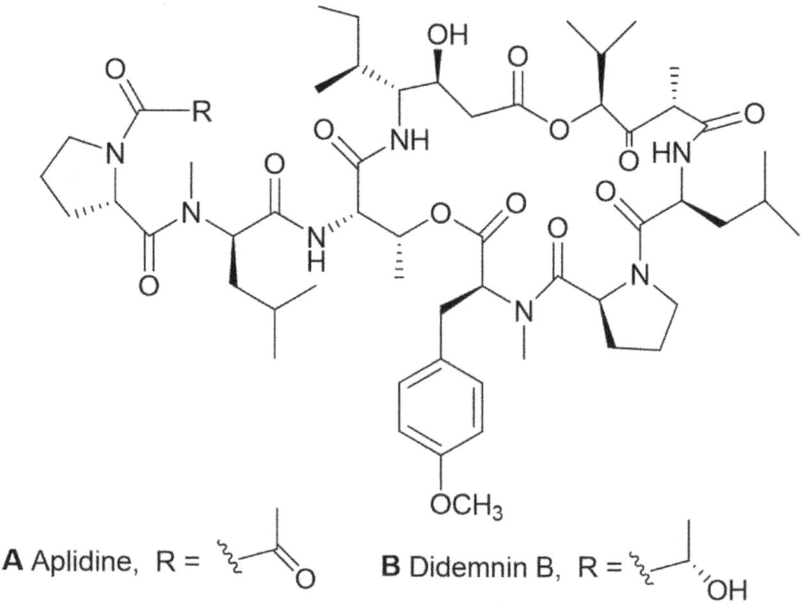

FIGURE 9 Structures of (A) aplidine, a drug lead for treatment of leukemia and lymphoma, and (B) didemnin B, a tunicate/prochloron–derived cyclic depsipeptide previously in clinical trials.

Recently, two bicyclic hexapeptides, *allo*-RA-V and *neo*-RA-V, and one cyclic hexapeptide, *O-seco*-RA-V, were isolated from the roots of *Rubia cordifolia* L.[98] Their structures were elucidated on the basis of spectroscopic analysis and X-ray crystallography. The absolute stereochemistry of these compounds was established by total syntheses and the absolute stereochemistry by chemical correlation with deoxybouvardin (RA-V) (**Figure 10**). Comparison of the 3D structures of highly active RA-VII (**Figure 10**) with the less-active compounds *allo*-RA-V and *neo*-RA-V, suggested that the orientation of the Tyr-5 and/or Tyr-6 phenyl rings plays an essential role in the cytotoxic activity.[98]

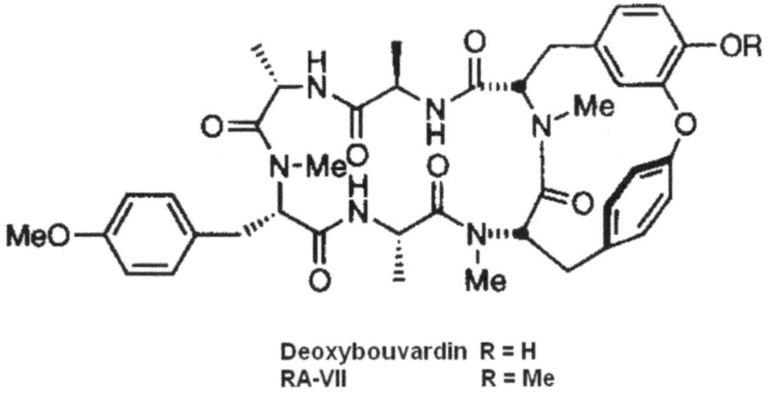

Deoxybouvardin R = H
RA-VII   R = Me

FIGURE 10   Structures of bicyclic peptides of deoxybouvardin (RA-V) and RA-VII.

The cyclic dodecapeptide, cycloleonurin (**Figure 11**), isolated from the fruits of *Leonurus heterophyllus* (Labiatae), showed potent immunosuppressive effect on human peripheral blood lymphocytes.[99]

Also, some cyclolinopeptides A-K (**Figure 12**),[100–102] isolated from seeds of the higher plant *Linum usitatissimum*, showed immunosuppressive activities against murine splenocytes. The conformational analysis of these cyclolinopeptides was performed by spectroscopic (NMR and X-ray analysis) and computational methods (MD and MM calculations), indicating that the conformation in solution was homologous to that in the solid state. Secondary and tertiary structures of these cyclolinopeptides have been recently elucidated in order to explain bioactivities [Pomilio *et al.*, unpublished results].

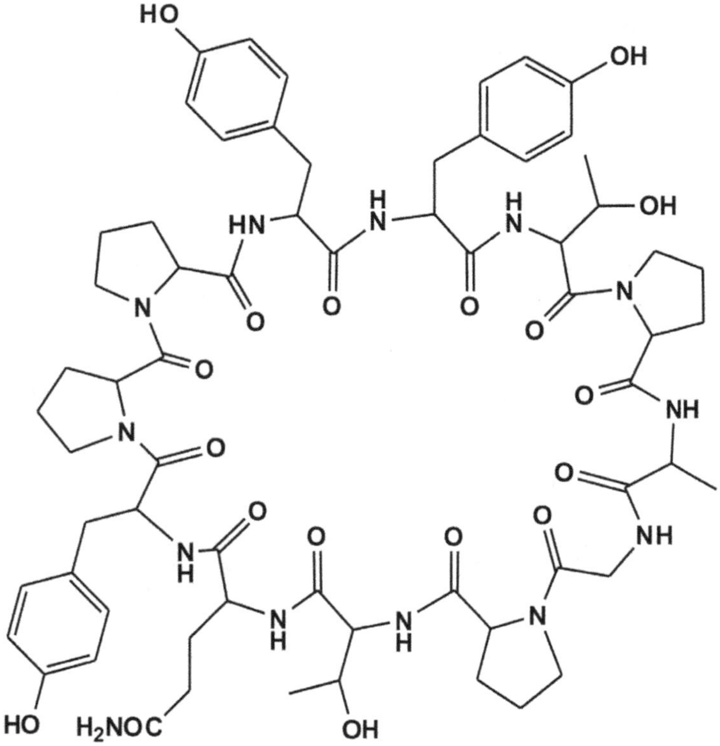

FIGURE 11   Structure of cycloleonurin.

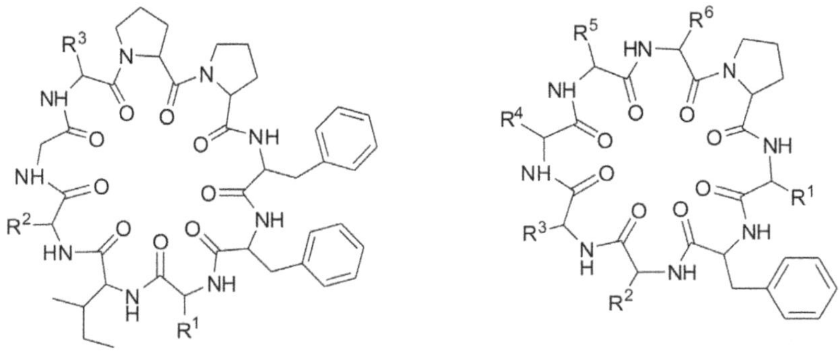

A R^1= i-Bu; R^2= s-Bu; R^3= i-Pr

B R^1= i-Pr; R^2= -$CH_2CH_2SCH_3$; R^3= s-Bu

C R^1= i-Pr; R^2= -$CH_2CH_2S(O)CH_3$; R^3= s-Bu

D R^1=-CH_2Ph; R^2 = indolyl; R^3 = s-Bu;
R^4= -$CH_2CH_2S(O)CH_3$; R_5=R_6= i-Bu

E R^1=R^4= i-Bu; R^2= s-Bu; R_3= -$CH_2CH_2S(O)CH_3$;
R^6= -CH_2Ph

FIGURE 12   Structures of cyclolinopeptides A, B, C, D, and E.

The cyclolinopeptides A, B, C, D, and E[101] (**Figure 12**) have shown a level of immunosuppressive activity similar to that of cyclosporin A (**Figure 7**). An analogue of cyclolinopeptide B was synthesized.[103]

The cyclolinopeptide A (**Figure 12**) mediates its bioactivity by inactivation of cyclophilin-dependent calcineurin. [104] Cyclolinopeptide A inhibits the calcium-dependent activation of T lymphocytes through direct binding to cyclophilin A, and subsequent inhibition of calcineurin action, which is a phosphatase that plays an important role in T lymphocyte signaling. This activity is comparable to the actions of cyclosporin A and FK506. However, the level of potency is about 10 times lower than that of cyclosporin A.[104]

The direct binding of cyclolinopeptide A to cyclophilin A was confirmed using tryptophan fluorescence studies, and peptidyl-propyl *cis–trans* isomerase (PPIase) assays. These results account for one of the examples of a natural product, which neutralizes calcineurin by a mechanism dependent on the primary binding to a PPIase.[104]

Recently, Ruchala *et al.,*[105] studied the synthesis, conformation, and immunosuppressive activity of cyclolinopeptides and its analogues.

Heart, liver, kidney, and bone marrow transplants are very often carried out, and survival is tightly related to the fungal metabolite, cyclosporin A (**Figure 7**). Cyclosporines A and B were tested not only for antibacterial and antifungal activities, but also for antiviral, cytostatic, and immunosuppressive activities. Cyclosporin A proved to have high potency combined with the absence of cytotoxicity, and this was a key discovery since most of the known immunosuppressants usually show cytotoxicity, since they inhibit mitosis in all fast dividing cells.

Cyclosporin A has a high degree of selectivity for T lymphocytes. Since 1978, it has been used in over 200,000 transplant operations. More than 750 analogues have since been prepared, but none of them has shown a higher activity than that of cyclosporin A.[106] Currently, its efficacy is also being evaluated for the treatment of autoimmune diseases, such as rheumatoid arthritis, systemic erythematosus lupus, and Crohn's disease.

For the past 14 years, research on these compounds has been directed toward elucidation of the mechanisms of their specific inhibition of T-cell activation and proliferation. [107] Results have provided important insights into the signaling pathways within T-cells, and a greater understanding of the role of these cells in the immune response.

The T lymphocyte is undoubtedly the most important cell for the initiation of an immune response. The glycoprotein antigen receptor on the T-cell surface can interact with foreign antigens that are presented by molecules of the major histocompatability complex (MHC) (positive selection). This association with foreign antigens will begin a cascade of intracellular signaling events leading to the activation and proliferation of T-cells and other cell types required for an immune response, and for the production of effector molecules, such as interleukin 2 (IL-2). It binds to IL-2 receptors on various cells, including T lymphocytes, and stimulates cells to progress from G_1 to S phase of the cell cycle.

The T-cell growth factor IL-2 is very important, and much of the immunosuppressive effect of cyclosporin A and FK506, can be attributed to their disruption of the activation of the gene for IL-2.

There is a chain of events after antigen binding. The increase in calcium ion concentrations within T-cells is caused by (1) ion release from intracellular stores via the inositol polyphosphate pathway;[108] and (2) release from the stores after the activation of protein kinase C (PKC) and the *Ras* pathways.[109]

At last, the association of the antigen with the receptor leads to the activation of several kinases with phosphorylation (and hence, activation) of various other enzymes, including phospholipase C*gamma*1 (PLCγ1), and guanine nucleotide releasing exchange factors that activate *Ras* proteins. In turn, PLCγ1 produces IP3, which acts directly on Ca^{2+} stores, while the activated *Ras* proteins initiate a cascade of kinase-mediated events, involving species such as *raf*, *map*-kinase, and *c-jun* kinase, thus resulting in the production of several transcription factors.

Cyclopeptides isolated from cyanobacteria, tunicates, and fungi also showed immunosuppressive activity.[110] The immunosuppressive properties of antamanide (**Figure 13**) from *A. phalloides* and a number of its analogues, including the symmetrical antamanide, were studied and compared with the activities of cyclosporin A (**Figure 7**) and cyclolinopeptide A (CLA) (**Figure 12**).[111] These peptides were analyzed by plaque-forming cells, graft *versus* host, delayed-type hypersensitivity, and autologous rosette forming cell tests. Antamanide and symmetrical antamanide exhibited a lower immunosupressive activity than that of CLA.

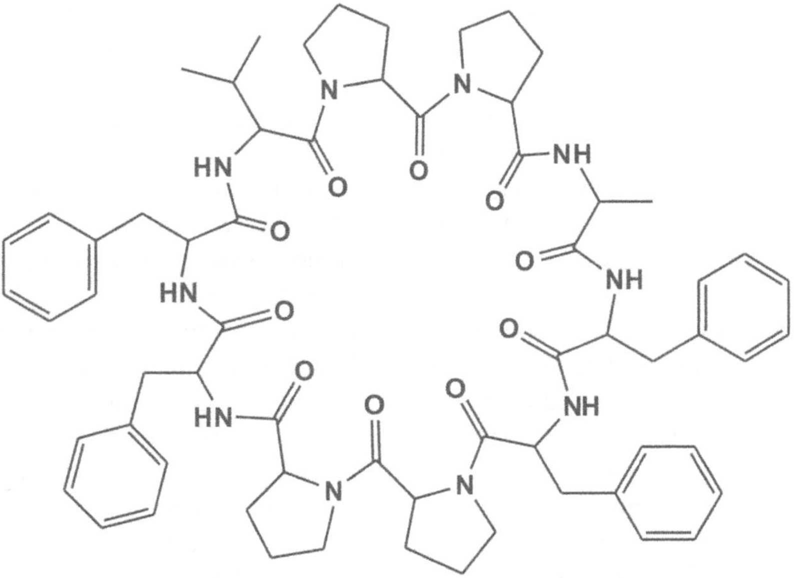

FIGURE 13 Structure of antamanide.

The immunosuppressive activities of the cycloamanides A, B, C, and D (**Figure 14**) from *A. phalloides*, and two of their D-amino acid-containing analogues, were analyzed[112] using plaque-forming cell and delayed-type hypersensitivity tests. Cycloamanide A and its D-Phe-containing analogue [*cyclo*(Phe-D-Phe-Ala-Gly-Pro-Val)] were the most potent immunosuppressants of the series.

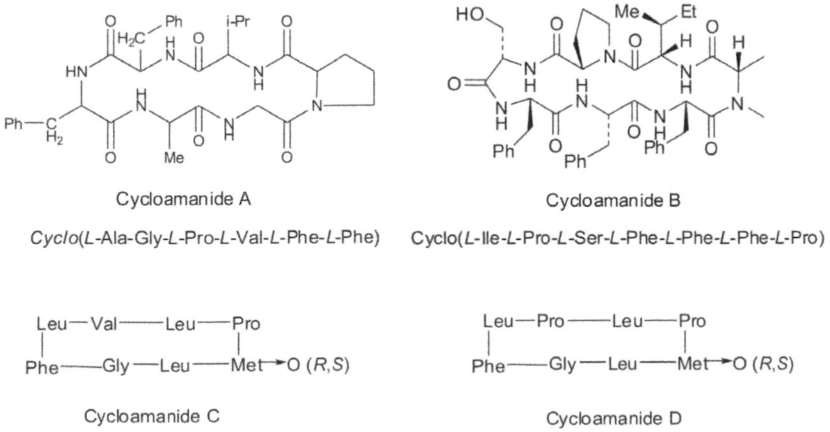

Cycloamanide A
Cyclo(L-Ala-Gly-L-Pro-L-Val-L-Phe-L-Phe)

Cycloamanide B
Cyclo(L-Ile-L-Pro-L-Ser-L-Phe-L-Phe-L-Phe-L-Pro)

Leu—Val——Leu—Pro
 | |
Phe——Gly—Leu——Met→O (R,S)

Cycloamanide C

Leu—Pro——Leu—Pro
 | |
Phe——Gly—Leu——Met→O (R,S)

Cycloamanide D

FIGURE 14 Structures of cycloamanides A, B, C, and D.

Cyclodepsipeptides comprise a wide variety of natural cyclopeptides that are characterized by the occurrence of at least one ester linkage, and display a variety of biological effects, such as immunosuppressive, antibiotic, antifungal, anti-inflammatory, or antitumoral activities. In addition, many of these cyclic depsipeptides represent useful tools for the research of biological processes involved in cellular regulation.[113] The didemnins, which belong to this family were first isolated from the marine tunicate *Trididemnum solidum*.[114] Since the discovery and isolation of the didemnin family of marine depsipeptides in 1981, the synthesis and biological activity of its congeners have been reviewed.[115–117] The didemnins have demonstrated antitumor, antiviral, and immunosuppressive activity at low nano- and femtomolar levels. Of the six marine-derived compounds that have reached clinical trials as antitumor agents three—didemnin B, aplidine, and ecteinascidin 743—are derived from tunicates.[118] Didemnin B (DB) (**Figure 9B**), a cyclic depsipeptide from the compound tunicate *T. solidum*, was the first marine-derived compound to enter phase I and II clinical trials. The phase II studies, sponsored by the U.S. National Cancer Institute, indicated complete or partial remissions with non-Hodgkins lymphoma, but cardiotoxicity caused didemnin B to be dropped from further study. The closely related dehydrodidemnin B (DDB, aplidine) (**Figure 9A**) was isolated in 1988 from a second colonial tunicate, *Aplidium albicans*, and spectroscopic studies assigned a structural formula in which a pyruvyl group in DDB replaced the lactyl group in DB and syntheses of DDB have been achieved. Aplidine is more active than DB and lacks DB's cardiotoxicity. It was introduced by PharmaMar into phase I clinical trials in January 1999. Aplidine's mechanism of action involves several pathways, including cell cycle arrest, inhibition of protein synthesis, and antiangiogenic activity. Phase I studies have been reported for a number of several schedules including 1-h, 3-h, and 24-h infusion. Evidences of antitumor activity and clinical benefit of aplidine in several tumor types were noted across phase I and phase II trials, particularly in advanced medullar thyroid carcinoma.[119,120] Plitidepsin (apladine) is currently in phase III clinical trials in multiple myeloma.[121] Within the entire phase I program, dose-limiting toxicities of aplidine were neuromuscular toxicity, asthenia, skin toxicity, and diarrhea. Interestingly, no hematological toxicity was observed. Aplidine displayed a very peculiar delayed neuromuscular toxicity that was found to be closely related to the symptoms described in the adult form of carnitine palmitoyl transferase deficiency type 2, which is a genetic disease treated with L-carnitine. Consistently, concomitant administration of L-carnitine allowed to improve aplidine-induced neuromuscular toxicity.[119]

Plitidepsin (aplidine) seems to be able to induce clinical benefit in patients with pretreated advanced medullary thyroid carcinoma (MTC), and its toxicity has been manageable at the recommended dose.[120]

The second family of tunicate-derived antitumor agents is the ecteinascidins from the mangrove tunicate *Ecteinascidia turbinata*, which were first described in 1969, but their small amounts prevented their isolation for over a decade. Phase II clinical trials with ET 743 are underway. Future supplies of ecteinascidins should be available from aquaculture or synthesis.[118]

About two decades later of DB trials, tamandarins A and B were isolated, and were found to have very similar structures and biological activities to that of the didemnin B (**Figure 15**). These compounds have shown impressive biological activity and some progress has been made in establishing SARs. However, their molecular mechanism of action still remains unclear.

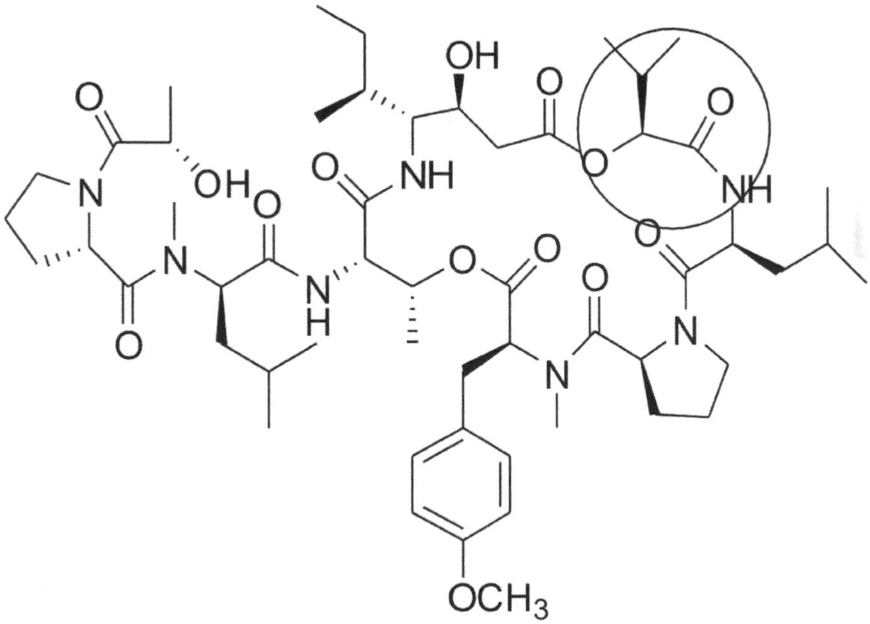

FIGURE 15   Structure of tamandarin A (difference with didemnin B is encircled).

The unusual structure of the didemnin congeners has led to several total syntheses by research groups from around the world. Some other anticancer peptides such as kahalalide F, hemiasterlin, dolastatins, cemadotin, and soblidotin have also entered the clinical trials.[122] Some progress was made in the molecular mechanism of action and in establishing SARs, but there is a lot to be performed in the future.[123] Didemnins, tamandarins (**Figure 15**), and related natural products have been recently reviewed.[124]

Bisintercalator natural products with potential therapeutic applications have been also reported.[125] Echinomycin (**Figure 16**) is the prototypical bisintercalator, a molecule that binds to DNA by inserting two planar chromophores between the base-pairs of duplex DNA, placing its cyclic depsipeptide backbone in the minor groove. This class of compounds shows biological antitumor and antiviral activities. One of the more recently identified marine natural product as bisintercalator that is close to clinical development is thiocoraline.

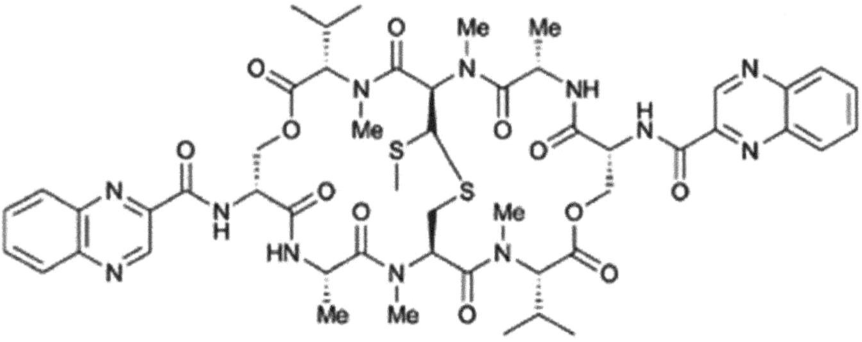

FIGURE 16   Structure of echinomycin.

Recently, the chemistry and biology of kahalalides have been also reviewed,[126] kahalalide F (**Figure 17**) being one of the most active compound of this family.[127] Recently, kahalalide Y (**Figure 17**) was isolated from *Bryopsis pennata.*[128] The application of a combination of MM and NOE distance constraint calculations was used to determine the conformation and the absolute configuration of the final stereogenic center of kahalalide Y. Using the Schrödinger suite, the structure was sketched in Maestro and minimized using the OPLS2005 force field in Macromodel. A conformational search was performed separately for structures having an *R* or *S* configuration at C-3 of the β-hydroxy fatty acid subunit that completes the cyclic scaffold, after which multiple minimizations for all generated conformers were carried out. The lowest energy conformers of *R* and *S* stereoisomers were then subjected to B3LYP geometry optimizations, including solvent effects. The *S* stereoisomer was shown to be in excellent agreement with the NOE-derived distance constraints and hydrogen-bonding stability studies.[128]

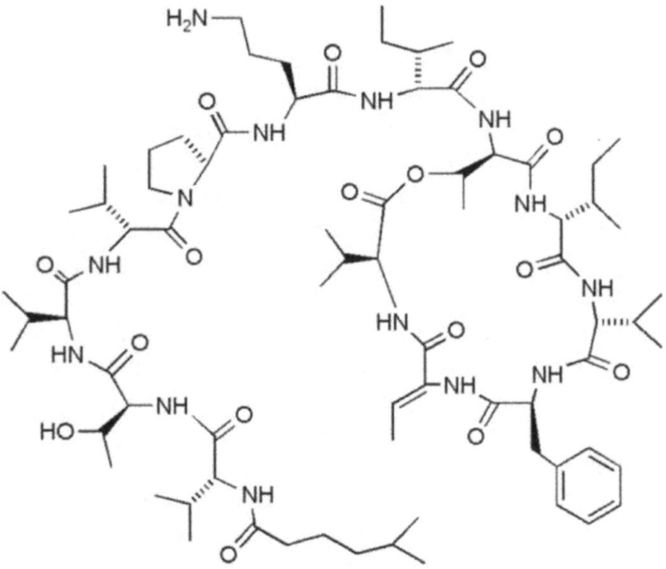

Kahalalide **F**

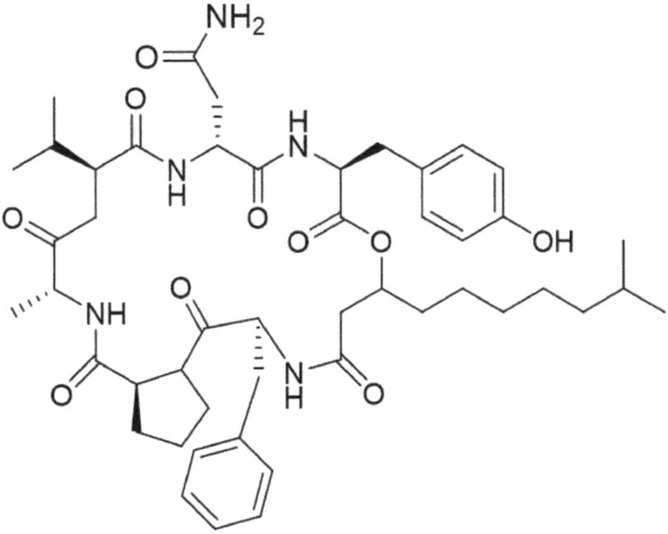

Kahalalide **Y**

FIGURE 17 Structures of kahalalides F and Y.

8.3.2 QSAR OF IMMUNOSUPPRESSIVE CYCLOPEPTIDES

One of the main strategies in current drug discovery is to reduce drug failures in early stages. Until 1985 poor pharmacokinetic properties were the main reason for drug failures, however, in the last 20 years safety and lack of efficacy have become major issues. Moreover, drugs have been withdrawn from the market mainly due to human adverse drug reactions (ADRs) over the past 20 years.[129] Rationalization of these failures led to the identification of a number of anti-targets, namely those targets which, upon interaction with therapeutic drugs, may result in severe ADRs.[130] P-glycoprotein (P-gp), also known as ABCB1 or MDR1, is a membrane protein member of the ATP-binding cassette (ABC) superfamily of transporters, which uses the released energy during the ATP hydrolysis to actively translocate a variety of structurally unrelated compounds across the cell membrane.[131] P-gp, together with hERG channel and CYP_3A_4, is probably the most widely studied antitarget.

P-gp is one of the most promiscuous efflux transporters, since it recognizes a number of structurally different and apparently unrelated xenobiotics; many of them are also CYP_3A_4 substrates. CYP_3A_4 and ABCB1 are often expressed in the same tissues, hence, for common substrates the amount of efflux determines the exposure to metabolism.[132] This interplay affects bioavailability of drugs coadministered with a P-gp inhibitor or inducer.[133,134]

P-gp can be found in different normal human tissues, including liver, kidney, small and large intestines, pancreas, brain, ovary, and testes. [135] It is preferentially expressed in organs and tissues that either function as a barrier (gastrointestinal tract; blood–brain barrier) or promote the removal of xenobiotics from the organism (liver and kidney).[136] As a result, P-gp has strong effects on the absorption, distribution, metabolism, excretion, and toxicity (ADME/Tox) of an administered drug.[137]

Furthermore, P-gp is involved in the multidrug resistance (MDR) in several diseases such as infectious diseases,[138] rheumatoid arthritis,[139] brain diseases,[140] and cancers.[141,142] Therefore, potent selective P-gp inhibitors have been rationalized as adjuvant therapy when coadministered with anticancer drugs. Therefore, several research groups all over the world search for effective P-gp inhibitors. Cyclosporine A, aureobasidin A, and related cyclopeptide analogues have shown potent P-gp inhibitory activities.

The inhibition of P-pg plays a clinically important role in modern chemotherapy since specific P-gp modulators can effectively reverse MDR in resistant cell lines, thus restoring sensitivity to chemotherapy, and improving treatment results.[143]

Until now, a number of candidates failed clinical trials due to poor selectivity. In particular, first-generation chemosensitizers, generally drugs known to be active toward other targets, were ineffective at nontoxic concentrations, while second-generation chemosensitizers often failed because of simultaneous P-gp and CYP_3A_4 inhibition.[144]

As P-gp limits drug bioavailability, the recognition of P-gp substrates (and inhibitors) at the early stages of drug development is essential for obtaining new chemotherapeutic agents that take into account MDR issues.[145,146] Di Ianni et al.,[147] have recently developed several classifier models based on topological descriptors to identify potential P-gp substrates, designed to be applied as secondary filter in virtual screenings. Receiver operating characteristic (ROC) curves showed that the combination of the individual models, through data fusion, in a three-model ensemble, allowed to attain higher areas under the curve, and an overall better behavior in terms of sensitivity or specificity. Individual discriminant functions (dfs) showed performances similar to those of previously reported models. These recent models only included low-dimensional (up to 2D) molecular descriptors, thus being suitable for virtual screening of increasingly large virtual chemical databases.[147]

MDR is highly associated with the overexpression of P-gp by cells, resulting in increased efflux of chemotherapeutical agents and reduction of intracellular drug accumulation. It is of clinical importance to develop P-gp inhibition predictive models in the process of drug discovery and development. Moreover, the integration of *in silico* and *in vitro* procedures can help to reduce costs. Therefore, a number of *in silico* models for recognition of P-gp substrates and inhibitors have been proposed in recent years. Lack of a high resolution crystal structure for human P-gp, together with the high flexibility of ABC transporters, justified the prevalence of ligand-based models.[148] Statistics and information gained from these models have been reviewed.[149,150] P-gp inhibition models generally agreed on the utility of pharmacophore descriptors, and stressed the importance of a hydrogen bond acceptor (HBA), together with some hydrophobic (HP) regions (between two and four). These models demonstrated diminished performance when tested against external validation sets. On the other hand, classification models using nonpharmacophore descriptors often showed better predictive power for P-gp substrate recognition, but were rarely used to discriminate inhibitors from noninhibitors.[151]

P-gp is involved in intestinal absorption, drug metabolism, and brain penetration, and its inhibition can seriously alter a drug's bioavailability and safety. Moreover, P-gp can be used to overcome MDR as mentioned above. Given this dual nature, reliable *in silico* procedures to predict P-gp inhibition are of great interest. *In silico* models must include an extensive data collection, thus allowing an appropriate chemical space coverage, combined with suitable molecular descriptors. Recently, Brocatelli et al.,[151] used a training set of 772 molecules from literature analysis, and two validation sets with different chemotypes, thus yielding more than 1,200 structures. In addition, different classes of molecular descriptors were evaluated, in order to account for nonspecific factors such as water solubility and membrane partitioning and for more specific pharmacophoric features responsible for ligand–protein interactions.

In particular, molecules described using GRID molecular interaction field (MIF) approaches resulted in a "composite model" for P-gp inhibition, based on an intuitive pipeline of preceding "local models" developed for competitive or noncompetitive binding. VolSurf+ descriptors were used to model physicochemical properties, whereas the pharmacophoric method FLAP[152,153] was used to superimpose molecules and evaluate their MIF similarity. With VolSurf+, a number of important parameters were detected for P-gp inhibition, while FLAP identified the most important pharmacophore features around the optimal molecular shape. All validations confirmed the robustness of the model and its suitability to help medicinal chemists in drug discovery. The information derived from the model was rationalized as a pharmacophore for competitive P-gp inhibition.[151] This model can be satisfactorily used to predict P-gp inhibition and to guide compound design.

There is a growing consensus in favor of using pharmacophore ensemble to accurately model the interactions between P-gp and substrates (and also inhibitors) in order to take into account the promiscuous nature of P-gp.[154] This promiscuous nature of P-gp and inhibitors can be resolved using a novel scheme recently derived by Leong,[155] in which a panel of plausible pharmacophore hypothesis candidates were adopted to construct a pharmacophore ensemble (PhE), which, in turn, was treated as input for regression analysis via support vector machines (SVM). Unlike any other analogue-base modeling scheme, each pharmacophore member in the PhE symbolizes a single protein conformation or a group of spatially similar protein conformations. It has been shown that the PhE/SVM model executed better than the consensus prediction of multiple pharmacophore models.[155] Consequently, a number of systems, whose target proteins are highly promiscuous, were also accurately modeled, including the case studies of the liability of hERG[155] as well as CYP_2A_6-[156] and CYP_2B_6-substrate interactions.[157] Leong et al.,[158] developed an accurate, fast and robust in silico model based on the PhE/SVM scheme to predict the binding affinity of P-gp inhibitors. EC_{50} values of 130 compounds were obtained from the literature.[159–162] Since 3D conformations of ligands are of critical importance in developing pharmacophore models,[163] all selected molecules were subjected to conformation search to generate the low-lying conformations, using the mixed Monte Carlo multiple minimum (MCMM)/low mode. MMFFs were chosen as force field and the truncated-Newton conjugated gradient method (TNCG) was set as the energy minimization method. Furthermore, the hydration effect and the solvation effect were taken into account by using the GB/SA algorithm[164] and water as solvent with a constant dielectric constant, respectively.

Further, 31 molecules, which totally consisted of 7,142 conformations, were selected for the training set for automatic pharmacophore generation and regression and their associated biological activities spanned seven orders of magnitude. The generated hypotheses were, in turn, validated by those remaining 88 molecules, whose biological activities varied over 5 log units.

In addition, 11 molecules, whose P-gp inhibition activities had been previously assayed,[165] were selected as the outlier set to assess the extrapolation capacity of the developed model. Similar to the observations found in the training set and test set, this PhE/SVM model performed better than any of the pharmacophore models in the ensemble in the outlier set as indicated by statistical parameters as well as the scatter plot of observed *versus* predicted pEC_{50} values.

The HypoGen module in Discovery Studio was used for automatic pharmacophore generation. It produced pharmacophore hypotheses, which quantitatively correlated the 3D arrangement of selected chemical features with the corresponding activities through three phases, namely construction, subtraction, and optimization as compared with any other QSAR techniques,[166,167] which normally rely on regression to generate predictive models. During the construction phase, HypoGen[168] generated common conformational alignment among those most active molecules in the training set. Pharmacophore hypotheses were further improved using the stimulated annealing scheme in the optimization phase. Hydrogen bond donor (HBD), HBA, and HP chemical features, which depicted the intermolecular interactions between an H atom on the ligand and a highly electronegative atom such as O, N, or F on the protein, between a highly electronegative atom on the ligand and an H atom on the protein, and between nonpolar moieties on both ligand and protein, respectively, were chosen for pharmacophore hypothesis development.

According to the results, of all generated pharmacophore models using various selections of chemical features and runtime parameters, three hypotheses, denoted by Hypo A, Hypo B, and Hypo C, were assembled to construct PhE based on their prediction performances on every single molecule in the training set and test set, and their corresponding statistical evaluations. These three candidate models in the ensemble consisted of a variety of combinations of chemical features, namely one HBD and four HPs in Hypo A; one HBA, one HBD, and two HPs in Hypo B and one HBD and three HPs in Hypo C.[158]

The final PhE/SVM model was generated by the SVM regression of those three pharmacophore hypotheses in the ensemble, yielding the number of the SVM input components (dimensionality) three. According to the results, the PhE/ SVM model executed better than all of those individual hypotheses in the

PhE for those molecules in the training set as further demonstrated by the scatter plot of observed versus the predicted pEC_{50} values. As a result, the PhE/SVM yielded the largest correlation coefficient (r^2) and the smallest root-mean-square error (RMSE), maximum residual (DMax), mean absolute error (MAE), and standard deviation (s) among those four predictive models.[158]

This PhE/SVM model showed to be suitable to predict the P-gp inhibition of structurally diverse compounds, as compared with any other conventional pharmacophore models, which adopted fixed selections of chemical features and can be only used to model molecules of specific chemical structures, substantially limiting their applicability as a result. Furthermore, the PhE/SVM model can elucidate the discrepancies among all reported pharmacophore models, thus showing to be better than the other theoretical models.[158]

In silico approaches were shown to be efficient for the evaluation of drug ADME/Tox.[169] By pharmacophore modeling a predictive model can be developed based on the combination of chemical features to mimic ligands/target protein interactions.[170] In fact, a number of pharmacophore hypotheses have been used to predict the P-gp inhibition, as we discuss hereunder.

P-gp is a highly flexible protein[171] since it can interact with a wide range of structurally diverse compounds.[172,173] According to Leong et al.,[158] a single pharmacophore hypothesis, for example, only a group of fixed chemical features, cannot be used because of the P-gp multiple binding sites,[174,175] suggesting that inhibitors can interact with P-pg using different chemical features. No single predictive model will accurately describe the interactions between P-gp and highly diverse inhibitors,[176] otherwise these predictive models can only be applied to some specific chemotypes.

Ekins *et al.*,[177,178] produced four pharmacophore hypotheses, which consisted of different combinations of chemical features, based on different sets of samples. The discrepancies in feature selections among these four models are consistent with the fact that Hypo A, Hypo B, and Hypo C in the PhE also used different chemical features, suggesting that different chemotypes of inhibitors can interact with P-gp using a variety of chemical interactions in agreement with Pajeva and Wiese,[179] and Pajeva et al.,[180] Furthermore, the four pharmacophore models developed by Ekins *et al.*, consisted of HBD, HBA, HP, and ring aromatic (RA) chemical features, indicating that the only qualitative difference between those four models and PhE/SVM was the absence of RA in the latter. Statistically, the lack of RA did not deteriorate the performance of PhE/SVM as compared with those four pharmacophore models, which gave rise to r^2 values in the range of 0.76–0.88 in the training set. PhE/SVM yielded instead a value of 0.89, suggesting that the chemical feature RA was not necessary to develop a predictive model. In fact, none of the reported predictive inhibition models enrolled the chemical feature RA, except those developed by Ekins et al.,[177,178] and Palmeira et al.,[181]

At least one HBA and one HP can be found among all reported pharmaco-phore hypotheses for P-gp inhibitors,[178–180,182–184] except for those models mentioned above.[177,181] However, only Hypo B in PhE/SVM adopted the chemical feature HBA in agreement with one of the predictive models developed by Ekins et al.,[177]

Langer et al.,[182] developed a pharmacophore hypothesis, which was composed of the chemical features (aromatic) HP, HBA, and positive ionizable (PI). Of the 106 samples in the test set, 34 molecules were projected as inactive. On the contrary, the PhE/SVM model—which comprised of HBD, HBA, and HP—chemical features yielded residuals of no more than 1 log unit for those same 34 molecules, thereby proving to be a much more accurate model.

The qualitative differences between both theoretical models may be attributed to the fact that Langer et al.,[182] enlisted PI as chemical feature without taking into account HBD, whereas PhE/SVM used HBD over PI, suggesting that HBD plays a key role in inhibitor–P-gp interaction.

Many studies have demonstrated the importance of HBD in determining the interaction between inhibitor and P-gp, for example, Ekins et al.,[177], Pajeva and Wiese[179], Pajeva et al.,[180], Wang et al.,[185], Zalloum and Taha[186], and Chen et al.,[187] used HBD related descriptor to construct their QSAR models; and even the CoMSIA model proposed by Labrie et al.,[188] also used the field HBD. Therefore, the chemical feature of HBD seems to play a critical role in the inhibitor/P-gp interaction, and therefore, must be included in any theoretical model.

Moreover, Zalloum and Taha[186] developed a predictive in silico model using receptor surface analysis (RSA) to construct two satisfactory receptor surface models (RSMs) for cyclosporine- and aureobasidin-based P-gp inhibitors. These pseudoreceptors were combined to achieve satisfactory 3D-QSAR for 68 different cyclosporine and aureobasidin derivatives. The resulting 3D-QSAR was used to probe the structural factors that control the inhibitory activities of cyclosporine and aureobasidin analogues against P-gp. Upon validation against an external set of 16 randomly selected P-gp inhibitors, the optimal 3D-QSAR was found to be self-consistent and predictive ($r^2_{LOO}=0.673$, $r^2_{PRESS}=0.600$).[186]

The discovery, bioactivity, mechanism, QSAR, and synthesis of the cyclo-peptides antibiotics gramicidin-S; vancomycin and daptomycin; immunosuppressive cyclosporin-A and astin-C; and antitumor aplidine, RA-V, and RA-VII have been recently reviewed.[97]

8.4   CONCLUSION

A predictive model can be greatly valuable to drug discovery and development. Nevertheless, few QSAR studies have been performed on cyclopeptides in comparison with small organic molecules. In this chapter we selected antimicrobial and immunosuppressive activities of the cyclopeptides from a variety of bioactivities. Structures and reported QSARs have been analyzed. Antimicrobial peptides have structural requirements, and their QSAR models have to take into account the hemolytic and cytotoxic activities.

Immunosuppressive activity refers to P-gp inhibition. Any *in silico* model has to take into account the promiscuous nature of P-gp. A quantitativepredictive model, derived from a novel scheme by assembling a panel of pharmacophore hypothesis candidates to construct PhE and SVM, which gives rise to a regression model, has been analyzed for prediction of P-gp inhibition. Different pharmacophore hypotheses have been discussed. All these models were developed to facilitate drug discovery and development by designing drug candidates with better pharmacokinetic profile in terms of better absorption, higher bioavailability, and more efficiency.

ACKNOWLEDGMENTS

Thanks are due to Universidad de Buenos Aires and CONICET (Argentina) for financial support; Ministerio de Ciencia, Tecnología e Innovación Productiva (MINCYT, Argentina) for electronic bibliography facilities. ABP and AAV are Research Members of the National Research Council (CONICET) of Argentina.

KEYWORDS

- **Antimicrobial cyclopeptides**
- **Cyclopeptides**
- **Lipopolysaccharide**
- **Minidefensins**
- **P-glycoprotein**
- **QSAR models**

REFERENCES

1. Moss, G. Pure Appl. Chem., Nomenclature of Cyclic Peptides. *Recomendación IUPAC*, PAC-REC-04-10-24, **2004**.

2. Soloshonok, V. A. *Enantioselective Synthesis of β-amino acids.* 2nd ed.; Juaristi, E., Ed.; Wiley: New York, **2005.**

3. Pomilio, A. B.; Battista, M. E.; Vitale, A. A. Naturally-Occurring Cyclopeptides: Structures and Bioactivity. *Curr. Org. Chem.* **2006,** 10, 2075–2121.

4. Battista, M. E.; Vitale, A. A.; Pomilio, A. B. Relationship Between the Conformation of the Cyclopeptides Isolated from the Fungus *Amanita Phalloides* (Vaill. Ex Fr.) Secr. and Its Toxicity. *Molecules* **2000,** 5, 489–490.

5. Pomilio, A. B.; Battista, M. E.; Vitale, A. A. Semiempirical AM1 and *Ab Initio* Parameters of the Lethal Cyclopeptides α-Amanitin and Its Related Thioether, *S*-Sulphoxide, Sulphone, and *O*-Methyl Derivative. *J. Mol. Struct.:Theochem* **2001,** 536, 243–262.

6. Pomilio, A. B.; Battista, S. M.; Vitale, A. A. 1. Quantitative Structure-Activity Relationship (QSAR) Studies on Bioactive Cyclopeptides. In *QSPR-QSAR Studies on Desired Properties for Drug Design;* Castro, E. A., Ed.; Research Signpost: Kerala, India, **2010;** Chapter 1.

7. Easton, D. M.; Nijnik, A.; Mayer, M. L.; Hancock, R. E. Potential of Immunomodulatory Host Defense Peptides as Novel Anti-Infectives. *Trends Biotechnol.* **2009,** 27, 582–590.

8. Zhang, L.; Falla, T. J. Potential therapeutic application of host defense peptides. *Methods Mol. Biol.* **2010,** 618, 303–327.

9. Kang, S. J.;Kim, D. H.; Mishig-Ochir, T.; Lee, B. J. Antimicrobial Peptides: Their Physico-chemical Properties and Therapeutic Application. *Arch. Pharm. Res.* **2012,** 35, 409–413.

10. Yeung, A. T.; Gellatly, S. L.; Hancock, R. E. Multifunctional Cationic Host Defence Peptides and Their Clinical Applications. *Cell. Mol. Life Sci.* **2011,** 68, 2161–2176.

11. Ahmad, A.; Ahmad, E.; Rabbani, G.; Haque, S.; Arshad, M.; Khan, R. H. Identification and Design of Antimicrobial Peptides for Therapeutic Applications. *Curr. Protein Pept. Sci.* **2012,** 13, 211–223.

12. Akamatsu, M.; Fujimoto, Y.; Kataoka, M.; Suda, Y.; Kusumoto, S.; Fukase, K. Synthesis of Lipid A Monosaccharide Analogues Containing Acidic Amino Acid: Exploring the Structural Basis for the Endotoxic and Antagonistic Activities. *Bioorg. Med. Chem.* **2006,** 14, 6759–6777.

13. Fujimoto, Y.; Adachi, Y.;Akamatsu, M.; Fukase, Y.; Kataoka, M.; Suda, Y.; Fukase, K.; Kusumoto, S. Synthesis of Lipid A and Its Analogues for Investigation of the Structural Basis for Their Bioactivity. *J. Endotoxin. Res.* **2005,** 11, 341–347.

14. Oyston, P. C.; Fox, M. A.; Richards, S. J.; Clark, G. C.Novel Peptide Therapeutics for Treatment of Infections. *J. Med. Microbiol.* **2009,** 58, 977–987.

15. Ahmad, A.; Yadav, S. P.; Asthana, N.; Mitra, K.; Srivastava, S. P.; Ghosh, J. K. Utilization of an Amphipathic Leucine Zipper Sequence to Design Antibacterial Peptides with Simultaneous Modulation of Toxic Activity Against Human Red Blood Cells. *J. Biol. Chem.* **2006,** 281, 22029–22038.

16. Kruse, T.; Kristensen, H. H. Using Antimicrobial Host Defense Peptides as Anti-Infective and Immunomodulatory Agents. *Expert Rev. Anti Infect. Ther.* **2008,** 6, 887–895.

17. Frecer, V.; Ho, B.; Ding, J. L. Interpretation of Biological Activity Data of Bacterial Endotoxins by Simple Molecular Models of Mechanism of Action. *Eur. J. Biochem.* **2000,** 267, 837–852.

18. Hong, M.; Su, Y. Structure and Dynamics of Cationic Membrane Peptides and Proteins: Insights from Solid-State NMR. *Protein Sci.* **2011,** 20, 641–655.

19. Boughton, A. P.; Nguyen, K.; Andricioaei, I.; Chen, Z. Interfacial Orientation and Secondary Structure Change in Tachyplesin I: Molecular Dynamics and Sum Frequency Generation Spectroscopy Studies. *Langmuir* **2011,** 27, 14343–14351.

20. Balhara, V.; Schmidt, R.; Gorr, S. U.; Dewolf, C. Membrane Selectivity and Biophysical Studies of the Antimicrobial Peptide GL13K. *Biochim. Biophys. Acta* **2013,** 1828, 2193–2203.

21. Mika, J. T.; Moiset, G.; Cirac, A. D.; Feliu, L.; Bardají, E.; Planas, M.; Sengupta, D.; Marrink, S. J.; Poolman, B. Structural Basis for the Enhanced Activity of Cyclic AntimicrobialPeptides: the Case of BPC194. *Biochim.Biophys.Acta* **2011**, 1808, 2197–2205.

22. Nguyen, L. T.; Haney, E. F.; Vogel, H. J. The Expanding Scope of Antimicrobial Peptide Structures and Their Modes of Action. *Trends Biotechnol.* **2011**, 29, 464–472.

23. Clifton, L. A.; Skoda, M. W. A.; Daulton, E. L.; Hughes, A. V.; Le Brun, A. P.; Lakey, J. H.; Holt, S. A. Asymmetric Phospholipid: Lipopolysaccharide Bilayers; A Gram-Negative Bacterial Outer Membrane Mimic. *J. R. Soc. Interface* **2013**, 10, 20130810.

24. El Ichi, S.; Leon, F.; Vossier, L.; Marchandin, H.; Errachid, A.; Coste, J.; Jaffrezic-Renault, N.; Fournier-Wirth, C. Microconductometric Immunosensor for Label-Free and Sensitive Detection of Gram-Negative Bacteria. *Biosens. Bioelectron.* **2014**, 54, 378–384.

25. Desai, P.; Ram, R.; Patlolla, R. R.; Singh, M. Interaction of Nanoparticles and Cell-Penetrating Peptides with Skin for Transdermal Drug Delivery. *Mol. Membr. Biol.* **2010**, 27, 247–259.

26. Hadley, E. B.; Hancock, R. E. Strategies for the Discovery and Advancement of Novel Cationic Antimicrobial Peptides. *Curr. Top. Med. Chem.* **2010**, 10, 1872–1881.

27. Kang, S. J.; Kim, D. H.; Mishig-Ochir, T.; Lee, B. J. Antimicrobial Peptides: Their Physicochemical Properties and Therapeutic Application. *Arch. Pharm. Res.* **2012**, 35, 409–413.

28. Jahnsen, R. D.; Frimodt-Møller, N.; Franzyk, H. Antimicrobial Activity of Peptidomimetics Against Multidrug-Resistant *Escherichia coli*: A Comparative Study of Different Backbones. *J. Med. Chem.* **2012**, 55, 7253–7261.

29. Allahverdiyev, A. M.; Kon, K. V.; Abamor, E. S.; Bagirova, M.; Rafailovich, M. Coping with Antibiotic Resistance: Combining Nanoparticles with Antibiotics and Other Antimicrobial Agents. *Expert Rev. Anti Infect. Ther.* **2011**, 9, 1035–1052.

30. Tran, N.; Tran, P. A. Nanomaterial-Based Treatments for Medical Device-Associated Infections. *Chemphyschem.* **2012**, 13, 2481–2494.

31. Milani, A.; Benedusi, M.; Aquila, M.; Rispoli, G. Pore Forming Properties of Cecropin-Melittin Hybrid Peptide in a Natural Membrane. *Molecules* **2009**, 14, 5179–5188.

32. Trabulo, S.; Cardoso, A.L.; Mano, M.; Pedroso de Lima, M. C. Cell-Penetrating Peptides—Mechanisms of Cellular Uptake and Generation of Delivery Systems. *Pharmaceuticals* **2010**, 3, 961–993.

33. Chen, Y.; Mant, C. T.; Farmer, S. W.; Hancock, R. E.; Vasil, M. L.; Hodges, R. S. Rational Design of *alpha*-Helical Antimicrobial Peptides with Enhanced Activities and Specificity/Therapeutic Index. *J. Biol. Chem.* **2005**, 280, 12316–12329.

34. Liu, F.; Lewis, R. N.; Hodges, R.S.; McElhaney, R. N. Effect of Variations in the Structure of a Polyleucine-Based *alpha*-Helical Transmembrane Peptide on Its Interaction with Phosphatidylglycerol Bilayers. *Biochemistry* **2004**, 43, 3679–3687.

35. Liu, F.; Lewis, R. N.; Hodges, R. S.; McElhaney, R. N. Effect of Variations in the Structure of a Polyleucine-Based *alpha*-Helical Transmembrane Peptide on Its Interaction With Phosphatidylethanolamine Bilayers. *Biophys. J.* **2004**, 87, 2470–2482.

36. Hoernke, M.; Schwieger, C.; Kerth, A.; Blume, A. Binding of Cationic Pentapeptides with Modified Side Chain Lengths to Negatively Charged Lipid Membranes: Complex Interplay of Electrostatic and Hydrophobic Interactions. *Biochim. Biophys. Acta* **2012**, 1818, 1663–1672.

37. Glukhov, E.; Burrows, L. L.; Deber, C. M. Membrane Interactions of Designed Cationic Antimicrobial Peptides: The Two Thresholds. *Biopolymers* **2008**, 89, 360–371.

38. McPhee, J. B., Hancock, R. E. Function and Therapeutic Potential of Host Defence Peptides. *J. Pept. Sci.* **2005**, 11, 677–687.

39. Afacan, N. J.; Yeung, A. T.; Pena, O. M.; Hancock, R. E. Therapeutic Potential of Host Defense Peptides in Antibiotic-Resistant Infections. *Curr. Pharm. Des.* **2012**, 18, 807–819.

40. Zikou, S.; Koukkou, A. I.; Mastora, P.; Sakarellos-Daitsiotis, M.; Sakarellos, C.; Drainas, C.; Panou-Pomonis, E. Design and Synthesis of Cationic Aib-Containing Antimicrobial Peptides: Conformational and Biological Studies. *J. Pept. Sci.* **2007**, 13, 481–486.

41. Hammami, R.; Ben Hamida, J.; Vergoten, G.; Fliss, I. PhytAMP: A Database Dedicated to Antimicrobial Plant Peptides. *Nucleic Acids Res.* **2009**, 37, D963–968.

42. Wang, G.; Li, X.; Wang, Z. APD2: The Updated Antimicrobial Peptide Database and Its Application in Peptide Design. *Nucleic Acids Res.* **2009**, 37, D933–937.

43. Dennison, S. R.; Morton, L. H.; Harris, F.; Phoenix, D. A. The Impact of Membrane Lipid Composition on Antimicrobial Function of an *alpha*-Helical Peptide. *Chem. Phys. Lipids* **2008**, 151, 92–102.

44. Mahalka, A. K.; Kinnunen, P. K. Binding of Amphipathic *alpha*-Helical Antimicrobial Peptides to Lipid Membranes: Lessons from Temporins B and L. *Biochim. Biophys. Acta* **2009**, 1788, 1600–1609.

45. Chen, Y., Guarnieri, M. T., Vasil, A. I., Vasil, M. L., Mant, C. T., Hodges, R. S. Role of Peptide Hydrophobicity in the Mechanism of Action of α-Helical Antimicrobial Peptides. *Antimicrob. Agents Chemother.* **2007**, 51, 1398–1406.

46. Huang, Y.; Huang, J.; Chen, Y. *alpha*-Helical Cationic Antimicrobial Peptides: Relationships of Structure and Function. *Protein Cell* **2010**, 1, 143–152.

47. Zhao, L. J.; Huang, Y. B.; Gao, S.; Cui, Y.; He, D.; Wang, L.; Chen, Y. X. Comparison on Effect of Hydrophobicity on the Antibacterial and Antifungal Activities of *alpha*-Helical Antimicrobial Peptides. *Scientia Sin. Chim.* **2013**, 43, 1041–1050.

48. Lehrer, R. I.; Lu, W. α-Defensins in Human Innate Immunity. *Immunol. Rev.* **2012**, 245, 84–112.

49. Fattorini, L.; Gennaro, R.; Zanetti, M.; Tan, D.; Brunori, L.; Giannoni, F.; Pardini, M.; with Isoniazid, Against *Mycobacterium tuberculosis*. *Peptides* **2004**, 25, 1075–1077.

50. Abraham, T.; Prenner, E. J.; Lewis, R. N.; Mant, C. T.; Keller, S.; Hodges, R. S.; McElhaney, R. N. Structure-Activity Relationships of the Antimicrobial Peptide Gramicidin S and Its Analogs: Aqueous Solubility, Self-Association, Conformation, Antimicrobial Activity and Interaction with Model Lipid Membranes. *Biochim. Biophys. Acta* **2014**, 1838, 1420–1429.

51. Sitaram, N. Antimicrobial Peptides with Unusual Amino Acid Compositions and Unusual Structures. *Curr. Med. Chem.* **2006**, 13, 679–696.

52. De Smet, K.; Contreras, R. Human Antimicrobial Peptides: Defensins, Cathelicidins and Histatins. *Biotechnol. Lett.* **2005**, 27, 1337–1347.

53. Mookherjee, N.; Rehaume, L.; Hancock, R. E. Cathelicidins and Functional Analogues as Antisepsis Molecules. *Expert Opin. Therap. Targets* **2007**, 11, 993–1004.

54. Yeung, A. T.; Gellatly, S. L.; Hancock, R. E. Multifunctional Cationic Host Defence Peptides and Their Clinical Applications. *Cell. Mol. Life Sci.* **2011**, 68, 2161–2176.

55. Hazlett, L.; Wu, M. Defensins in Innate Immunity. *Cell Tissue Res.* 2011, 343, 175–188.

56. Cole, A. M.; Lehrer, R. I. Minidefensins: Antimicrobial Peptides with Activity against HIV-1. *Curr. Pharm. Des.* **2003**, 9, 1463–1473.

57. Redman, J. E.; Wilcoxen, K. M.; Ghadiri, M. R. Automated Mass Spectrometric Sequence Determination of Cyclic Peptide Library Members. *J. Comb. Chem.* **2003**, 5, 33–40.

58. Boddy, C. N. Sweetening Cyclic Peptide Libraries. *Chem. Biol.* **2004**, 11, 1599–1600. Comment on: *Chem. Biol.* **2004**, 11, 1635.

59. Devine, D. A.; Hancock, R. E. W. Cationic Peptides: Distribution and Mechanisms of Resistance. *Curr. Pharm. Des.* **2002**, 8, 703–714.

60. Jin, Y.; Hammer, J.; Pate, M.; Zhang, Y.; Zhu, F.; Zmuda, E.; Blazyk, J. Antimicrobial Activities and Structures of Two Linear Cationic Peptide Families with Various Amphipathic *beta*-Sheet and *alpha*-Helical Potentials. *Antimicrob. Agents Chemother.* **2005**, 49, 4957–4964.

61. Muhle, S. A.; Tam, J. P. Design of Gram-Negative Selective Antimicrobial Peptides. *Biochemistry* **2001**, 40, 5777–5785.
62. Ramamoorthy, A.; Thennarasu, S.; Tan, A.; Gottipati, K.; Sreekumar, S.; Heyl, D. L.; An, F. Y.; Shelburne, C. E. Deletion of All Cysteines in Tachyplesin I Abolishes Hemolytic Activity and Retains Antimicrobial Activity and Lipopolysaccharide Selective Binding. *Biochemistry* **2006**, 45, 6529–6540.
63. Schmitt, M. A.; Weisblum, B.; Gellman, S. H. Interplay among Folding, Sequence, and Lipophilicity in the Antibacterial and Hemolytic Activities of *alpha/beta*-Peptides. *J. Am. Chem. Soc.* **2007**, 129, 417–428.
64. Oren, Z.; Shai, Y. Cyclization of a Cytolytic Amphipathic *alpha*-Helical Peptide and Its Diastereomer: Effect on Structure, Interaction with Model Membranes, and Biological Function. *Biochemistry* **2000**, 39, 6103–6114.
65. Kondejewski, L. H.; Lee, D. L.; Jelokhani-Niaraki, M.; Farmer, S. W.; Hancock, R. E. W.; Hodges, R. S. Optimization of Microbial Specificity in Cyclic Peptides by Modulation of Hydrophobicity within a Defined Structural Framework. *J. Biol. Chem.* **2002**, 277, 67–74.
66. Lee, D. L.; Powers, J. P. S.; Pflegerl, K.; Vasil, M. L.; Hancock, R. E. W.; Hodges, R. S. Effects of Single *D*-Amino Acid Substitutions on Disruption of *beta*-Sheet Structure and Hydrophobicity in Cyclic 14-Residue Antimicrobial Peptide Analogs Related to Gramicidin S. *J. Pept. Res.* **2004**, 63, 69–84.
67. Frecer, V.; Ho, B.; Ding, J. L. *De Novo* Design of Potent Antimicrobial Peptides. *Antimicrob. Agents Chemother.* **2004**, 48, 3349–3357.
68. Jenssen, H.; Hamill, P.; Hancock, R. E. W. Peptide Antimicrobial Agents. *Clin. Microbiol. Rev.* **2006**, 19, 491–511.
69. Lee, D. L.; Mant, C. T.; Hodges, R. S. A Novel Method to Measure Self-Association of Small Amphipathic Molecules: Temperature Profiling in Reversed-Phase Chromatography. *J. Biol. Chem.* **2003**, 278, 22918–22927.
70. Brown, K. L.; Mookherjee, N.; Hancock, R. E. W. *Antimicrobial, Host Defence Peptides and Proteins. Encyclopedia of Life Sciences.* John Wiley: Chichester, **2007**.
71. Abraham, T.; Lewis, R. N. A. H.; Hodges, R. S.; McElhaney, R. N. Isothermal Titration Calorimetry Studies of the Binding of a Rationally Designed Analogue of the Antimicrobial Peptide Gramicidin S to Phospholipid Bilayer Membranes. *Biochemistry* **2005**, 44, 2103–2112.
72. Mei, H.; Liao, Z. H.; Zhou, Y.; Li, S. Z. A New Set of Amino Acid Descriptors and Its Application in Peptide QSARs. *Biopolymers* **2005**, 80, 775–786.
73. Feder, R.; Dagan, A.; Mor, A. Structure-Activity Relationship Study of Antimicrobial Dermaseptin S4 Showing the Consequences of Peptide Oligomerization on Selective Cytotoxicity. *J. Biol. Chem.* **2000**, 275, 4230–4238.
74. Rotem, S.; Radzishevsky, I.; Mor, A. Physicochemical Properties That Enhance Discriminative Antibacterial Activity of Short Dermaseptin Derivatives. *Antimicrob. Agents Chemother.* **2006**, 50, 2666–2672.
75. Lazaridis, T.; He, Y.; Prieto, L. Membrane Interactions and Pore Formation by the Antimicrobial Peptide Protegrin. *Biophys. J.* **2013**, 104, 633–642.
76. Skalicky, J. J.; Selsted, M. E.; Pardi, A. Structure and Dynamics of the Neutrophil Defensins NP-2, NP-5, and HNP-1: NMR Studies of Amide Hydrogen Exchange Kinetics. *Proteins* **1994**, 20, 52–67.
77. Robinson, J. A.; Shankaramma, S. C.; Jetter, P.; Kienzl, U.; Schwenderer, R. A.; Vrijbloed, J. W.; Obrecht, D. Properties and Structure-Activity Studies of Cyclic *beta*-Hairpin Peptidomimetics Based on the Cationic Antimicrobial Peptide Protegrin I. *Bioorg. Med. Chem.* **2005**, 13, 2055–2064.
78. Chen, J.; Falla, T. J.; Liu, H.; Hurst, M. A.; Fujii, C. A.; Mosca, D. A.; Embree, J. R.; Loury, D. J.; Radel, P. A.; Chang, C. C.; Gu, L.; Fiddes, J. C. Development of Protegrins for the

Treatment and Prevention of Oral Mucositis: Structure-Activity Relationships of Synthetic Protegrin Analogues. *Biopolymers* **2000**, 55, 88–98.

79. Shankaramma, S. C.; Athanassiou, Z.; Zerbe, O.; Moehle, K.; Mouton, C.; Bernardini, F.; Vrijbloed, J. W.; Obrecht, D.; Robinson, J. A. Macrocyclic Hairpin Mimetics of the Cationic Antimicrobial Peptide Protegrin I: A New Family of Broad-Spectrum Antibiotics. *ChemBioChem.* **2002**, 3, 1126–1133.

80. Shankaramma, S. C.; Moehle, K.; James, S.; Vrijbloed, J. W.; Obrecht, D.; Robinson, J. A. A Family of Macrocyclic Antibiotics with a Mixed Peptide-Peptoid *beta*-Hairpin Backbone Conformation. *Chem. Commun. (Camb.)* **2003**, 1842–1843.

81. Descours, A.; Moehle, K.; Renard, A.; Robinson, J. A. A New Family of *beta*-Hairpin Mimetics Based on a Trypsin Inhibitor from Sunflower Seeds. *Chembiochem.* **2002**, 3, 318–323.

82. Athanassiou, Z.; Dias, R. L. A.; Moehle, K.; Dobson, N.; Varani, G.; Robinson, J. A. Structural Mimicry of Retroviral Tat Proteins by Constrained *beta*-Hairpin Peptidomimetics: Ligands with High Affinity and Selectivity for Viral TAR RNA Regulatory Elements. *J. Am. Chem. Soc.* **2004**, 126, 6906–6913.

83. Fasan, R.; Dias, R.L.A.; Moehle, K.; Zerbe, O.; Vrijbloed, J.W.; Obrecht, D.; Robinson, J.A. Using a *beta*-Hairpin to Mimic an *alpha*-Helix: Cyclic Peptidomimetic Inhibitors of the P53-HDM2 Protein-Protein Interaction. *Angew. Chem., Int. Ed.* **2004**, 43, 2109–2112.

84. Frecer, V. QSAR Analysis of Antimicrobial and Haemolytic Effects of Cyclic Cationic Antimicrobial Peptides Derived from Protegrin-1. *Biorg. Med. Chem.* **2006**, 14, 6065–6074.

85. Dawson, R. M. C.; Elliott, D. C.; Elliott, W. H.; Jones, K. M. *Data for Biochemical Research;* 3rd ed.; Oxford Science Publications, 1, **1986**.

86. Jenssen, H.; Lejon, T.; Hilpert, K.; Fjell, C.; Cherkasov, A.; Hancock, R. E. W. Evaluating Different Descriptors for Model Design of Antimicrobial Peptides with Enhanced Activity toward *P. aeruginosa*. *Chem. Biol. Drug Design* **2007**, 70, 134–142.

87. Rogers, D.; Hopfinger, A. J. Application of Genetic Function Approximation to Quantitative Structure-Activity Relationships and Quantitative Structure-Property Relationships. *J. Chem. Inf. Comput. Sci.* **1994**, 34, 854–866.

88. Tam, J. P.; Wu, C.; Yang, J.-L. Membranolytic Selectivity of Cystine-Stabilized Cyclic Protegrins. *Eur. J. Biochem.* **2000**, 267, 3289–3300.

89. Lai, J. R.; Huck, B. R.; Weisblum, B.; Gellman, S. H. Design of Non-Cysteine-Containing Antimicrobial *beta*-Hairpins: Structure-Activity Relationship Studies with Linear Protegrin-1 Analogues. *Biochemistry* **2002**, 41, 12835–12842.

90. Mani, R.; Waring, A. J.; Lehrer, R. I.; Hong, M. Membrane-Disruptive Abilities of *beta*-Hairpin Antimicrobial Peptides Correlate with Conformation and Activity: A ^{31}P And ^{1}H NMR Study. *Biochim. Biophys. Acta* **2005**, 1716, 11–18.

91. Bhonsle, J. B.; Venugopal, D.; Huddler, D. P.; Magill, A. J.; Hicks, R. P. Application of 3D-QSAR for Identification of Descriptors Defining Bioactivity of Antimicrobial Peptides. *J. Med. Chem.* **2007**, 50, 6545–6553.

92. Sundriyal, S.; Sharma, R. K.; Jain, R.; Bharatam, P. V. Minimum Requirements of Hydrophobic and Hydrophilic Features in Cationic Peptide Antibiotics (CPAs): Pharmacophore Generation and Validation with Cationic Steroid Antibiotics (CSAs). *J. Mol. Model.* **2008**, 14, 265–278.

93. Hilpert, K.; Fjell, C.D.; Cherkasov, A. Short Linear Cationic Antimicrobial Peptides: Screening, Optimizing, and Prediction. *Methods Mol. Biol.* **2008**, 494, 127–159.

94. Fjell, C. D.; Jenssen, H.; Hilpert, K.; Cheung, W. A.; Pante, N.; Hancock, R. E.; Cherkasov, A. Identification of Novel Antibacterial Peptides by Chemoinformatics and Machine Learning. *J. Med. Chem.* **2009**, 52, 2006–2015.

95. Cruz-Monteagudo, M.; Romero, Y.; Cordeiro, M. N.; Borges F. Desirability-Based Multi-Criteria Virtual Screening of Selective Antimicrobial Cyclic *beta*-Hairpin Cationic Peptidomimetics. *Curr. Pharm. Des.* **2013**, 19, 2148–2163.

96. Mann, J. Natural Products as Immunosuppressive Agents. *Nat. Prod. Rep.* **2001**, 18, 417–430.
97. Xu, W. Y.; Zhao, S. M.; Zeng, G. Z.; He, W. J.; Xu, H. M.; Tan, N. H. [Progress in the Study of Some Important Natural Bioactive Cyclopeptides]. *Yao Xue Xue Bao* **2012**, 47, 271–279. Article in Chinese.
98. Hitotsuyanagi, Y.; Odagiri, M.; Kato, S.; Kusano, J.; Hasuda, T.; Fukaya, H.; Takeya, K. Isolation, Structure Determination, and Synthesis of *Allo*-RA-V and *Neo*-RA-V, RA-Series Bicyclic Peptides from *Rubia cordifolia* L. *Chem.-Eur. J.* **2012**, 18, 2839–2846.
99. Morita, H.; Gonda, A.; Takeya, K.; Itokawa, H.; Hirano, T.; Oka, K.; Shirota, O. Solution State Conformation of an Immunosuppressive Cyclic Dodecapeptide, Cycloleonurinin. *Tetrahedron* **1997**, 53, 7469–7478.
100. Morita, H.; Shishido, A.; Matsumoto, T.; Takeya, K.; Itokawa, H.; Hirano, T.; Oka, K. A New Immunosuppressive Cyclic Nonapeptide, Cyclolinopeptide B from *Linum usitatissimum*. *Bioorg. Med. Chem. Lett.* **1997**, 7, 1269–1272.
101. Picur, B.;Cebrat, M.; Zabrocki, J.;Siemion, I. Z. Cyclopeptides of *Linum usitatissimum*. *J. Pept. Sci.* **2006**, 12, 569–574.
102. Rempel, B.; Gui ,B.; Maley, J.; Reaney, M.; Sammynaiken, R. Biomolecular Interaction Study of Cyclolinopeptide A with Human Serum Albumin. *J. Biomed. Biotechnol.* **2010**, 2010, 737289.
103. Witkowska, R.; Donigiewicz, A.; Zimecki, M.; Zabrocki, J. New Analogue of Cyclolinopeptide B Modified by Amphiphilic Residue of *alpha*-Hydroxymethylmethionine. *Acta Biochim. Polonica* **2004**, 51, 67–72.
104. Gaymes, T. J.; Cebrat, M.; Siemion, I. Z.; Kay, J. E. Cyclolinopeptide A (CLA) Mediates Its Immunosuppressive Activity Through Cyclophilin-Dependent Calcineurin Inactivation. *FEBS Lett.* **1997**, 418, 224–227.
105. Ruchala, P.; Picur, B.; Lisowski, M.; Cierpicki, T.; Wieczorek, Z.; Siemion, I. Z. Synthesis, Conformation, and Immunosuppressive Activity of CLX and Its Analogues. *Biopolymers,* **2003**, 70, 497–511.
106. Wenger, R. M. Pharmacology of Cyclosporin (Sandimmune). II. Chemistry. *Pharmacol. Rev.* **1990**, 41, 243–247.
107. Rao, A.; Luo, C.; Hogan, P. G. Transcription Factors of the NFAT Family: Regulation and Function. *Annu. Rev. Immunol.* **1997**, 15, 707–747.
108. Krauss, G. *Biochemistry of Signal Transduction and Regulation*, Wiley VCH: Weinheim, **1999**, 220.
109. Hinterding, K.; Alonso-Díaz, D.; Waldmann, H.Organic Synthesis and Biological Signal Transduction. *Angew. Chem., Int. Ed.* **1998**, 37, 688–749.
110. Simmons, T. L.; Andrianasolo, E.; McPhail, K.; Flatt, P.; Gerwick, W. H. Marine Natural Products as Anticancer Drugs. *Mol. Cancer Ther.* **2005**, 4, 333–342.
111. Siemion, I. Z.; Pedyczak, A.; Trojnar, J.; Zimecki, M.; Wieczorek, Z. Immunosuppressive Activity of Antamanide and Some of Its Analogues. *Peptides* **1992**, 13, 1233–1237.
112. Wieczorek, Z.; Siemion, I. Z.; Zimecki, M.; Bolewska-Pedyczak, E.; Wieland T. Immunosuppressive activity in the series of cycloamanide peptides from mushrooms. *Peptides* **1993**, 14, 1–5.
113. Sarabia, F.; Chammaa, S.; Ruiz, A. S.; Ortiz, L. M.; Herrera, F. J. Chemistry and Biology of Cyclic Depsipeptides of Medicinal and Biological Interest. *Curr. Med. Chem.* **2004**, 11, 1309–1332.
114. Rinehart, K. L.; Kishore, V.; Bible, K. C.; Sakai, R.; Sullins, D. W.; Li, M. Didemnins and Tunichlorin: Novel Natural Products from the Marine Tunicate *Trididemnum solidum*. *J. Nat. Prod.* **1988**, 51, 1–21. Erratum in: *J. Nat. Prod.* **988**, 51, 624.

115. Jimeno, J., López-Martín, J. A.; Ruiz-Casado, A.; Izquierdo, M. A.; Scheuer, P. J., Rinehart, K. Progress in the Clinical Development of New Marine-Derived Anticancer Compounds. *Anticancer Drugs* **2004**, 15, 321–329.

116. Hamada, Y.; Shioiri, T. Recent Progress of the Synthetic Studies of Biologically Active Marine Cyclic Peptides and Depsipeptides. *Chem. Rev.* **2005**, 105, 4441–4482.

117. Singh R.; Sharma M.; Joshi P.; Rawat D. S. Clinical Status of Anti-Cancer Agents Derived from Marine Sources. *Anticancer Agents Med. Chem.* **2008**, 8, 603–617.

118. Rinehart, K. L. Antitumor Compounds from Tunicates. *Med. Res. Rev.* **2000**, 20, 1–27.

119. Le Tourneau, C.; Raymond, E.; Faivre, S. Aplidine: A Paradigm of How to Handle the Activity and Toxicity of a Novel Marine Anticancer Poison. *Curr. Pharm. Des.* **2007**, 13, 3427–3439.

120. Le Tourneau, C.; Faivre, S.; Ciruelos, E.; Domínguez, M. J.; López-Martín, J. A.; Izquierdo, M. A.; Jimeno, J.; Raymond, E. Reports of Clinical Benefit of Plitidepsin (Aplidine), a New Marine-Derived Anticancer Agent, in Patients with Advanced Medullary Thyroid Carcinoma. *Am. J. Clin. Oncol.* **2010**, 33, 132–136.

121. Muñoz-Alonso, M. J.; Álvarez, E.; Guillén-Navarro, M. J.; Pollán, M.; Avilés, P.; Galmarini, C. M.; Muñoz, A. c-Jun N-Terminal Kinase Phosphorylation Is a Biomarker of Plitidepsin Activity. *Mar Drugs* **2013**, 11, 1677–1692.

122. Rawat , D. S.; Joshi, M. C.; Joshi, P.; Atheaya, H. Marine Peptides and Related Compounds in Clinical Trial. *Anticancer Agents Med .Chem.* **2006**, 6, 33–40.

123. Vera, M. D.; Joullié M. M. Natural Products as Probes of Cell Biology: 20 Years of Didemnin Research. *Med. Res. Rev.* **2002**, 22, 102–145.

124. Lee, J.; Currano, J. N.; Carroll, P. J.; Joullié, M. M. Didemnins, Tamandarins and Related Natural Products. *Nat. Prod. Rep.* **2012**, 29, 404–424.

125. Dawson, S.; Malkinson, J. P.; Paumier, D.; Searcey, M. Bisintercalator Natural Products with Potential Therapeutic Applications: Isolation, Structure Determination, Synthetic and Biological Studies. *Nat. Prod. Rep.* **2007**, 24, 109–126.

126. Gao, J.; Hamann, M. T. Chemistry and Biology of Kahalalides. *Chem. Rev.* **2011**, 111, 3208–3235.

127. Jimeno, J.; Aracil, M.; Tercero, J. C. Adding Pharmacogenomics to the Development of New Marine-Derived Anticancer Agents. *J. Trans. Med.* **2006**, 4, 3.

128. Albadry, M. A.; Elokely, K. M.; Wang, B.; Bowling, J. J.; Abdelwahab, M. F.; Hossein, M. H.; Doerksen, R. J.; Hamann, M. T. Computationally Assisted Assignment of Kahalalide Y Configuration Using an NMR-Constrained Conformational Search. *J. Nat. Prod.* **2013**, 76, 178–185.

129. Schuster, D.; Laggner, C.; Langer, T. Why Drugs Fail – A Study on Side Effects in New Chemical Entities. In *Antitargets Prediction and Prevention of Drug Side Effects*. Vaz, R. J.; Klabunde, T., Eds.; Wiley-VCH: Weinheim, **2008**; pp. 3–22.

130. Mannhold, R.; Kubinyi, H.; Folkers, G. Preface, In *Antitargets Prediction and Prevention of Drug Side Effects*; Vaz, R. J.; Klabunde, T., Eds.; Wiley-VCH: Weinheim, 2008; pp. XIX–XX.

131. Schinkel, A. H.; Jonker, J. W. Mammalian Drug Efflux Transporters of the ATP Binding Cassette (ABC) Family: An Overview. *Adv. Drug Deliver. Rev.* **2003**, 55, 3–29.

132. Benet, L. Z. The Drug Transporter-Metabolism Alliance: Uncovering and Defining the Interplay. *Mol. Pharmaceutics* **2009**, 6, 1631–1643.

133. Grover, A.; Benet, L. Z. Effects of Drug Transporters on Volume of Distribution. *AAPS J.* **2009**, 11, 250–261.

134. Shutgarts, S.; Benet, L. Z. The Role of Transporters in the Pharmacokinetics of Orally Administered Drugs. *Pharm. Res.* **2009**, 26, 2039–2054.

135. Ambudkar, S. V.; Kimchi-Sarfaty, C.; Sauna, Z. E.; Gottesman, M. M. P-Glycoprotein: From Genomics to Mechanism. *Oncogene* **2003**, 22, 7468–7485.

136. Gottesman, M. M.; Pastan, I. Biochemistry of Multidrug Resistance Mediated by the Multidrug Transporter. *Ann. Rev. Biochem.* **2003**, 62, 385–427.
137. Bansal, T.; Jaggi, M.; Khar, R. K.; Talegaonkar, S. Status of Flavonols as P-Glycoprotein Inhibitors in Cancer Chemotherapy. *Curr. Cancer Ther. Rev.* **2009**, 5, 89–99.
138. Ambudkar, S. V,; Dey, S.; Hrycyna, C. A,; Ramachandra, M.; Pastan, I.; Gottesman, M. M.Biochemical, Cellular, and Pharmacological Aspects of the Multidrug Transporter. *Annu. Rev. Pharmacol. Toxicol.* **1999**, 39, 361–398.
139. Jansen, G.; Scheper, R.; Dijkmans, B. Multidrug Resistance Proteins in Rheumatoid Arthritis, Role in Disease-Modifying Antirheumatic Drug Efficacy and Inflammatory Processes: An Overview. *Scand. J. Rheumatol.* **2003**, 32, 325–336.
140. Löscher W, Potschka, H. Drug Resistance in Brain Diseases and the Role of Drug Efflux Transporters. *Nat. Rev. Neurosci.* **2005**, 6, 591–602.
141. Leonard, G. D.; Fojo, T.; Bates, S. E. The Role of ABC Transporters in Clinical Practice. *Oncologist* **2003**, 8, 411–424.
142. Szakacs, G.; Paterson, J. K.; Ludwig, J. A.; Booth-Genthe, C.; Gottesman, M. M. Targeting Multidrug Resistance in Cancer. *Nat. Rev. Drug Discov.* **2006**, 5, 219–234.
143. Crowley, E.; McDevitt, C. A.; Callaghan, R. Generating inhibitors of P-glycoprotein: Where to, Now? In *Multi-Drug Resistance in Cancer*; Zhou, J., Ed.; Humana Press: New York, **2010**; pp 405–432.
144. Choi, S. ABC Transporters as Multidrug Resistance Mechanisms and the Development of Chemosensitizers for their Reversal. *Cancer Cell Int.* **2005**, 5, 30. Online.
145. Broccatelli, F.; Carosati, E.; Cruciani, G.; Oprea, T. I. Transporter-Mediated Efflux Influences CNS Side Effects: ABCB1, from Antitarget to Target. *Mol. Inf.* **2010**, 29, 16–26.
146. Food and Drug Administration, Advisory Committee for Pharmaceutical Science [accessed January 2014]. http://www.fda.gov/ohrms/dockets/ac/04/slides/2004-4079s1.htm.
147. Di Ianni, M.; Alan Talevi, A.; Castro, E. A.; Bruno-Blanch, L. E. Development of a Highly Specific Ensemble of Topological Models for Early Identification of P-Glycoprotein Substrates. *J. Chemometrics* **2011**, 25, 313–322.
148. Klepsch, F.; Ecker, G. F. Impact of the Recent Mouse P-Glycoprotein Structure for Structure-Based Ligand Design. *Mol. Inf.* **2010**, 29, 276–286.
149. Demel, M. A.; Schwaha, R.; Krämer, O.; Ettmayer, P.; Haaksma, E. E. J.; Ecker, G. F. *In Silico* Prediction of Substrate Properties for ABC-Multidrug Transporters. *Expert. Opin. Drug. Metab. Toxicol.* **2008**, 4, 1167–1180.
150. Crivori, P. Computational Models for P-Glycoprotein Substrates and Inhibitors. In *Antitargets Prediction and Prevention of Drug Side Effects;* Vaz, R. J.; Klabunde, T., Eds.; Wiley-VCH: Weinheim, **2008**; pp. 367–397.
151. Broccatelli, F.; Carosati, E.; Neri, A.; Frosini, M.; Goracci, L.; Oprea, T. I.; Cruciani, G. A Novel Approach for Predicting P-glycoprotein (ABCB1) Inhibition Using Molecular Interaction Fields. *J. Med. Chem.* **2011**, 54, 1740–1751.
152. Perruccio, F.; Mason, J.; Sciabola, S.; Baroni, M. FLAP: 4 Point Pharmacophore Fingerprints from GRID. In *Molecular Interaction Fields: Applications in Drug Discovery and ADME Prediction*; Cruciani, G, Ed.; Wiley-VCH: Weinheim, **2005**; Vol. 27; pp. 83–102.
153. Baroni, M.; Cruciani, G.; Sciabola, S.; Perruccio, F.; Mason, J. S. A Common Reference Framework for Analyzing/Comparing Proteins and Ligands. Fingerprints for Ligands and Proteins (FLAP): Theory and Application. *J. Chem. Inf. Model.* **2007**, 47, 279–294.
154. Li, W.-X.; Li, L.; Eksterowicz, J.; Ling, X. B.; Cardozo, M. Significance Analysis and Multiple Pharmacophore Models For Differentiating P-Glycoprotein Substrates. *J. Chem. Inf. Model.* **2007**, 47, 2429–2438.
155. Leong, M. K. A Novel Approach Using Pharmacophore Ensemble/Support Vector Machine (PhE/SVM) for Prediction of hERG Liability. *Chem. Res. Toxicol.* **2007**, 20, 217–226.

156. Leong, M. K.; Chen, Y.-M.; Chen, H.-B.; Chen, P.-H. Development of a New Predictive Model for Interactions with Human Cytochrome P450 2A6 Using Pharmacophore Ensemble/Support Vector Machine (PhE/SVM) Approach. *Pharm. Res.* **2009**, 26, 987–1000.

157. Leong, M. K.; Chen, T.-H. Prediction of Cytochrome P450 2B6-Substrate Interactions Using Pharmacophore Ensemble/Support Vector Machine (PhE/SVM) Approach. *Med. Chem.* **2008**, 4, 396–406.

158. Leong, M. K.; Chen, H.-B.; Shih, Y.-H. Prediction of Promiscuous P-Glycoprotein Inhibition Using ä Novel Machine Learning Scheme. *PLoS ONE* **2012**, 7, e33829.

159. Chiba, P.; Holzer, W.; Landau, M.; Bechmann, G.; Lorenz, K.; Plagens, B.; Hitzler, M.; Richter E.; Ecker, G. Substituted 4-Acylpyrazoles and 4-Acylpyrazolones: Synthesis and Multidrug Resistance-Modulating Activity. *J. Med. Chem.* **1998**, 41, 4001–4011.

160. Hiessböck, R.; Wolf, C.; Richter, E.; Hitzler, M.; Chiba, P.;Kratzel, M.; Ecker, G. Synthesis and *In Vitro* Multidrug Resistance Modulating Activity of a Series of Dihydrobenzopyrans and Tetrahydroquinolines. *J. Med. Chem.* **1999**, 42, 1921–1926.

161. Klein, C.; Kaiser, D.; Kopp, S.; Chiba, P.; Ecker, G. F. Similarity Based SAR (SIBAR) as Tool for Early ADME Profiling. *J. Comput.-Aided Mol. Des.* **2002**, 16, 785–793.

162. Langer, T.; Eder, M.; Hoffmann, R. D.; Chiba, P.; Ecker, G. F. Lead Identification for Modulators of Multidrug Resistance Based on *In Silico* Screening with a Pharmacophoric Feature Model. *Arch. Pharm.* **2004**, 337, 317–327.

163. Foloppe, N.; Chen, I. -J. Conformational Sampling and Energetics of Drug-Like Molecules. *Curr. Med. Chem.* **2009**, 16, 3381–3413.

164. Still, W. C.; Tempczyk, A.; Hawley, R. C.; Hendrickson, T. Semianalytical Treatment of Solvation for Molecular Mechanics and Dynamics. *J. Am. Chem. Soc.* **1990**, 112, 6127–6129.

165. Labrie, P.; Maddaford, S. P.; Lacroix, J.; Catalano, C.; Lee, D. K. H.; Rakhit, S.; Gaudreault, R. C. *In Vitro* Activity of Novel Dual Action MDR Anthranilamide Modulators with Inhibitory Activity at CYP-450. *Bioorg. Med. Chem.* **2006**, 14, 7972–7987.

166. Kurogi,Y.; Güner, O. F. Pharmacophore Modeling and Three-dimensional Database Searching for Drug Design Using Catalyst. *Curr. Med. Chem.* **2001**, 8, 1035–1055.

167. Evans, D. A.; Doman, T. N.; Thorner, D. A.; Bodkin, M. J. 3D QSAR Methods: Phase and Catalyst Compared. *J. Chem. Inf. Model.* **2007**, 47, 1248–1257.

168. Li, H.; Sutter, J.; Hoffmann, R. HypoGen: An Automated System for Generating 3D Predictive Pharmacophore Models. In *Pharmacophore Perception, Development, and Use in Drug Design;* Güner, O. F., Ed.; International University Line: La Jolla, California, **2000**; pp 171–189.

169. Ekins, S.; Mestres, J.; Testa, B. *In Silico* Pharmacology for Drug Discovery: Applications to Targets and Beyond. *Br. J. Pharmacol.* **2007**, 152, 21–37.

170. Chang, C.; Ekins, S. Pharmacophores for Human ADME/Tox-related Proteins. In *Pharmacophores and Pharmacophore Searches;* Langer T.; Hoffmann, R. D., Eds.; Wiley: Weinheim, Germany, **2006**; pp 299–324.

171. Pleban, K.; Kaiser, D.; Kopp, S.; Peer, M.; Chiba, P.; Ecker, G. F. Targeting Drug Efflux Pumps—A Pharmacoinformatic Approach. *Acta Biochim. Pol.* **2005**, 52, 737–740.

172. Loo, T. W.; Bartlett, M. C.; Clarke, D. M. Substrate-Induced Conformational Changes in the Transmembrane Segments of Human P-Glycoprotein. Direct Evidence for the Substrate-Induced Fit Mechanism for Drug Binding. *J. Biol. Chem.* **2003**, 278, 13603–13606.

173. Ekins, S. Predicting Undesirable Drug Interactions with Promiscuous Proteins *In Silico. Drug Discov. Today* **2004**, 9, 276–285.

174. Ecker, G. F. QSAR Studies on ABC Transporter – How to Deal with Polyspecificity. In *Transporters as Drug Carriers: Structure, Function, Substrates;* Ecker, G.; Chiba, P., Eds.; Wiley-VCH: Weinheim, Germany, **2010**; pp 195–214.

175. Gutmann, D. A. P.:, Ward, A.; Urbatsch, I. L.; Chang, G.; van Veen, H. W. Understanding Polyspecificity of Multidrug ABC Transporters: Closing in on the Gaps in ABCB1. *Trends Biochem. Sci.* **2010**, 35, 36–42.

176. Chang, C.; Bahadduri, P. M.; Polli, J. E.; Swaan, P. W.; Ekins, S. Rapid Identification of P-glycoprotein Substrates and Inhibitors. *Drug Metab. Dispos.* **2006**, 34, 1976–1984.

177. Ekins, S.; Kim, R. B.; Leake, B. F.; Dantzig, A. H.; Schuetz, E. G.;Lan, L. B.; Yasuda, K.; Shepard, R. L.;Winter, M. A.; Schuetz, J. D.; Wikel, J. H.; Wrighton, S. A. Three-Dimensional Quantitative Structure-Activity Relationships of Inhibitors of P-Glycoprotein. *Mol. Pharmacol.* **2002**, 61, 964–973.

178. Ekins, S.; Kim, R. B.; Leake, B. F.; Dantzig, A. H.; Schuetz, E. G.; Lan, L. B.; Yasuda, K.; Shepard, R. L.;Winter, M. A.; Schuetz, J. D.; Wikel, J. H.; Wrighton, S. A. Application of Three-Dimensional Quantitative Structure-Activity Relationships of P-Glycoprotein Inhibitors and Substrates. *Mol. Pharmacol.* **2002**, 61, 974–981.

179. Pajeva, I. K.; Wiese, M. Pharmacophore Model of Drugs Involved in P-Glycoprotein Multidrug Resistance: Explanation of Structural Variety (Hypothesis). *J. Med. Chem.* **2002**, 45, 5671–5686.

180. Pajeva, I.; Globisch, C.; Fleischer, R.; Tsakovska, I.; Wiese, M. Molecular Modeling of P-Glycoprotein and Related Drugs. *Med. Chem. Res.* **2005**, 14, 106–117.

181. Palmeira, A.; Rodrigues, F.; Sousa, E.; Pinto, M.; Vasconcelos, M. H.; Fernandes, M. X. Pharmacophore-Based Screening as a Clue for the Discovery of New P-glycoprotein Inhibitors. In *Advances in Bioinformatics*; Rocha, M.; Riverola, F.; Shatkay, H.; Corchado, J.; Eds.; Springer: Berlin/Heidelberg, **2010**; pp 175–180.

182. Langer, T.; Eder, M.; Hoffmann, R. D.; Chiba, P.; Ecker, G. F. Lead Identification for Modulators of Multidrug Resistance Based on *In Silico* Screening with a Pharmacophoric Feature. *Model. Arch. Pharm.* **2004**, 337, 317–327.

183. Chang, C:, Bahadduri, P. M.; Polli, J. E.; Swaan, P. W.; Ekins, S. Rapid Identification of P-glycoprotein Substrates and Inhibitors. *Drug Metab. Dispos.* **2006**, 34, 1976–1984.

184. Zhou, H.; Wu, S.; Zhai, S.; Liu, A.; Sun, Y.; Li, R.; Zhang, R. Y.; Ekins, S.; Swaan, P. W.; Fang, B.; Zhang, B.; Yan, B. Design, Synthesis, Cytoselective Toxicity, Structure-Activity Relationships, and Pharmacophore of Thiazolidinone Derivatives Targeting Drug-Resistant Lung Cancer Cells. *J. Med. Chem.* **2008**, 51, 1242–1251.

185. Wang,Y.-H.; Li, Y.; Yang, S.-L.; Yang, L. An *In Silico* Approach for Screening Flavonoids as P-Glycoprotein Inhibitors Based an a Bayesian-Regularized Neural Network. *J. Comput.-Aided Mol. Des.* **2005**, 19, 137–147.

186. Zalloum, H. M.; Taha, M. O. Development of Predictive *In Silico* Model for Cyclosporine- and Aureobasidin-Based P-Glycoprotein Inhibitors Employing Receptor Surface Analysis. *J. Mol. Graph. Model.* **2008**, 27, 439–451.

187. Chen, L.; Li, Y.; Zhao, Q.; Peng, H.; Hou, T. ADME Evaluation in Drug Discovery. 10. Predictions of P-Glycoprotein Inhibitors using Recursive Partitioning and Naïve Bayesian Classification Techniques. *Mol. Pharmaceutics* **2011**, 8, 889–900.

188. Labrie, P.; Maddaford, S. P.; Fortin, S.; Rakhit, S.; Kotra, L. P.; Gaudreault, R. C. A Comparative Molecular Field Analysis (CoMFA) and Comparative Molecular Similarity Indices Analysis (CoMSIA) of Anthranilamide Derivatives that Are Multidrug Resistance Modulators. *J. Med. Chem.* **2006**, 49, 7646–7660.

CHAPTER 9

ON THE USE OF QUANTITATIVE STRUCTURE–ACTIVITY RELATIONSHIPS AND GLOBAL REACTIVITY DESCRIPTORS TO STUDY THE BIOLOGICAL ACTIVITIES OF POLYCHLORINATED BIPHENYLS

NAZMUL ISLAM

Theoretical and Computational Chemistry Research Laboratory,
Techno Global-Balurghat, Balurghat, Dakshin Dinajpur district,
West Bengal 733103, India; E-mail: nazmul.islam786@gmail.com

CONTENTS

ABSTRACT

In the present chapter, we found a linear relationship between density functional theory (DFT) global descriptors and an experimental biological activity (pIC) of some selected polychlorinated biphenyls (PCB). We have also proposed some ansatz to calculate the biological activity of the PCBs using the DFT descriptors invoked in the present study.

The work establishes that the global reactivity descriptors have significant reliability to predict/correlate the biological activity (toxic nature) of some polychlorinated biphenyls. We also found that the global reactivity descriptors are dependent on the number of chlorination in the biphenyl moiety.

9.1   INTRODUCTION

Nowadays, several scientists are engaged to understand and then to synthesize some novel pharmacologically active molecules with reduced toxicity. The ultimate objective of such attempts is to predict some novel pharmacologically active molecules prior to their laboratory synthesis. The observations led to the development of the modern "reactivity theory". The prime interest of this theory, the so-called "reactivity indices", has been proven to be important analytical tools for seemingly very incongruent phenomena in contemporary chemistry [1]. Such theory provides the analysis of activity and/or toxicity of a diverse class of systems using the reactivity or selectivity descriptors based on conceptual density functional theory (CDFT).

Recently, quantitative structure–activity relationships (QSAR) have gained importance in the field of pharmacological sciences [2]. Also it is observed that QSAR can be used as "predictive tools" for a preliminary evaluation of the activity of chemical compounds by using computer-aided models.

The polychlorinated biphenyls (PCBs) are a class of organic compounds with 1 to 10 chlorine atoms attached to biphenyl moiety. PCB congeners are odorless, tasteless, clear pale-yellow in colour, and viscous liquids. The PCBs are very stable compounds and do not degrade readily. Their destruction by chemical, thermal, and biochemical processes is extremely difficult. For such reasons, the PCBs have been used for various individual and commercial purposes. The PCBs are used as insulating fluids or dielectric fluids in transformers capacitors and coolants especially in components of early fluorescent light fittings, heat transfer, hydraulic fluids or vacuum pump fluids, plasticizers in paints and cements and fire retardants stabilizing additives in flexible PVC coatings of electrical wiring and electronic components, etc. Moreover, they were used as pesticide extenders, cutting oils, reactive flame retardants, lubricating oils, hydraulic fluids, sealants for caulking in schools and commercial buildings, adhesives, wood floor finishes, water-proofing compounds, fixatives in microscopy, surgical implants, and in carbonless copy ("NCR") paper and many others [3].

PCBs are very highly toxic and present the risk of generating extremely toxic dibenzodioxins and dibenzofurans through partial oxidation. PCBs are responsible for several adverse health effects on the immune, reproductive, nervous, endocrine system, and cancer. PCB is an electron acceptor and the lipophilicity of PCBs contributes to their magnification in the food chain. Toxic effects in humans include chlorance, pigmentation of the skin and nails, excessive eye discharge, swelling, of the eyelids, distinctive hair follicles, and gastrointestinal disturbances. PCBs are listed as a carcinogen by the Environmental Protection Agency (EPA) [4–8]. Because of their toxicity and persistence in the environment, the manufacture of PCBs was discontinued in 1976.

The chlorination pattern or position in the biphenyl ring strongly affects the absolute hardness values of the PCBs. That is, planer PCBs are soft and nonplaner PCBs are hard. These findings show that: (a) soft PCBs have small absolute hardness (η) values and potent induction ability and (b) the measured absolute hardness (η) values predict the toxic potency and induction ability.

Bacteria play a fundamental role in the removal of waste chemical compounds from the environment. Bioremediation is a promising technology for the treatment of PCB-contaminated environments [8] but the process of bioremediation of PCBs is still not well understood and its microbial and molecular basis needs further study. The biodegradation performance of bacteria can be affected by the toxicity of the pollutants or metabolites derived from them [9].

9.2 STRUCTURE–ACTIVITY RELATIONSHIP

The notion of an inherent chemical reactivity of a molecule implies that the way the molecule reacts with other molecules is predetermined by its own structure [10]. This of course, is only part of the truth [11] that chemical reactions are dependent on all the partners and two molecules together have unique features that neither molecule posses alone. However, in considering a single molecule in reactions with partners of a given family, single molecule reactivity concepts have been proved to be fruitful [10]. Density functional theoretical [11] methods are in general capable of generating a variety of isolated molecular properties. The commercial exploitation of organic compounds as a medicinal drug or daily required substances likely to require, at some stage of its development, the determination of biological or chemical activities or properties related to the intended end use of the compound. It is desirable, therefore, to have at hand relatively straightforward and inexpensive procedures enabling the efficient and accurate prediction of a molecular activity or property especially when its direct measurement by experiment is, for one reason or another, to be avoided if at all possible. The procedures that are conventionally used for indirect determinations of activities make use of molecular "descriptors" which include suitable molecular properties and physical-organic constructs obtained from both experimental and computational sources. Molecular descriptors are ultimately related to molecular structure. Hence the relationships between activities and the descriptors on which they depend are generally known as quantitative structure–activity relationships (QSARs) or quantitative structure–property relationships (QSPRs) [2] depending upon whether the property of interest is to be characterized as biological or nonbiological, respectively.

The structure of a molecule determines its electronic wave function, which in turn determines many of its physico-chemical properties. It is reasonable to suppose that the biological activity of molecules or its potency as a drug will also be dependent upon the molecular electronic wave function. Given that it is now possible to perform accurate ab initio calculations routinely on molecules of moderate size at reasonable cost, it would clearly be advantageous to have available a procedure for estimating a molecular activity or property from descriptors which are derived from, and in turn characterize the electronic wave function of a molecule.

It is possible in principle to determine any molecular property that is ultimately dependent upon the molecule's electronic ground state wave function. In practice, this determination can sometimes be achieved using rigorous procedures. It can, for instance, be achieved for certain properties using quantum-mechanical expectation values. When rigorous procedures are tedious or difficult or virtually impossible, then it is necessary to resort either to less rigorous model calculations or to the use of QSAR or QSPR methods. QSAR techniques increase the probability of success, reduce time, and cost involvement in drug discovery process.

SARs are the traditional practices of medicinal chemistry which try to modify the effect or the potency (i.e., activity) of bioactive chemical compounds by modifying their chemical structure. Medicinal chemists use the techniques of chemical synthesis to insert new chemical groups into the biomedical compound and test the modifications for their biological effects. This enables the identification and determination of the chemical groups responsible for evoking a target biological effect in the organism. The basic assumption for all molecule-based hypotheses is that similar molecules have similar activities. This is the so-called SAR.

One of the major goals of SARs for the design of drugs in medicinal chemistry and pharmacology is to understand molecular mechanism for a drug–enzyme complex in living systems. Many useful and important quantum mechanical methods have been widely used for SARs studies [13, 14(a)–14(b)].

The nature of the interaction of substrate with enzyme and receptor also can be investigated by more rigorous quantum mechanical methods. In a recent study, an important relationship between absolute hardness and biological activity exists for environmental pollutants, such as dioxins [15], was reported.

It is now well established [4, 16, 17] that the absolute hardness-absolute electronegativity $(\eta-\chi)$ activity diagrams play an important role as a new coordinate of bioactivity in the study of SARs. For example, Kobayashi *et al.,* [4] successfully used the absolute hardness–absolute electronegativity $(\eta-\chi)$ activity diagrams to discuss the potency of bioactivities for PCBs. It was found that the diagram plays an important role as a new coordinate of bioactivity in SARs.

According to the hardness concept, a hardness controlled acid or base prefers to interact with a hardness controlled base or acid. An electronegativity controlled acid (or base) prefers to interact with an electronegativity controlled base (or acid) [18(a)–18(b)]. Therefore, the chemical characteristics of drugs (or chemicals) based on absolute hardness or absolute electronegativity are an extremely useful tool for drug design, toxicity prediction, and analysis of mechanisms of bioactive compounds.

In their study, Waller *et al.,* [19] have utilized comparative molecular field analysis (CoMFA), a three-dimensional (3D) QSAR paradigm, to explore the physico-chemical requirements for binding to the Ah receptor.

Ever since the power of QSAR-based techniques has been highlighted, several descriptors have been proposed from time to time in developing QSAR models [20–26] for understanding various aspects of pharmacological sciences including drug design and the possible ecotoxicological characteristics of the drug molecules. Specific quantitative structure–toxicity relationship (QSTR) models have also been developed. In these studies the toxicity of various chemicals has been understood via corresponding molecular structures.

The possibility of an electron transfer between a toxic molecule and a biosystem has been considered as one of the major reasons of toxic behavior of these molecules. Accordingly, the related descriptors like electron affinity, ionization potential, planarity, electrophilicity, etc have been turned out to be useful QSTR descriptors.

In this chapter, we explore the efficacy of three very important DFT descriptors—the global hardness, the electronegativity, and the electrophilicity index for the studies of the toxicity of various PCBs via corresponding molecular structures.

9.3 QUANTUM CHEMICAL METHODS OF COMPUTATION

9.3.1 HARTREE–FOCK AND SEMIEMPIRICAL MOLECULAR ORBITAL METHODS

Quantum mechanical methods [27] for the study of molecules can be divided into two categories: ab initio and semiempirical methods. Ab initio methods refer to quantum chemical methods in which all the integrals are exactly evaluated in the course of a calculation. Ab initio methods include Hartree–Fock (HF) or molecular orbital (MO) theory, configuration interaction (CI) theory, perturbation theory (PT), and density functional theory (DFT). Ab initio methods that include correlation can have accuracy comparable with experiment in structure and energy predictions. However, a drawback is that ab initio calculations are extremely demanding in computer resources, especially for large molecular systems. Semiempirical quantum chemical methods lie between ab initio and molecular mechanics (MM). Like MM, they use experimentally derived parameters to strive for accuracy, like ab initio methods; they are quantum-mechanical in nature. Semi empirical methods are computationally fast because many of the difficult integrals are neglected. The error introduced is compensated through the use of several useful parameters. Thus, semiempirical procedure can often produce greater accuracy than ab initio calculations at a similar level.

9.4 GLOBAL REACTIVITY DESCRIPTORS OF CDFT

Electronegativity is a measure of the attraction of an atom for the electrons in a chemical bond. Parr et al., [28] discovered a new fundamental quantity as a new index of chemical reactivity known as the electronic chemical potential (μ). The chemical potential (μ) is a characteristic property of atoms, molecules, ions, and radicals and is the first derivative of energy with respect to the number of electron. Within the DFT formalism, Parr et al., [28] showed that the slope, $[\partial E(r)/\partial N]_v$ of the energy E(r) versus the number of electrons (N) curve at a constant external potential (v), is the chemical potential, μ, and this property, like thermodynamic chemical potential [29] measures the escaping tendency of electrons in the species. Then following Iczkowski and Margrave [30], Parr et al., [28] defined the electronegativity as the additive inverse of the chemical potential:

$$\chi = -\mu \tag{1}$$

$$\text{or, } \chi = -[\,\partial E/\partial N\,]_v \tag{2}$$

Parr and Pearson [18(a)], using the DFT as a basis, have rigorously defined the term hardness as the second-order derivative of energy with respect to the number of electron, that is,

$$\eta = \frac{1}{2}[(\delta^2 E/\delta N^2)_V]$$ (3)

The softness (S) is the reciprocal of the hardness; $S = 1/\eta$ (4)

Invoking finite difference approximation, Parr and Pearson [18(a)] gave approximate and operational formulae for electronegativity and hardness as

$$\chi = \frac{(I+A)}{2}$$ (5)

$$\eta = \frac{(I-A)}{2}$$ (6)

where I and A are the first ionization potential and electron affinity of the chemical species.

According to Koopmans' theorem the orbital energies of the frontier orbitals can be written as

$$-\varepsilon_{HOMO} = I$$ (7)

and

$$-\varepsilon_{LUMO} = A$$ (8)

In 1986, within the limitations of Koopmans' theorem, Pearson [31] placed electronegativity and hardness into an MO framework as follows:

$$\chi = (\partial E/\partial N)v = (I+A)/2$$

$$\text{or } \chi = -(\varepsilon_{LUMO} + \varepsilon_{HOMO})/2$$ (9)

and

$$\eta = (\partial^2 E/\partial N^2)v = (I-A)/2$$

$$\text{or, } \eta = (\varepsilon_{LUMO} - \varepsilon_{HOMO})/2 \tag{10}$$

He again pointed out that a hard species has a large HOMO–LUMO gap and a soft species has a small HOMO–LUMO gap [31].

The electrophilicity, ω, is a descriptor of reactivity that allows a quantitative classification of the global electrophilic nature of a molecule within a relative scale. Parr *et al.*, [32] suggested that electronegativity squared divided by hardness measures the electrophilic power of a ligand its prosperity to "soak up" electrons.

Thus,

$$\omega = \mu^2/2\eta = \chi^2/2\eta \tag{11}$$

It is further anticipated that electrophilicity, ω, should be related to electron affinity, because both ω and electron affinity measures capacity of an agent to accept electrons. Electron affinity reflect capability of an agent to accept only one electron from the environment, whereas electrophilicity index measures the energy lowering of a ligand due to maximal electron flow between the donor and acceptor. The electron flows may be either less or more than one. Thus, the electrophilicity index provides the direct relationship between the rates of reaction and the electrophilic power of the inhibitors [33].

9.5 METHOD OF COMPUTATION

The semiempirical computational procedure, AM1 [34 (a), 34(b)] was adopted to compute the orbital energies (HOMO, LUMO) of the PCBs under study. The planar structure of each of the substituted biphenyls was drawn on the program Argus Lab 4.0.1[35] and the optimization of geometry was carried out at the restricted Hartree–Fock level (RHF) using STO-3G minimal basis set. The ionization energies and electron affinities were calculated using the Koopman's theorem. Then using I and A, we computed the hardness and electronegativity of the molecules under study invoking Parr and Pearson [18(a)] formulae $\eta=(I-A)/2$ and $\chi=(I+A)/2$, respectively. The electrophilicity index was calculated using the formula $\omega=\chi^2/2\eta$ of Parr *et al.*, [32].

Then we have plotted the computed hardness values with the observed pIC value of 14 PCB congeners and have found a linear correlation. We found a linear relationship between hardness and experimental biological activity (pIC) [36] of the PCBs. Theoretical biological activity (potency of benzopyrene 3-hydroxylation activity) was computed using least square fitting method. The proposed relationship is

$$\text{pIC (theoretical)} = 50.13\eta - 1.810 \qquad (12)$$

We further plotted the computed electronegativity values with the observed pIC value of the 14 PCB congeners. We found a linear correlation between the electronegativities and the potency of benzopyrene 3-hydroxylation activity of those compounds. The theoretical biological activity was computed using least square fitting method. The relationship is

$$\text{pIC (theoretical)} = 14.50\chi + 2.869 \qquad (13)$$

Then we plotted the computed electrophilicity values with the observed pIC value and have found a good correlation. A linear relationship between electrophilicity and the experimental biological activity (pIC) of the PCBs was observed. Theoretical biological activities were computed using least square fitting method. The relationship is

$$\text{pIC (theoretical)} = 5.998\omega + 4.916 \qquad (14)$$

9.6   RESULTS AND DISCUSSIONS

In **Table 1** we have summarized computed HOMO and LUMO orbital energies obtained from AM1 calculations and absolute hardness, absolute and electronegativity index values of some selected PCBs.

TABLE 1   Computed hardness, electronegativity, and electronegativity index of some selected PCBs

Chlorination Sites	Absolute Hardness, η (au)	Absolute Electronegativity, χ (au)	Electrophilicity Index, ω (au)
2,0	0.155957	0.172303	0.095181
2,3	0.155346	0.178103	0.102097
2,2'	0.154194	0.177194	0.101812
2,3'	0.155631	0.17878	0.102686
2,4'	0.152888	0.177421	0.102945
2,5'	0.155711	0.178928	0.102803
2,6'	0.154986	0.177704	0.101876
2,3,4	0.151871	0.182652	0.109836
2,3,4,5	0.150774	0.187919	0.117108
2,5,2',5'	0.152281	0.188346	0.116476

TABLE 1   (*Continued*)

2,5,3',6'	0.153092	0.188961	0.116617
2,5,4',5'	0.151487	0.188389	0.11714
2,6,2',4'	0.150563	0.187226	0.116408
2,6,2',3'	0.153168	0.188115	0.115518
2,3,2',5'	0.152927	0.188255	0.115872
2,3,2',6'	0.153168	0.188115	0.115523
2,4,3',5'	0.152411	0.189977	0.118401
2,4,3',4'	0.149503	0.187565	0.117659
3,4,2',5'	0.150617	0.187846	0.117139
3,4,2',4'	0.149502	0.187566	0.117661
3,4,2',3'	0.150097	0.188183	0.117966
3,4,3',4'	0.150093	0.18813	0.117903
3,4,4',6'	0.149563	0.1877	0.117781
3,4,5',6'	0.151858	0.187859	0.116197
3,5,2',4'	0.152411	0.189977	0.118401
3,5,2',3'	0.155162	0.190513	0.116959
3,6,2',6'	0.15211	0.18768	0.115784
3,6,2',5'	0.153092	0.188961	0.116617
4,5,3',5'	0.152758	0.190182	0.118387
4,5,3',4'	0.150097	0.188183	0.118387
4,6,3',6'	0.150617	0.187846	0.117139
4,6,4',5'	0.149503	0.187567	0.117661
5,6,4',6'	0.151126	0.187575	0.116407
5,6,5',6'	0.153608	0.188107	0.115177
5,6,2',3'	0.154399	0.188483	0.115045
3,4,5,4'	0.150011	0.188345	0.118237
3,3',4',5'	0.151775	0.187959	0.116384
2,4,4',6'	0.149256	0.187431	0.117685
2,3,4,5,6	0.148932	0.191819	0.123528
2,3,4,3',4'	0.148837	0.191601	0.123326
3,4,5,3',4'	0.149531	0.192996	0.124547
3,4,3',4',5'	0.149531	0.192996	0.124547
3,3',4',5'	0.151775	0.187959	0.116384
2,4,5,4',5'	0.148905	0.191761	0.123475
2,4,5,4',5'	0.148595	0.192342	0.124484

TABLE 1   (*Continued*)

2,3,4,5,4'	0.14828	0.191861	0.124125
3,4,5,3',4',5'	0.149087	0.197588	0.130933
2,4,5,2',4',5'	0.14717	0.195885	0.130362
2,3,4,5,4',5'	0.147987	0.196302	0.130195
2,4,5,3',4'5'	0.148254	0.196844	0.130679
2,4,5,3',4',6'	0.147538	0.196124	0.130355
2,4,6,3',4',5'	0.147939	0.196437	0.130417
2,3,4,5,3',4',5'	0.147739	0.200637	0.136237

We have presented the computed pIC values using global hardness vis-á-vis their observed pIC values, the computed pIC values using elctronegativity vis-á-vis their observed pIC value and the computed pIC values using electrophilicity index vis-á-vis their observed pIC value in **Tables 2 to 4**, respectively.

TABLE 2 Computed pIC values of some selected PCBs using their global hardness data vis-à-vis their observed pIC value

Chlorination	Hardness, η (au)	pIC (calculated)	pIC (observed)
3,4,3',4'	0.150093	5.714162	7.028
3,4,5,4'	0.150011	5.710026	5.204
3,4,5,3',4'	0.149531	5.685964	7.871
3,3',4',5'	0.151775	5.798456	5.584
2,4,5,4',5'	0.148905	5.654583	6.134
2,4,5,4',5'	0.148595	5.639042	5.762
2,3,4,5,4'	0.14828	5.623276	6.157
2,3,4,5,4',5'	0.147987	5.608588	6.057
2,4,5,3',4'5'	0.148254	5.621948	5.482
2,3,4,5,3',4',5'	0.147739	5.596131	5.885
2,4,4',6'	0.149256	5.672203	4.442
2,4,5,3',4',6'	0.147538	5.58608	4.689
2,3,4,5	0.150774	5.748301	4.405
2,4,6,3',4',5'	0.147939	5.606157	4.577

TABLE 3 Computed pIC values of some selected PCBs using their electronegativity data vis-à-vis their observed pIC value

Chlorination	Absolute Electronegativity, χ (au)	pIC (calculated)	pIC (observed)
3,4,3',4'	0.18813	5.596885	7.028
3,4,5,4'	0.188345	5.599995	5.204
3,4,5,3',4'	0.192996	5.667435	7.871
3,3',4',5'	0.187959	5.594398	5.584
2,4,5,4',5'	0.191761	5.649527	6.134
2,4,5,4',5'	0.192342	5.657952	5.762
2,3,4,5,4'	0.191861	5.650985	6.157
2,3,4,5,4',5'	0.196302	5.715379	6.057
2,4,5,3',4'5'	0.196844	5.723231	5.482
2,3,4,5,3',4',5'	0.200637	5.778229	5.885
2,4,4',6'	0.187431	5.58675	4.442
2,4,5,3',4',6'	0.196124	5.712798	4.689
2,3,4,5	0.187919	5.593826	4.405
2,4,6,3',4',5'	0.196437	5.717329	4.577

TABLE 4 Computed pIC values of some selected PCBs using their electrophilicity data vis-à-vis their observed pIC value

Chlorination	Electrophilicity Index, ω (au)	pIC (calculated)	pIC (observed)
3,4,3',4'	0.117903	5.623184	7.028
3,4,5,4'	0.118237	5.625187	5.204
3,4,5,3',4'	0.124547	5.663035	7.871
3,3',4',5'	0.116384	5.614074	5.584
2,4,5,4',5'	0.123475	5.656606	6.134
2,4,5,4',5'	0.124484	5.662655	5.762
2,3,4,5,4'	0.124125	5.660504	6.157
2,3,4,5,4',5'	0.130195	5.696912	6.057
2,4,5,3',4'5'	0.130679	5.699815	5.482
2,3,4,5,3',4',5'	0.136237	5.733152	5.885
2,4,4',6'	0.117685	5.621875	4.442
2,4,5,3',4',6'	0.130355	5.697869	4.689

(Continued)

2,3,4,5	0.117108	5.618411	4.405
2,4,6,3',4',5'	0.130417	5.698239	4.577

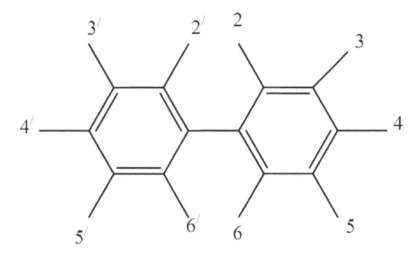

FIGURE 1   Structure of PCB.

From the calculated results (**Table 1**), it is transparent that the hardness of hexacholorobiphenyl is less than that of pentacholobiphenyl and the hardness of pentacholobiphenyl is less than that of tetracholorobiphenyl ($\eta_{3,4,5,3',4',5'\text{-PCB}} < \eta_{3,4,5,3',4'\text{-PCB}} < \eta_{3,4,3',4'\text{-PCB}}$). Experimentally [1] it is found that 3,4,5,3',4',5'-hexachlorobiphenyl, 3,4,5,3',4'-pentachlorobiphenyl compounds are more toxic and 2,5,2',5'-tetrachlorobiphenyl is less toxic and the toxicity order is 3,4,5,3',4',5'-PCB, 3,4,5,3',4'-PCB. From **Table 1** it is clear that electronegativity of 3,4,5,3',4',5'-PCB>3,4,5,3',4'-PCB, hardness of 3,4,5,3',4',5'-PCB<3,4,5,3',4'-PCB and electrophilicity index of 3,4,5,3',4',5'-PCB<3,4,5,3',4'-PCB.

A look on **Table 1** reveals that the order of absolute electronegativity (χ) is 2,0< 2,3 -PCB<2,3,4-PCB<2,3,4,5-PCB<2,3,4,5,6-PCB, the absolute hardness (η) is 2,0 >2,3-PCB>2,3,4-PCB>2,3,4,5-PCB>2,3,4,5,6-PCB, and the electrophilicity index (ω) is 2,0< 2,3-PCB<2,3,4-PCB<2,3,4,5-PCB<2,3,4,5,6-PCB. Thus, it is transparent from the computed value of the three global reactivity descriptors that with increase in chlorination in the same ring,   absolute electronegativity (χ) value of the compound increases, the absolute hardness (η) value of compound decreases, and electrophilicity index (ω) value of the compound increases.

A look on **Table 1** reveals that the order of absolute electronegativity (χ) is 2,2'-PCB<2,3'-PCB>2,4'-PCB, and <the absolute electronegativity (χ) of 2,5'-PCB>2 ,6'-PCB. It is also transparent from Table 1 that the absolute electronegativity (χ) of 2,5'-PCB<2,4'-PCB.

The order absolute hardness (η) data is 2,2'-PCB<2,3'-PCB, and 2,4'-PCB<2,5'-PCB.

The order of electrophilicity index (ω) is 2,2'-PCB<2,3'-PCB and that of 2,4'-PCB>2,5'-PCB.

Thus it is the theoretical observation of this work that when the position of the chlorination in one ring is fixed and the position of the chlorination in another ring is changed (number of chlorines in both the rings are fixed) the value of absolute electronegativity (χ) and absolute hardness (η) decreases, but the value of electrophilicity index (ω) increases.

From **Table 1** it is evident that the biphenyl ring containing only one chlorine atom at position 2 has the highest hardness. The compound 2,4,5,2',4',5'-PCB has the lowest hardness; compound 2,3,4,5,3',4',5'-PCB has the highest absolute electronegativity; compound with chlorination at position 2 has the lowest absolute electronegativity value; compound 2,3,4,5,3',4',5'-PCB has the highest electrophilicity index; and compound with chlorination at position 2 has the lowest electrophilicity index value.

From **Table 2** we can say that for 8 cases among 14 PCB congeners, the pIC values calculated using proposed ansatz and the hardness data of the PCBs under study have a very good correlation (standard deviation [SD] is less than 10%).

From **Table 3** we can notice that in 8 cases among 14 PCB congeners, the pIC values calculated using proposed ansatz and the electronegativity data of the PCB compounds under study have a very good correlation (SD is less than 10%).

From **Table 4** we can notice that for 8 cases among 14 PCB congeners, the pIC values calculated using proposed ansatz and electrophilicity data of the PCB congeners under study have a very good correlation (SD<10%).

Thus, we can say that the theoretically predicted pIC values using three very important global reactivity descriptors fairly correlate with their experimental counter parts.

It has been reported [37] that chlorination at both para and at least, two meta positions resulted in maximum activity, whereas at the ortho position in decreased activity. This observation is not that much reflected in the theoretically calculated potency of benzopyrene 3-hydroxylation activity (pIC) values. In this work, we found a nice correlation in 8 cases among 14 PCB compounds between the theoretically and experimentally observed pIC values. We use the simple linear correlation model for the QSAR study. Thus, it is our hope that the result of the work [37] may improve using the linear correlation model for the QSAR study of those compounds.

9.7 CONCLUSIONS

In the present chapter, we found a linear relationship between DFT global descriptors and experimental biological activity (pIC) of some selected PCB. We have also proposed some ansatz to calculate the biological activity of the PCBs using the DFT descriptors invoked in the present study.

This work showed that the global reactivity descriptors have significant reliability to predict or correlate the biological activity (toxic nature) of some polychlorinated biphenyls and the value of global reactivity descriptors are dependent on the number of chlorination in the biphenyl moiety.

ACKNOWLEDGMENTS

The authors would like to thank the management of Techno Global-Balurghat and Techno India Group for providing research facility.

KEYWORDS

- **DFT descriptors**
- **HOMO–LUMO**
- **PCBs**
- **pIC value**
- **QSAR**
- **QSPR**

REFERENCES

1. Mineva, T. Selectivity study from the density functional local reactivity indices, *J. Mole. Struct. THEOCHEM*, **76**, 279–86(2006).
2. Karelson, M. *Molecular Descriptors in QSAR/QSPR*, Wiley-Interscience, USA (2000).
3. Rudel R. A., Seryak L. M, Brody J. G, PCB-containing wood floor finish is a likely source of elevated PCBs in residents' blood, household air and dust: a case study of exposure, *Environ. Health*, **7**, 2–9(2008).
4. Kobayashi, S.; Hamashjima, H.; Kurihara, M.; Miyata, N.; Tanaka, A. Hardness controlled enzymes and electronegativity controlled enzymes: role of an absolute hardness-electronegativity (eta-chi) activity diagram as a coordinate for biological activities. *Chem. Pharm. Bull.* **46** (7), 1108–1115(1998).

5. Drinker, C. K.; Warren, M. F.; Bennet, G. A. The problem of possible systemic effects from certain chlorinated hydrocarbons, *J. Ind. Hyg. Toxicol.***19**, 283–311(1937).

6. Brouwer, A.; Longnecker, M. P.; Birnbaum, L. S.; Cogliano, J.; Kostyniak, P.; Moore, J.; Schantz, S.; Winneke, G. Characterization of potential endocrine-related health effects at low-dose levels of exposure to PCBs. *Environ. Health Perspect.***107**, 639–649(1999).

7. Aoki, Y. Polychlorinated biphenyls, polychlorinated dibenzo-p-dioxins, and polychlorinated dibenzofurans as endocrine disrupters--what we have learned from Yusho disease. *Environ. Res.***86**, 2–11(2001).

8. Harkness, M. R.; McDermott, J. B.; Abramowicz, D. A.; Salvo, J. J.; Flanagan, W. P.; Stephens, M. L.; Mondello, F. J.; May, R. J.; Lobos, J. H.; Carroll, K. M.; Brennan, M. J.; Bracco, A. A.; Fish, K. M.; Warner, G. L.;Wilson, P. R.; Dietrich, D. K.; Lin, D. T.; Morgan, C. B.; Gately, W. L. In situ stimulation of aerobic PCB biodegradation in Hudson River sediments, *Science* **259**, 503–507(1993).

9. Blasco, R., Mallavarapu, M., Wittich, R. M., Timmis, K. N., Pieper, D. H. Evidence that formation of protoanemonin from metabolites of 4-chlorobiphenyl degradation negatively affects the survival of 4-chlorobiphenyl-cometabolizing microorganisms. *Appl. Environ. Microbiol.* **63**, 427–434(1997).

10. Lee, C.; Yang, W.; Parr, R. G. Local softness and chemical reactivity in the molecules CO, SCN⁻ and H₂CO, *J. Mol. Struct. (Theochem)***163**, 305–313(1988).

11. Salem, L. *Electrons in chemical reaction: First principles*, John Wiley, New York, (1982)

13. Parr, R. G.; Yang, W. *Density Functional Theory of Atoms and Molecules*, Oxford University Press, (1989).

13. Patani, G. A.; LaVoie, E. J. Bioisosterism: *Chem. Rev.***96**, 3147–3176(1996).

14. (a)Hansch, C. Quantitative structure-activity relationships and the unnamed science, *Acc. Chem. Res.***26**, 147–153(1993); (b) Wagener, M.; Sadowski, J.; Gasteiger, J. Autocorrelation of molecular surface properties for modeling corticosteroid binding globulin and cytosolic Ah receptor activity by neural networks. *J. Am. Chem. Soc.***117**, 7769–7775(1995).

15. Kobayashi, S.; Saito, A.; Ishii, Y.; Tanaka, A.; Tobinaga, S. Relationship between the biological potency of polychlorinated dibenzo-p-dioxins and their electronic states, *Chem. Pharm. Bull.*, **39**, 2100–2105(1991).

16. Kobayashi, S.; Hamashima, H.; Kurihara, M.; Miyata, N.; Tanaka, A., Hardness controlled enzymes and electronegativity controlled enzymes: role of an absolute hardness-electronegativity (η–χ) activity diagram as a coordinate for biological activities. *Pharm. Bull.***46**, 1108–1115(1998).

17. Poland A., Kuntson J. C., 2,3,7,8-Tetrachlorodibenzo-thorn-dioxin and related halogenated aromatic hydrocarbons: examination of the mechanism of toxicity, *Ann. Rev. Pharmacol. Toxicol.***22**, 517–554(1982).

18. a)Parr, R. G, Pearson, R. G., Absolute hardness: Companion parameter to absolute electronegativity, *J. Am. Chem. Soc.***105**,7512–7516(1983).
    b) Pearson, R. G., The principle of maximum hardness, *Acc. Chem. Res.***26**, 250–255(1993).

19. Waller, C. L.; McKinney, J. D., Three-dimensional quantitative structure-activity relationships of dioxins and dioxin-like compounds: model validation and Ah receptor characterization, *Chem. Res. Toxicol.* **8**, 847–858(1995).

20. Smeyers,Y. G.; Bouniam, L.; Smeyers, N. J.; Ezzamarty, A.; Hernandez-Laguna,A.; Sainz-Diaz, C. I. Quantum mechanical and QSAR study of some α-arylpropionic acids as anti-inflammatory agents, *Eur. J. Med. Chem.***33**, 103–112(1998).

21. Busse, W. D.; Ganellin, C. R.; Mitscher, L. A. Vocational training for medicinal chemists: views from industry, *Eur. J. Med. Chem.***31**, 747–760(1996).

22. Hansch, C.; Hoekman, D.; Leo, A.; Weininger D.; Selassie, C. Chem-bioinformatics: comparative QSAR at the interface between chemistry and biology, *Chem. Rev.***102**, 783–812(2002).

23. Hansch, C.; Kurup, A.; Garg, R.; Gao, H. Chem-Bioinformatics and QSAR: A review of QSAR lacking positive hydrophobic terms, *Chem. Rev.* **101**, 619–672(2001).
24. Hansch, C.; Li, R. I.; Blaney, J. M.; Langridge, R. J. Comparison of the inhibition of Escherichia coli and Lactobacillus casei dihydrofolate reductase by 2,4-diamino-5-(substituted-benzyl)pyrimidines: quantitative structure-activity relationships, x-ray crystallography, and computer graphics in structure-activity analysis, *J. Med. Chem.* **25**, 777–784(1982).
25. Leach, A. R.; Gillet, V. J., An Introduction to Chemoinformatics, Kluwer: Dordrecht, (2003).
26. Ormerod, A.; Willett, P.; Bawden, D. Comparison of fragment weighting schemes for substructural analysis, *Quant Struct-Act Relat.* **8**, 115–129(1989).
27. Hasanein, A. A.; Evans, M. W, *Computational methods in Quantum Chemistry: Quantum Chemistry Vol. 2*, World Scientific, Singapore (1996).
28. Parr, R. G.; Donnelly, R.A.; Levy, M.; Palke, W.E. Electronegativity: the density functional viewpoint, *J. Chem. Phys.* **68**, 3801–3807(1978).
29. Gyftpoulous, E. P.; Hatsopoulos, G. N. Quantum-thermodynamic definition of electronegativity, *Proc. Natl. Acad. Sci.* **60**, 786–793(1968).
30. Iczkowski, R. P.; Margrave, J. L. Electronegativity, *J. Am. Chem. Soc.* **83**, 3547–3551(1961).
31. Pearson, R. G., Absolute electronegativity and hardness correlated with molecular orbital theory, *Proc. Natl. Acad. Sci.* **83**, 8440–8441(1986).
32. Parr, R. G.; Szentpaly, L. V.; Liu, S. Electrophilicity Index, *J. Am. Chem. Soc.* **121**, 1922–1924(1999).
33. Maynard, A. T.; Covell, D. G. Reactivity of zinc finger cores: analysis of protein packing and electrostatic screening, *J. Am. Chem. Soc.* **123**, 1047–1058(2001).
34. (a) Dewar, M. J. S.; Zoebisch, E. G.; Healy, E. F.; Stewart, J. J. P. Development and use of quantum mechanical molecular models. 76. AM1: a new general purpose quantum mechanical molecular model. *J. Am. Chem. Soc.* **107**, 3902–3909(1985). (b) Dewar M. J. S., Thiel W., Ground states of molecules. 38. The MNDO method. Approximations and parameters, *J. Am. Chem. Soc.* **99**, 4899–4907(1977).
35. ArgusLab 4.0 Mark A. Thompson Planaria Software LLC, Seattle, WA (2010).
36. Waller C. L., McKinney J. D., Three-dimensional quantitative structure-activity relationships of dioxins and dioxin-like compounds: model validation and Ah receptor characterization, *Chem. Res. Toxicol*, **8**, 847–858(1995).
37. Matsumoto, J.; Miyamoto, T.; Minamida, A.; Nishimura, Y.; Egawa, H.; Nishimura, H. 1,4-Dihydro-4-oxopyridinecarboxylic acids as antibacterial agents. 2. Synthesis and structure-activity relationships of 1,6,7-trisubstituted 1,4-dihydro-4-oxo-1,8-naphthyridine-3-carboxylic acids, including enoxacin, a new antibacterial agent, *J. Med. Chem.* **27**, 292–301(1984).

CHAPTER 10

APPLICATIONS OF QUANTITATIVE STRUCTURE–RELATIVE SWEETNESS RELATIONSHIPS IN FOOD CHEMISTRY

CRISTIAN ROJAS[2*], PABLO R. DUCHOWICZ[1],
REINALDO PIS DIEZ[3], and PIERCOSIMO TRIPALDI[4]

[1]Instituto de Investigaciones Fisicoquímicas Teóricas y Aplicadas INIFTA (CCT La Plata-CONICET, UNLP), Diag. 113 y 64, C.C. 16, Sucursal 4, 1900 La Plata, Argentina

[2]Decanato General de Investigaciones. Universidad del Azuay, Av. 24 de Mayo 7-77 y Hernán Malo. Apartado Postal 01.01.981, Cuenca, Ecuador

[3]CEQUINOR, Centro de Química Inorgánica (CONICET, UNLP), Departamento de Química, Facultad de Ciencias Exactas, UNLP, C.C. 962, 1900 La Plata, Argentina

[4]Laboratorio de Química-Física de Alimentos, Facultad de Ciencia y Tecnología, Universidad del Azuay, Av. 24 de Mayo 7-77 y Hernán Malo., Apartado Postal 01.01.981, Cuenca, Ecuador

*Corresponding author. E-mail: crojasvilla@gmail.com. Telephone: (+54)(221) 4257430 Fax: (+54)(221) 4254642.

CONTENTS

ABSTRACT

This chapter reviews multicriteria quantitative structure–relative sweetness relationships (QSRSR) applications published during the period 2004–2014. It includes QSRSR models for different series of sugars and sweeteners, comparative studies, and advances in methodologies. This period was marked by an increase in the number of studies regarding quantitative structure–activity relationships/ quantitative structure–property relationships (QSAR/QSPR) applications for both understanding the sweetness mechanism and synthesizing novel sweetener compounds for the food additive industry. To improve such applications, it is recommended that food chemists generate larger sweetness databases to help in the development of stronger predictive models for achieving better sweeteners, both as raw material and as food additives for food processing.

10.1   BACKGROUND

Sucrose (saccharose), [*α-D-glucopyranosyl β-D-fructofuranoside,* **Figure 1**] is the most inexpensive and common sugar [1]. It is widely distributed in nature, and has the largest production around the world [1, 2]. It is distinguished from other sugars and sweeteners by its pleasant taste even at high concentrations, and is the sweetener most often chosen for all applications. The main sources for industrial production of sucrose are sugar cane (*Saccharum officinarum*) [3] and sugar beets (*Beta vulgaris ssp. vulgaris var. altissima*) [4]. Sweeteners are defined as natural or synthetic compounds which imprint upon the brain a sweet sensation without bringing any nutritional value. The rise in obesity has established a trend for a nutrition regimen based on caloric intake. Thus, there is considerable interest in developing new sweeteners [2].

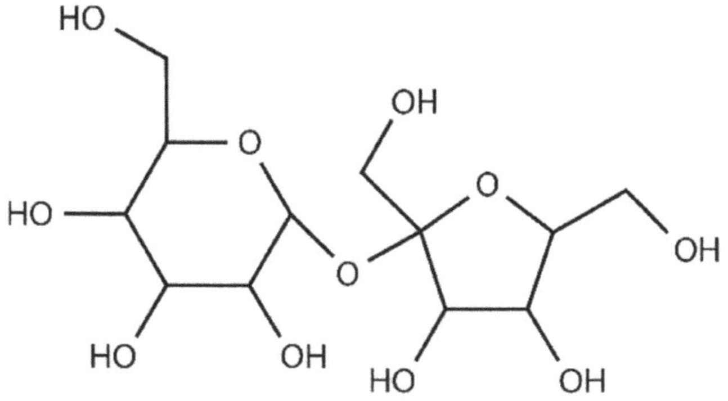

FIGURE 1   Molecular structure of sucrose.

Sweetness is one of the most important tastes of mankind. Sweet substances produce a pleasant sensation, and sucrose is the standard substance used as a sweetener [5]. As the sweet taste is an important property of a sweetener, the relative sweetness (*RS*) factor is a key criterion for comparing different sweeteners. RS is defined as the ratio of the standard sugar concentration and the iso-sweet concentration of sweetener [6], that is, a solution of sucrose has a sweetness perception rating of 1 (or 100), and the sweetness of another substance is rated relative to this one. It is supposed that the sweet perception is generated from the interaction of the sugar molecule with the G-protein-coupled taste receptor, which is identified as the T1R receptor at the taste receptor cells. However, the mechanism of the selective interaction of the ligand–receptor complex is not yet fully understood [7–13].

The search for new sweeteners is complicated. On the one hand, the relationship between chemical structure and sweetness perception is not yet satisfactorily resolved. Some other criteria should also be investigated, for example, solubility, stability at wide pH and temperature ranges, clean sweet taste without postflavor effects, sweetening effect as compared to low-cost sucrose, and finally their safety for human health [2]. On the other hand, due to the high cost for determining the RS, and the importance for understanding the relationships between sweeteners and their structures it has been necessary to build quantitative structure models for modeling this activity, which, in turn, are useful for both developing and synthesizing new potent sweeteners [14, 15].

The first theory regarding the structure–sweet taste relationship was proposed in 1919 by Oertly and Myers [16]. They intended to explain the production of sweetness by the relationship between two functional groups labeled as *glucophores* and *auxoglucs*. Subsequently, Shallenberger and Acree [17] proposed in 1967 the AH-B theory, which states that a compound to be sweet needs to contain a hydrogen bond donor (AH) and a Lewis base (B) separated by a distance of about 3 Å. In this way, the AH-B unit of a sweetener binds with the analogous AH-B unit presented in the biological sweetness receptor. Lemont Kier [18] proposed in 1972 the B-X theory in which a sweetener must have a third binding site, labeled as X that interacts via London dispersion forces with the biological sweet receptor. However, these theories were demonstrated to be very simplistic for both explaining and understanding structure–taste relationships [19]. More recently, Tinti and Nofre [20–22] proposed the most accepted theory, which is designated as the multipoint attachment (MPA) theory. This theory involves a total of eight interaction sites for the sweetness receptor; however, not all the sweeteners compounds interact with all sites.

Edna W. Deutsch and Corwin Hansch [23] are considered pioneers for publishing the first quantitative structure–activity relationships (QSAR) study of sweeteners using some series of 2-amino-4-nitrobencene derivatives. They have concluded that RS is correlated with hydrophobicity and with the Hammett constant, σ, of the substituent. Since that study, there were several applications of this theory in order to understand the interaction between the sweetener and the receptor mechanism as well as modeling, and predicting the RS for sweetener compounds [6, 24–43].

The QSAR/QSPR theory depends on the main assumption that the biological activity of a chemical compound is solely determined by its molecular structure. This theory does not offer specific details of the usually complex mechanism/ path of action involved. However, it is possible to get some insight into the underlying mechanism by means of the QSAR-based predicted activities [44–48]. In the realms of QSAR/QSPR, the molecular structure is quantified by using a set of suitable molecular descriptors, which are numbers carrying information on the constitutional, topological, geometrical, hydrophobic, and/or electronic aspects of the chemical structure [49–52]. Then, a set of appropriate descriptors can be statistically correlated to different experimental biological activities resulting in a model which will be used to predict the biological activity of new chemicals.

Altogether, QSAR/QSPR models are affected by various factors from which the most important are (a) the selection of molecular descriptors that should include maximum information of structures and minimum collinearity between them, (b) the use of suitable multicriteria modeling methods, (c) the number of descriptors to be included in the model, (d) the composition of the training and test sets, and (e) the employment of validation techniques to verify the predictive performance of the developed models [53–61].

LIST OF ABBREVIATIONS

AC: accuracy; aug-MIA-QSPR: augmented multivariate image analysis applied to quantitative structure–activity relationship; ANN: artificial neural network; CART: classification and regression tree analysis; COIN: combined outlier index criterion; CoMSIA: comparative molecular similarity indices analysis; CoMFA: comparative molecular field analysis; d: number of descriptors; DA: discriminant analysis; E_R: relative edulcoration; F: Fisher function; FDA: Food and Drug Administration; GFA: genetic functional algorithm; HOMO: highest occupied molecular orbital; K: Kendall rank correlation; K_{cv}: Kendall cross-validated rank correlation; KohNN: Kohone's self-organizing neural network; LDA: linear discriminant analysis; log-(RS): logarithm of relative sweetness; LOO: leave-one-out; LUMO: lowest unoccupied molecular orbital; LV: latent variables; MLR: multivariable linear regression; MPA: multipoint attachment;

PLS: partial least squares; PRECLAV: property evaluation by class variables; QDA: quadratic discriminant analysis; QSAR: quantitative structure–activity relationships; QSPR: quantitative structure–property relationships; QSRSR: quantitative structure–relative sweetness relationships; R^2: coefficient of determination; R_{cv}^2: coefficient of determination of cross-validation; R_{rand}^2: coefficient of determination of Y-randomization; RMSEC: root mean square error of calibration; $RMSE_{cv}$: root mean square error of cross-validation; RMSEP: root mean square error of prediction; RS: relative sweetness; SD: standard deviation; SI: sweet index; SVM: support vector machine; 3D-QSAR: three dimensional quantitative structure–activity relationships; U: relative utility.

10.2 MULTICRITERIA QSAR/QSPR STUDIES ON RELATIVE SWEETNESS

In the last 10 years, many multicriteria QSAR/QSPR models have been developed for applications to understand and model the RS of a series of sweetener compounds by using different modeling approaches. This section summarizes such studies in a chronological way.

In 2005, Kelly et al., [62] synthesized 19 monosubstituted phenylsulfamates (cyclamates) (refer to **Figure 2** for the structure of sodium phenylsulfamate), which were tasted by an experienced panel of five people using a sip and spit method. In addition, another 63 sweeteners were considered in order to study a total of 83 compounds. The sweetness was categorized into three classes, that is, sweet, nonsweet, and sweet/nonsweet. The data set was randomly split into a training and test set of 75 and 8 compounds, respectively. PC SPARTAN PRO software [63] was used in order to calculate nine molecular descriptors. Spatial parameters such as x, y, and z that provide the length, height, and width of the molecule, respectively, were used as descriptors. Subsequently, the V_{CPK} volume was calculated as the xyz product. Moreover, HOMO and LUMO energies, the aqueous solvation energy E_{solv} as well as the volume $V_{Spartan}$ were also used as descriptors. Finally, the Hammett constant σ, was also used.

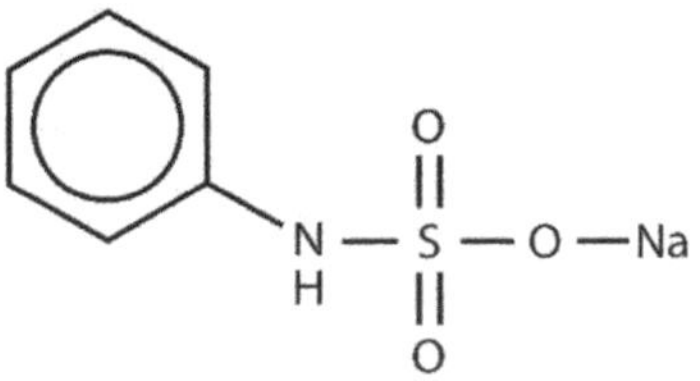

FIGURE 2 Molecular structure of sodium phenylsulfamate salt.

DA was carried out considering eight molecular descriptors such as x, y, z, HOMO, LUMO, E_{solv}, $V_{Spartan}$, and σ. For the training set, LDA and QDA showed that the accuracy (AC) of the classification models were not satisfactory. Moreover, Sensitivity (Sn) of each class was also reported. In fact, results presented in **Table 1** indicated a low prediction capability. The authors suggested that the low prediction capability for both methods was due to the lack of incorporation of the panel-derived sweetness values. To achieve better models, the CART methodology has been applied. In a first step, a classification tree is constructed using the three classes mentioned above, and in a second step, a regression tree was established considering only the most significant descriptors, that is, x, HOMO, LUMO, E_{solv}, $V_{Spartan}$, and σ. Model efficiency was evaluated by means of the regression coefficient ($R^2=0.627$), which suggested the presence of a real model. S-Plus software [64] was used to perform both DA and CART.

TABLE 1 QSAR models' results for calibration and validation sets for both DA and CART performed by Kelly *et al.*, (2005)

Method	$Sn_{nonsweet}$	$Sn_{sweet/nonsweet}$	Sn_{sweet}	AC_{train}	AC_{cv}	AC_{test}
LDA	51.2	61.1	56.3	54.7	41.3	50.0
QDA	61.0	100.0	93.8	77.3	49.3	25.0
CART classification	--	--	--	77.0	--	--
CART regression	--	--	--	81.3	--	75.0

In a subsequent project of the same year, Tarko *et al.*, [65] worked with three data sets containing 41 diverse sweeteners such as sugars and halosugars (data set 1), guanidine derivatives (data set 2), and 3-aminosuccinamic acid derivatives (data set 3) (refer to **Figure 3**). Initially, a QSAR analysis was performed for the three data sets separately. Subsequently, these groups were considered together for building a more consistent QSAR model (data set 4). The response considered by those authors was the logarithm of RS, $\log(RS)$. The geometry of the minimum energy conformer was obtained using the MMX force field and GMMX algorithms implemented in the PCMODEL molecular mechanics program [66]. The quantum mechanics software MOPAC (Molecular Orbital PACkage) [67] was used in order to refine the optimized structures. Moreover, molecular descriptors calculations were carried out in both MOPAC and PRECLAV (property evaluation by class variables) [68].

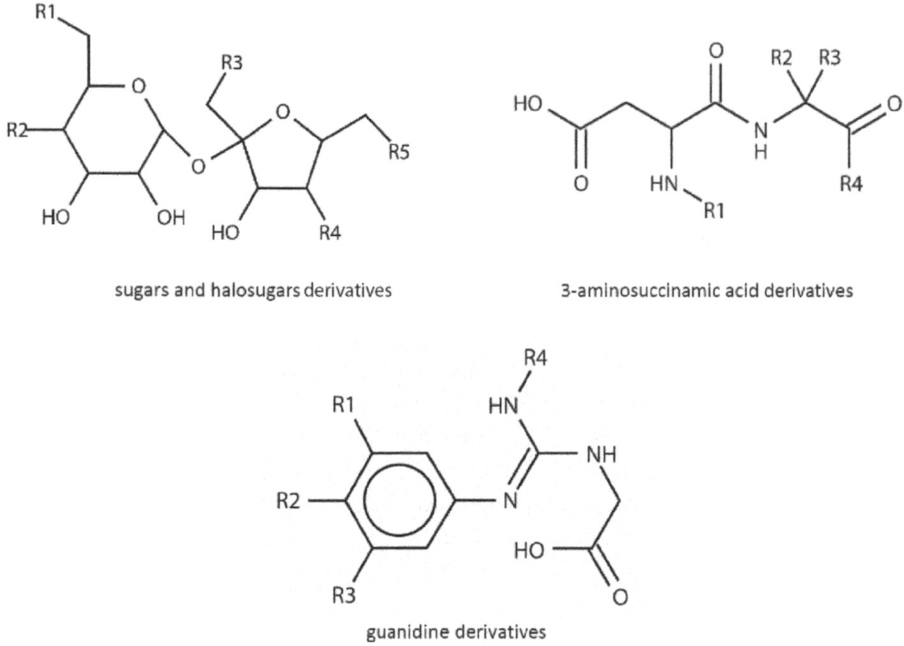

sugars and halosugars derivatives

3-aminosuccinamic acid derivatives

guanidine derivatives

FIGURE 3 Molecular structures for some sweeteners derivatives: sugars and halosugars, 3-aminosuccinamic acid, and guanidine derivatives.

The four data sets were split into training and test sets by a standard procedure. The best model was selected from thousands of MLR models. Results were classified into three categories such as recommended, uncertain, or unrecommended for synthesis. The Kendall rank correlation (K) was used in order to measure the quality of predictions. **Table 2** shows the results achieved in that study for the four models, where d is the number of descriptors considered in a model, and SD is the standard deviation. In QSAR model 1, the most important descriptor is the "*QSAR of molecular orbital energies*". Meanwhile, in model 2 the descriptors having the highest influence are the "*grid descriptor A33*", and the "*bond orders sum*". On the other hand, "*E(LUMO+1)-E(HOMO-1)gap*" and "*Platt topological index/Heavy atoms number ratio*" are the most important descriptors for model 3. Finally, for the model considering all three groups, the "*Molecular weight*", and "*Percentage of oxygen × Maximum charge of oxygen atoms product*" were found to be the most relevant descriptors.

TABLE 2   QSAR models parameters for calibration and validation sets proposed by Tarko *et al.*, (2005)

Data set	d	N_{train}	N_{test}	SD_{train}	K_{cv}	K_{train}	SD_{test}	K_{test}
1	3	33	8	0.338	0.8788	139.9	0.489	0.7143
2	3	33	8	0.356	0.5758	24.4	0.393	0.7857
3	5	33	8	0.193	0.9129	120.3	0.715	0.5714
4	5	98	25	0.485	0.7921	172.5	0.507	0.7933

One year later, the same group [69] presented a new QSAR study for modeling the log(1+*RS*) of 136 derivatives of the 3-aminosuccinamic acid (refer to **Figure 3**) by using PRECLAV software. Molecular geometry optimization is described earlier. The calibration set was obtained by eliminating outliers identified by a COIN criterion. Molecules were divided into virtual fragments, which were considered significant when the R^2 parameter was greater than a previously established limit. They considered only PRECLAV descriptors. Moreover, the program calculated the relative utility (U) of the descriptors when only a training set was considered. Thus, a useful descriptor was retained when its U value is greater than 400.

Model 1 is constructed by considering the total number of molecules. Meanwhile, model 2 is performed by excluding the 15 outliers. The elimination of the outliers clearly suggests an improvement in the quality of the model. Only 33 virtual molecular fragments are identified in model 2 and, among them, the –*CN* (cyano) and –$C_6H_4NHCONH$ (aryl-substituted urea) fragments lead to a significant increase of the RS. On the other hand, the nonconjugated or weakly conjugated fragment –NH_2 produces a significant decrease of the RS. A third QSAR model is performed, in which the data set is obtained by splitting the second one into training and validation sets, and a class function is used to select the significant descriptors. Parameters for both calibration and validation sets are close, which clearly suggest that PRECLAV identify in an accurate way the molecules suggested for synthesis. Table 3 shows a comparison of these three models, where F is the Fisher function.

TABLE 3   QSAR quality parameters for the models developed by Tarko *et al.*, (2006) using 3-amino-succinamic acid

Model	N_{train}	N_{test}	d	SD_{train}	R^2_{train}	F_{train}	K_{train}	K_{cv}	SD_{test}	R^2_{test}	K_{test}
1	136	0	4	0.652	0.655	62.6	0.677	0.664	--	--	--
2	121	0	5	0.399	0.847	128.2	0.782	0.770	--	--	--
3	97	24	5	0.425	0.830	89.9	0.773	0.756	0.384	0.858	0.761

Spillane *et al.,* [70] published a second study in 2006 in which they synthesized 42 new disubstituted phenylsulfamates, which were considered together with the 40 mono-substituted phenylsulfamates already synthesized in their previously work [62] in order to study a data set of 82 molecules. Due to the fact that the sweetness values were in the range 0–100, they split this response into three classes, that is, nonsweet (0–39), sweet/nonsweet (40–60), and sweet (61–100). The PC SPARTAN PRO software was used for molecular geometry optimizations as well as for the calculation of nine molecular descriptors [62]. Then, the data set was randomly split into a training set and a test set of 70 and 12 molecules, respectively. Molecules in the test set were only the newly synthesized compounds, that is, 11 nonsweet and 1 sweet/nonsweet compounds. The four newly synthesized compounds classified as sweet are considered in the training set.

According to the results achieved in their previously work, LDA and QDA analysis were not considered, and only a CART analysis was performed by using S-Plus statistical program. In a first approach, the whole data set was analyzed as a training set (Model 1); after that, 70 compounds were used as a training set for Model 2 (refer to **Table 4**). Both models were constructed with 13 and 11 terminal nodes, respectively, and the 6 molecular descriptors x, y, σ, V_{Spartan}, HOMO, and LUMO energies. As an alternative to improve the quality of the results, the authors considered the sweetness value to perform a regression tree (Model 3). For this, 7 molecular descriptors (x, z, V_{Spartan}, HOMO, LUMO, E_{solv}, and σ), 16 terminal nodes and 10-fold-cross-validation were used to obtain a regression coefficient of $R^2=0.757$.

TABLE 4 Statistical results for CART models on the disubstituted phenylsulfamates proposed by Spillane *et al.,* (2006)

Model	AC_{train}	AC_{test}	$Sn_{nonsweet}$	$Sn_{sweet/nonsweet}$	Sn_{sweet}
1	89	--	95	81	50
2	87	58	93	75	75
3	89	83	100	67	75

In 2007, Birta and Doca [71] studied seven alcoholic sweeteners; namely, sorbitol, sucrose, mannitol, xylitol, erytritol, glycerin and fructose. The molecular design, 3D visualization, the identification of the most stable structure, as well as the calculation of five molecular descriptors (stearical energy, heat of formation, dipole moment, electrostatic potential, and a chiral parameter) were performed with the aid of the ChemOffice Ultra 2000 software [72]. The authors were able to identify four groups of compounds from the dependency of the relative edulcoration (ER) relative edulcoration (E_R) and on the heat of formation on the one hand, and on the electrostatic potential on the other. The first group was formed by maltitol and sucrose, that have similar chemical structure with respect to the imposed condition, that is, maltitol sweetness is lower than sucrose sweetness. In the next group, sorbitol and mannitol reflected a similar behavior, as well as erytritol and glycerine. In contrast, xylitol and fructose were different.

Those authors also established a close correlation between the heat of formation and the electrostatical potential for almost all the sweeteners, with the exception of maltitol and sucrose. Moreover, they have proposed that the sweetness is connected to an asymmetric center. For this reason, a chiral parameter was calculated. They performed a series of mono-parametric QSAR models in which, the stearical energy had the better correlation ($R^2 = 0.74$). The dipole moment, on the other hand, reflected a low correlation ($R^2 = 0.43$) that disagreed with the remarkable conclusions achieved by Deutsch and Hansch [23]. Additionally, there is clearly a lack of correlation of the descriptors chiral parameter ($R^2 = 0.10$), heat of formation ($R^2 = 0.04$), and electrostatical potential ($R^2 = 0.00$).

A subsequent study by Lee et al., [73] was published in 2007. In this case, a QSAR study was carried out to analyze the effect of artificial sweeteners containing six-membered rings, such as saccharin, sucralose, and aspartame (refer to **Figures 4 and 5**), on the T1R2 and T1R3 glutamate receptors on the tongue measured as sweet index (SI). The molecules were built on the WebMO system [74] and their geometries were optimized with the aid of both semiempirical and ab initio methods as implemented in GAUSSIAN [75].

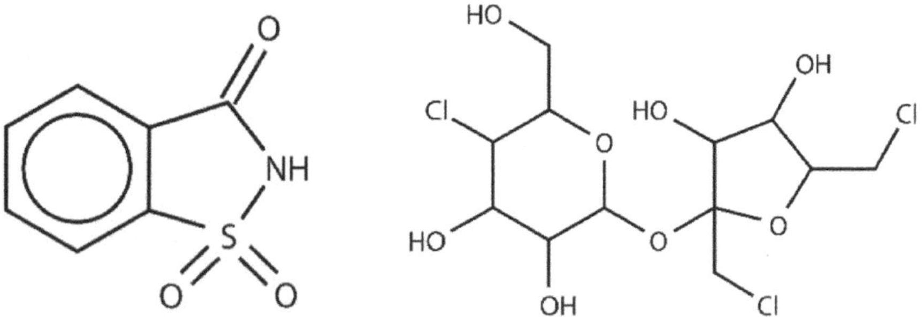

FIGURE 4 Molecular structures for saccharin (left) and sucralose (right).

The authors calculated seven molecular descriptors such as RHF energy, dipole moment, HOMO, and LUMO energies, HOMO/LUMO gap, and electrostatic potential maxima and minima. The two best models were selected among 12 MLRs (**Table 5**) involving the RHF energy, dipole moment, and HOMO energy descriptors. Molecules containing higher values of RHF energy were more probable to bond well to the receptor. In the case of dipole moment, the receptor was more likely to accept polar molecules, that is, the active sites of the receptor may accept atoms with high electron affinities, and attract the negatively charged end of a polar molecule. Furthermore, a low value of the HOMO energy suggested that the molecule is more capable of binding to the receptor.

TABLE 5 Best descriptors selected for the construction of the two QSAR models in the work of Lee *et al.*, (2007)

Model	Descriptors	R^2_{train}
1	RHF energy, dipole moment	0.994
2	RHF energy, dipole moment, HOMO energy	1.000

Vepuri *et al.,* [76] also published a work in 2007 regarding a 3D-QSAR. They studied 53 molecules of aspartame analogues and chemically modified derivatives (**Figure 5**), in which log(RS) was reported. The data set was split into a training set and a test set containing 43 and 10 molecules, respectively. Cerius2 software [77] was used to obtain a 3D-QSAR model with GFA, which included four molecular descriptors. In a further analysis, CoMFA, and CoMSIA were used. The van der Waals potential and coulombic terms representing the steric and electrostratic fields, respectively, were calculated by using CoMFA modeling by means of PLS. In addition, the steric, electrostatic, hydrophobic, hydrogen-bond donor, and hydrogen-bond acceptor potential fields are calculated for CoMSIA analysis.

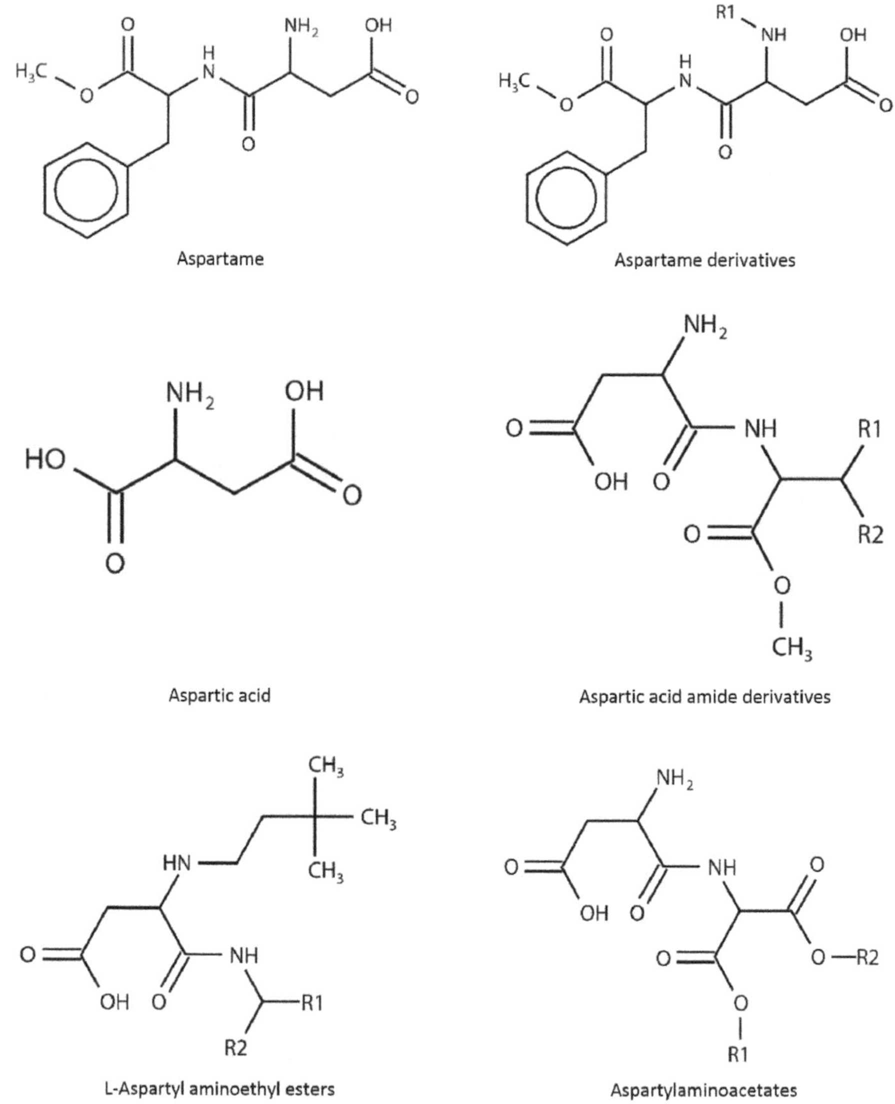

FIGURE 5   Molecular structures for aspartame, aspartic acid, and their analogues.

Results for the three models are presented in **Table 6**. All the three models have the same standard deviation ($SD = 5.148$). The GFA model shows that the descriptors hydrophobicity and molecular volume are important for modeling the log(RS). On the other hand, the hydrophobicity interactions of a molecule favor the formation of a receptor/molecule complex with low free energy due to the increase of the entropy. The molecular volume that belongs to a 3D spatial descriptor represents the contact area inside the binding pocket. The best results for CoMSIA were achieved using a combination of steric, electrostatic, hydrophobic, hydrogen-bond donor, and hydrogen-bond acceptor fields. As a remarkable conclusion, the authors indicated that contributions of CoMFA and CoMSIA are the same.

TABLE 6 Results for the three QSAR models developed by Vepuri *et al.,* (2007) for modeling the Sweetness Potency of Aspartic Acid Analogues

Model	d	R^2_{train}	R^2_{cv}	R^2_{test}
3D-GFA-QSAR	4	0.753	0.660	0.375
3D-CoMFA-QSAR	3	0.768	0.390	0.535
3D-CoMSIA-QSAR	6	0.927	0.585	0.596

In 2009, Spillane *et al.,* [78] published a third study using 28 new five-membered aromatic ring thiazolyl-, benzothiazolyl-, and thiadiazolylsulfamates as well as 30 well-known similar heterocyclic sulfamates. The data set was divided into three clases, that is, nonsweet, sweet/nonsweet, and sweet. In order to find a reliable QSAR model, a total of nine molecular descriptors such as HOMO and LUMO energies, length of the molecule, area of the molecule, volume of the molecule, dipole moment, E_{solv}, and Hammett constant σ were considered. Furthermore, the partition coefficient descriptor (Log *P*) was calculated using the HyperChem software [79]. Both LDA and QDA analyses were carried out for the 58 molecules using Minitab software [80]. LDA was used in order to discriminate between two classes, that is, sweet and nonsweet. For this, the six sweet/nonsweet compounds were divided into these two classes.

Due to the success of the classification models achieved previously [62, 70], CART methodology was used to improve the quality of the models with the S-Plus statistical software.The data set was split into a training set and a test set containing 48 and 10 compounds, respectively. Initially, CART was used considering only the two classes constructed for DA (CART-1). In a second step, the three classes were considered and a new tree was performed (CART-2). The test set was constructed according to the taste and to the molecular structure. CART-2 was found to be superior with respect to the other tools, and was successful for classifying the three considered classes (refer to **Table 7**).

TABLE 7 DA and CART models obtained in the research of Spillane *et al.*, (2009)

Method	d	AC_{train}	AC_{cv}	AC_{test}	$Sn_{nonsweet}$	$Sn_{sweet/nonsweet}$	Sn_{sweet}
LDA	2	66.0	60.0	--	--	--	--
QDA	3	76.0	60.0	--	--	--	--
CART-1		95.8	--	70	97.0	--	84
CART-2		93.8	--	80	87.5	83.3	100

In 2011, Yang *et al.*, [14] used 29 sugars and 74 common sweeteners to develop three QSAR models. MDL ISIS DRAW/BASE [81] was used for structure management, editing, comparing, and data extraction. Geometry optimizations were performed with CORINA software [82]. Afterward, ADRIANA. Code program [83] allowed the calculation of 154 molecular descriptors. These descriptors had 19 global molecular descriptors, 8 shape descriptors, 88 2D autocorrelation vectors, and 39 autocorrelation of surface properties [84, 85]. Subsequently, 6,776 new descriptors were computed based on 2D autocorrelations vectors, and four of them were selected for analysis together with the other 66 descriptors from the other blocks.

Three molecular descriptors were selected by analyzing the pairwise correlation coefficient between each descriptor and the log(RS), as well as the pairwise correlation among the descriptors. In order to split the data set, SONNIA software [86] was used for building a rectangular Kohone's self-organizing neural network (KohNN). One object of each occupied neuron was used for the training set, that is, 58 molecules, and the remaining constituted the test set. The ANN was developed within the ASNN software [87]. The SVM model was constructed with the aid of the LIBSVM program [88]. The authors demonstrated that both nonlinear methods provide better results than the MLR method (refer to **Table 8**).

TABLE 8 Statistical results for the best linear and nonlinear models achieved by Yang *et al.*, (2011)

Method	R^2_{train}	SD_{train}	F	R^2_{rand}	R^2_{test}	SD_{test}
MLR	0.885	1.023	139.047	0.269	0.856	1.205
ANN	0.899	1.049	--	--	0.869	1.162
SVM	0.910	1.037	--	--	0.889	1.192

In a work published in 2013, Zhong *et al.,* [15] studied 320 unique compounds. For this, they extended their previous data set [14] by adding 157 L-aspartyl dipeptide analogues, 23 isovanillic, and some other compounds. The 2D structures were designed using the MOE software [89]. The CORINA program was used to obtain the 3D structure of the compounds. Subsequently, 1,235 molecular descriptors were calculated with the ADRIANA.Code software, which included 5 categories, that is, 19 global molecular descriptors, 8 shape descriptors, 88 2D autocorrelation vectors, 88 3D autocorrelation vectors, and 1,024 3D property-weighted radial distribution function descriptors. Furthermore, 6,776 new combinations of descriptors were calculated from the 2D autocorrelation descriptors according to the Yang's method [14].

Further, 12 descriptors were selected using the stepwise lineal regression variable selection method. Nine of those descriptors were based on atom RDF properties. In addition, the data set was randomly split into a training set and a test set containing 214 and 106 molecules, respectively. Then, QSAR models were performed by means of MLR and SVM analysis. According to the results presented in **Table 9**, those two models have strong predictive capabilities and, moreover, they provide very similar results. It was demonstrated that the sweetness of a compound was correlated to descriptors based on atom charges, vectorial molecular descriptors based on radial distribution functions of atom pair properties, and 3D autocorrelation π charge, as well as to descriptors related to atomic electronegativity and polarizability.

TABLE 9 Comparison of the best two QSAR models performed by Zhong *et al.,* (2013)

Model	R^2_{train}	SD_{train}	F	R^2_{test}	SD_{test}
MLR	0.814	0.958	73.275	0.773	1.029
SVM	0.830	0.979	--	0.778	0.994

In a subsequent work published in 2013, Nunes and Freitas [90] used 40 sucrose derivatives previously studied by Barker *et al.,* [25] (refer to **Figure 3**). The authors applied the aug-MIA-QSPR. The ChemSketch program [91] was used for drawing purposes. The Kennard-Stone algorithm [92] was used for splitting the data set into a training set and a test set of 30 and 10 compounds, respectively. The aug-MIA-QSPR model was constructed by means of PLS using six latent variables (LV). They confirmed the reliability of the model by using its squared correlation coefficient ($R^2_{train} = 0.970$), the cross-validation leave-one-out ($R^2_{cv} = 0.86$), and the root mean square error of cross-validation

($RMSE_{cv} = 0.39$). Moreover, the external validation was statistically evaluated by means of $R^2_{test} = 0.94$, and the root mean square error in prediction ($RMSEP = 0.30$). Model robustness was also validated by Y-randomization ($R^2_{rand} = 0.63$). Chemoface software [93] was used for these calculations. These results show a very satisfactory model for regression and prediction purposes.

In 2013, Nunes and Freitas [94] used again the aug-MIA-QSPR for modeling the RS of 47 guanidine derivatives (refer to **Figure 3**). These compounds were previously studied by Barker *et al.,* [25]. For comparison purposes, the data set is split into a training set and a test set containing 38 and 9 molecules, respectively. The molecular design of the compounds was described in their previous work [90].

The authors were able to identify four outliers within the data set. These compounds were excluded for further analysis. In this way, the new calibration set of 43 molecules was analyzed by means of PLS regression using 6 LV. Satisfactory results were achieved, as can be deduced from $R^2 = 0.96$, $RMSEC = 0.11$, $R^2_{cv} = 0.73$, $RMSE_{cv} = 0.27$, $R^2_{test} = 0.57$, ($R^2_{test} \geq 0.50$ was recommended), and the $R^2_{rand} = 0.7 \pm 0.02$. Additionally, the statistical difference between R^2 and R^2_{rand} was evaluated by means of a special parameter $^c R^2_p = 0.50$ ($^c R^2_p \geq 0.50$ was recommended) [95]. This aug-MIA-QSPR model demonstrates that 2D molecular descriptors are enough to understand the RS; and these descriptors are used to predict the log(RS) of two new guanidine derivatives (refer to **Figure 6**).

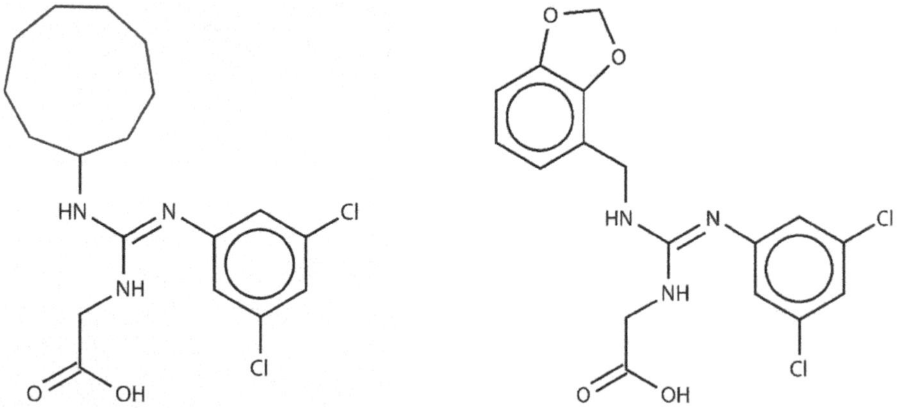

FIGURE 6   Molecular structures for the two new guanidine derivatives proposed by Nunes and Freitas (2013) as potential sweeteners.

Recently, Singh *et al.,* [5] published a QSAR study using 31 sucrose derivatives and 30 guanidine derivatives (**Figure 3**). Geometry optimizations and the calculation of molecular descriptors were carried out with CACHe Pro software. Descriptors such as electron affinity (EA), ionization potential (IP), electrophilicity index (ω), and total energy (TE) were obtained from calculations based on the generalized gradient approximation version of the DFT. Calculation of heat of formations (ΔH_f) and steric energies (SE) were performed by using the PM3 method. Solvent accessible surface area (SASA) was obtained from the implicit conductor-like screening model (COSMO) and the PM3 method. The atom typing scheme of Ghose *et al.,* [96] was used for the calculation of the molar refractivity (MR) descriptor.

Two and three outliers were removed from the sucrose and guanidine databases, respectively. Subsequently, MLR analysis was performed, and a triparametric model was selected as the best model for both cases. They found that the IP descriptor plays an important role for modeling the sucrose–receptor interaction. The MR descriptor was the most important one for modeling the guanidine–receptor interaction, which is related to the molecular volume and to the London forces. According to the results presented in **Table 10** (SEE is the standard error of the estimate), it is concluded that these two models have predictive power, and they can be used in order to predict the RS of any new sucrose or guanidine derivative.

TABLE 10 A brief of the QSAR models for sucrose and guanidine derivatives proposed by Singh *et al.,* (2014)

Family	N_{train}	R^2_{train}	SD_{train}	R^2_{cv}	SEE	Descriptors
Sucrose	29	0.865	0.076	0.817	0.354	IP, MR, and SASA
Guanidine	27	0.778	0.107	0.616	0.276	IP, MR, and ΔH_f

10.3 CONCLUSIONS

Although the main applications of the QSAR/QSPR theory are found in the field of drug design, there is a notable increase in the application of this theory in food science, particularly for studying the chemistry of sweeteners.

In this review, the successful applications of the QSAR/QSPR theory are presented regarding the study and prediction of the RS of sweeteners. Models presented above complement previous reported results from the literature, and in some cases, produce more general and predictive quantitative structure–relative sweetness relationships.

It is expected that the QSRSR method will become an important tool in food science for understanding sweetener–receptor interactions and for discovering more potent and commercially feasible sweeteners to be used both as raw material and as additives for food processing.

Finally, our recommendation to food chemists is to develop larger sweeteners databases in order to establish more predictive QSRSR models, because the RS prediction of unknown compounds should not be limited to the same derivatives.

10.4 ACKNOWLEDGMENTS

Cristian Rojas is grateful for his Ph.D. fellowship from the National Secretary of Higher Education, Science, Technology, and Innovation (SENESCYT) from the Republic of Ecuador. Pablo R. Duchowicz wishes to thank the National Scientific and Technical Research Council of Argentina (CONICET) for the project grant PIP11220100100151, and the Minister of Science, Technology, and Productive Innovation for the use of the electronic library facilities. Pablo R. Duchowicz and Reinaldo Pis Diez are members of the Scientific Researcher Career of CONICET.

KEYWORDS

- **Molecular descriptors**
- **QSAR/QSPR theory**
- **Relative sweetness**
- **Sucrose**
- **Sweeteners.**

REFERENCES

1. Cooper, J.M., *Sucrose*, in *Optimising sweet taste in foods*, W.J. Spillane, Editor 2006, CRC Press.
2. Belitz, H.-D., W. Grosch, and P. Schieberle, *Food Chemistry.* 4th ed, 2009. Springer-Verlag.
3. Hugot, E. and G.H. Jenkins, *Handbook of cane sugar engineering.* Vol. 114. 1972: Elsevier.
4. Asadi, M., *Beet-sugar handbook,* 2006. John Wiley & Sons.
5. Singh, R.K., M.A. Khan, and P.P. Singh, *Rating of sweetness by molar refractivity and ionization potential: QSAR study of sucrose and guanidine derivatives.* South African Journal of Chemistry, 2014. 67: p. 12–20.
6. Bassoli, A., *et al.,, Quantitative structure-activity relationships of sweet isovanillyl derivatives.* Quantitative Structure-Activity Relationships, 2001. 20(1): p. 3–16.

7. Li, X., *et al.,*, *Human receptors for sweet and umami taste.* Proceedings of the National Academy of Sciences, 2002. 99(7): p. 4692–4696.
8. Lindemann, B., *Taste reception.* Physiological Reviews, 1996. 76(3): p. 719–766.
9. Lindemann, B., *Receptors and transduction in taste.* Nature, 2001. 413(6852): p. 219–225.
10. Margolskee, R.F., *Molecular mechanisms of bitter and sweet taste transduction.* Journal of Biological Chemistry, 2002. 277(1): p. 1–4.
11. Nie, Y., *et al.,*, *Distinct contributions of T1R2 and T1R3 taste receptor subunits to the detection of sweet stimuli.* Current Biology, 2005. 15(21): p. 1948–1952.
12. Sainz, E., *et al.,*, *Identification of a novel member of the T1R family of putative taste receptors.* Journal of Neurochemistry, 2001. 77(3): p. 896–903.
13. Zhao, G.Q., *et al.,*, *The receptors for mammalian sweet and umami taste.* Cell, 2003. 115(3): p. 255–266.
14. Yang, X., *et al.,*, *In-silico prediction of sweetness of sugars and sweeteners.* Food Chemistry, 2011. 128(3): p. 653–658.
15. Zhong, M., *et al.,*, *Prediction of sweetness by multilinear regression analysis and support vector machine.* Journal of Food Science, 2013. 78(9): p. S1445–S1450.
16. Oertly, E. and R.G. Myers, *A new theory relating constitution to taste. Simple relations between the constitution of aliphatic compounds and their sweet taste.* Journal of the American Chemical Society, 1919. 41(6): p. 855–867.
17. Shallenberger, R.S. and T.E. Acree, *Molecular theory of sweet taste.* Nature, 1967. 216: p. 480–482.
18. Kier, L.B., *A molecular theory of sweet taste.* Journal of Pharmaceutical Sciences, 1972. 61(9): p. 1394–1397.
19. Crosby, G.A., G.E. DuBois, and R.E. Wingard Jr, *The design of synthetic sweeteners*, in *Drug design*, E.J. Ariëns, Editor. 1979. Academic Press: New York. p. 215–310.
20. Nofre, C. and J.-M. Tinti, *Sweetness reception in man: the multipoint attachment theory.* Food Chemistry, 1996. 56(3): p. 263–274.
21. Nofre, C. and J.M. Tinti, *In quest of hyperpotent sweeteners*, in *Sweet Taste Chemoreception*, M. Mathlouthi, J.A. Kanters, and G.G. Birch, Editors. 1993. Elsevier Science Publishers: p. 205–236.
22. Nofre, C., J.M. Tinti, and D. Glaser, *Evolution of the sweetness receptor in primates. II. Gustatory responses of non-human primates to nine compounds known to be sweet in man.* Chemical senses, 1996. 21(6): p. 747–762.
23. Deutsch, E.W. and C. Hansch, *Dependence of relative sweetness on hydrophobic bonding.* Nature, 1966. 211: p. 75.
24. Arnoldi, A., *et al.,*, *Isovanillyl sweeteners. Synthesis, conformational analysis, and structure-activity relationship of some sweet oxygen heterocycles.* Journal of the Chemical Society, Perkin Transactions 2, 1991. (9): p. 1399–1406.
25. Barker, J.S., C.K. Hattotuwagama, and M.G.B. Drew, *Computational studies of sweet-tasting molecules.* Pure and applied chemistry, 2002. 74(7): p. 1207–1217.
26. Bassoli, A., *et al.,*, *General pseudoreceptor model for sweet compounds: a semiquantitative prediction of binding affinity for sweet-tasting molecules.* Journal of Medicinal Chemistry, 2002. 45(20): p. 4402–4409.
27. Drew, M.G.B., *et al.,* *Quantitative structure-activity relationship studies of sulfamates RNH-SO3Na: distinction between sweet, sweet-bitter, and bitter molecules.* Journal of Agricultural and Food Chemistry, 1998. 46(8): p. 3016–3026.
28. Hansch, C., *Use of σ^+ in structure-activity correlations.* Journal of Medicinal Chemistry, 1970. 13(5): p. 964–966.

29. Iwamura, H., *Structure-taste relationship of perillartine and nitro-and cyanoaniline derivatives*. Journal of Medicinal Chemistry, 1980. 23(3): p. 308–312.
30. Iwamura, H., *Structure-sweetness relationship of L-aspartyl dipeptide analogs. A receptor site topology*. Journal of Medicinal Chemistry, 1981. 24(5): p. 572–583.
31. Katritzky, A.R., *et al.,, A QSPR study of sweetness potency using the CODESSA program*. Croatica Chemica Acta, 2002. 75(2): p. 475–502.
32. Pietrzycki, W., *QSAR computational model of Nofre-Tinti theory on sweetness of mono- and disaccharides composed by pyranose units*. Polish Journal of Chemistry, 2001. 75(10): p. 1569–1582.
33. Rao, M. and N. Kumar, *Quantitative correlation between steric factors and the relative sweetness of 2-substituted 5-nitroanilines*. Indian Drugs, 1986. 23: p. 35–38.
34. Spillane, W.J., *Quantitative structure-taste relationship studies of sulphamate sweeteners*. Chemistry and Industry 1983. p. 16–19.
35. Spillane, W.J. and G. McGlinchey, *Structure-activity studies on sulfamate sweeteners II: Semiquantitative structure-taste relationship for sulfamate (RNHSO-3) sweeteners-the role of R*. Journal of Pharmaceutical Sciences, 1981. 70(8): p. 933–935.
36. Spillane, W.J., *et al.,, Structure-activity studies on sulfamate sweetners III: Structure-taste relationships for heterosulfamates*. Journal of Pharmaceutical Sciences, 1983. 72(8): p. 852–856.
37. Spillane, W.J., *et al.,, Development of structure-taste relationships for sweet and non-sweet heterosulfamates*. Journal of the Chemical Society, Perkin Transactions 2, 2000. (7): p. 1369–1374.
38. Spillane, W.J., *et al.,, Sulfamate sweeteners*. Food Chemistry, 1996. 56(3): p. 255–261.
39. Spillane, W.J. and M.B. Sheahan, *Semi-quantitative and quantitative structure-taste relationships for carboand hetero-sulphamate (RNHSO$_3^-$) sweeteners*. Journal of Chemical Society, Perkin Transactions. 2, 1989. (7): p. 741–746.
40. van der Heijden, A., L.B.P. Brussel, and H.G. Peer, *Quantitative structure-activity relationships (QSAR) in sweet aspartyl dipeptide methyl esters*. Chemical Senses, 1979. 4: p. 141–152.
41. Walters, D.E., *Genetically Evolved Receptor Models (GERM) as a 3D QSAR tool*, in *3D QSAR in drug design. Recent Advances*, H. Kubinyi, G. Folkers, and Y.C. Martin, Editors. 2002. Kluwer Academic Publishers. p. 159–166.
42. Walters, D.E. and R.M. Hinds, *Genetically evolved receptor models: A computational approach to construction of receptor models*. Journal of Medicinal Chemistry, 1994. 37(16): p. 2527–2536.
43. Walters, D.E., *Analysing and predicting properties of sweet-tasting compounds*, in *Optimising Sweet Taste in Foods*, W.J. Spillane, Editor. 2006. p. 283–291.
44. Consonni, V. and R. Todeschini, *structure-activity relationships by autocorrelation descriptors and genetic algorithms*, in *Chemoinformatics and Advanced Machine Learning Perspectives: Complex Computational Methods and Collaborative Techniques*, H. Lodhi and Y. Yamanishi, Editors. 2010. IGI Global Publishers: Hershey. p. 60–93.
45. Duchowicz, P.R. and E.A. Castro, *On applications of macromolecular QSAR theory*, in *Advanced Methods and Applications in Chemoinformatics: Research Progress and New Applications*, E.A. Castro and A.K. Haghi, Editors. 2012. Engineering Science Reference. p. 219–228.
46. Kubinyi, H., *QSAR: Hansch Analysis and Related Approaches* 2008. Wiley-Interscience.
47. Puzyn, T., Leszczynski, J., Cronin. M. T., *Recent Advances in QSAR Studies: Methods and Applications*. First ed., 2009. New York: Springer.

48. Mercader, A.G. and E.A. Castro, *Partial-order ranking and linear modeling: their use in predictive QSAR/QSPR studies*, in *Statistical Modelling of Molecular Descriptors in QSAR/QSPR*, M. Dehmer, K. Varmuza, and D. Bonchev, Editors. 2012. Wiley-VCH. p. 149–174.
49. Diudea, M.V., *QSPR/QSAR Studies by Molecular Descriptors*, 2001. Nova Science Publishers.
50. Katritzky, A.R., Lobanov, V. S., Karelson, M., *QSPR: the correlation and quantitative prediction of chemical and physical properties from structure*. Chemical Society Reviews, 1995. 24: p. 279–287.
51. Todeschini, R., Consonni, V., *Molecular Descriptors for Chemoinformatics*. 2009. Wiley-VCH.
52. Trinajstic, N., *Chemical Graph Theory*, 1992. Boca Raton (FL): CRC Press.
53. Chicu, S.A., Putz, M. V., *Köln-Timişoara Molecular Activity Combined Models toward Interspecies Toxicity Assessment*. International Journal of Molecular Science, 2009. 10: p. 4474–4497.
54. Golbraikh, A., Tropsha, A., *Beware of q2!* Journal of Molecular Graphics and Modelling, 2002. 20: p. 269–276.
55. Goodarzi, M., Duchowicz, P. R., Wu, C. H., Fernández, F. M., Castro, E. A., *New hybrid genetic based support vector regression as QSAR approach for analyzing flavonoids-GABA(A) complexes*. Journal of Chemical Information and Modeling, 2009. 49: p. 1475–1485.
56. Hawkins, D.M., Basak, S. C., Mills, D., *Assessing model fit by cross validation*. Journal of Chemical Information and Modeling, 2003. 43: p. 579–586.
57. Lacrămă, A.M., Putz, M. V., Ostafe, V., *A spectral-SAR model for the anionic-cationic interaction in ionic liquids: application to Vibrio fischeri ecotoxicity*. International Journal of Molecular Science, 2007. 8: p. 842–863.
58. Putz, M.V., Putz, A. M., Lazea, M., Lenciu, L., Chiriac, A., *Quantum-SAR extension of the spectral-SAR algorithm. Application to polyphenolic anticancer bioactivity*, International Journal of Molecular Science, 2009. 10: p. 1193–1214.
59. Putz, M.V., Ionaşcu, C., Putz, A. M., Ostafe, V., *Alert-QSAR. Implications for electrophilic theory of chemical carcinogenesis*. International Journal of Molecular Science, 2011. 12: p. 5098–5134.
60. Putz, M.V., *Residual-QSAR. Implications for genotoxic carcinogenesis*. Chemistry Central Journal, 2011. 5: p. doi: 10.1186/1752-153X-5-29.
61. Consonni, V. and R. Todeschini, *Multivariate analysis of molecular descriptors*, in *Statistical Modelling of Molecular Descriptors in QSAR/QSPR*, M. Dehmer, K. Varmuza, and D. Bonchev, Editors. 2012. Wiley-VCH. p. 111–147.
62. Kelly, D.P., W.J. Spillane, and J. Newell, *Development of structure-taste relationships for monosubstituted phenylsulfamate sweeteners using Classification and Regression Tree (CART) analysis*. Journal of Agricultural and Food Chemistry, 2005. 53(17): p. 6750–6758.
63. *PC Spartan Pro '14*, 1999. Wavefunction, Inc., http://www.wavefun.com/.
64. *S-Plus 8.2 for Windows*, 2010. Solution Metrics, Inc., http://www.solutionmetrics.com.au/.
65. Tarko, L., I. Lupescu, and D. Groposila-Constantinescu, *Sweetness power QSARs by PRECLAV software*. Arkivoc, 2005. 10: p. 254–271.
66. *PCMODEL*, 2014. Serena Software, Inc., http://www.serenasoft.com/.
67. *MOPAC (Molecular Orbital PACkage)* 2012. Stewart Computational Chemistry, Inc., http://openmopac.net/.
68. *PRECLAV (Property Evaluation by Class Variables)*, 2006. Center of Organic Chemistry (CCO)-Bucharest: Bucharest.
69. Tarko, L., I. Lupescu, and D. Constantinescu-Groposila, *QSAR Studies on amino-succinamic acid derivatives sweeteners*. Arkivoc, 2006. 13: p. 22–40.

70. Spillane, W.J., et al.,, Structure-taste relationships for disubstituted phenylsulfamate tastants using Classification and Regression Tree (CART) analysis. Journal of Agricultural and Food Chemistry, 2006. 54(16): p. 5996–6004.

71. Birta, N. and N. Doca, Quantitative evaluation of sorbitol with other alcoholic sweeteners trough QSAR studies. Annals of West University of Timisoara. Series Chemistry, 2007. 16(1): p. 91–96.

72. ChemOffice Ultra 2000, 2001. Perkin Elmer, http://www.cambridgesoft.com/.

73. Lee, K., K. Cooper, and C. Kennedy, QSAR Analysis of artificial sweeteners. Journal of Student Computational Chemistry, 2007. 1: p. 8–12.

74. WebMO Pro, 2014. WebMO, LLC, Inc., http://www.webmo.net/.

75. Gaussian 09, 2009. Gaussian, Inc., http://www.gaussian.com/.

76. Vepuri, S.B., N.R. Tawari, and M.S. Degani, Quantitative structure-activity relationship study of some aspartic acid analogues to correlate and predict their sweetness potency. QSAR & Combinatorial Science, 2007. 26(2): p. 204–214.

77. Cerius2, 1997. Laboratory for molecular simulation, Inc., http://lms.chem.tamu.edu/.

78. Spillane, W.J., et al.,, Development of structure-taste relationships for thiazolyl-, benzothiazolyl-, and thiadiazolylsulfamates. Journal of Agricultural and Food Chemistry, 2009. 57(12): p. 5486–5493.

79. HyperChem, 2008. Hypercube, Inc., http://www.hyper.com.

80. Minitab 17, 2010. Minitab, Inc., www.minitab.com.

81. MDL ISIS DRAW/BASE, 2005. MDL Information Systems, Inc.

82. CORINA – Fast Generation of High-Quality 3D Molecular Models, 2010. Molecular Networks, Inc., http://www.molecular-networks.com/.

83. ADRIANA.Code - Calculation of Molecular Descriptors, 2009. Molecular Networks, Inc., http://www.molecular-networks.com/.

84. Teckentrup, A., H. Briem, and J. Gasteiger, Mining high-throughput screening data of combinatorial libraries: development of a filter to distinguish hits from nonhits. Journal of chemical information and computer sciences, 2004. 44(2): p. 626–634.

85. Wagener, M., J. Sadowski, and J. Gasteiger, Autocorrelation of molecular surface properties for modeling corticosteroid binding globulin and cytosolic Ah receptor activity by neural networks. Journal of the American Chemical Society, 1995. 117(29): p. 7769–7775.

86. SONNIA - Self-Organizing Neural Network Package, 2008. Molecular Networks, Inc., http://www.molecular-networks.com/.

87. Tetko, I., et al.,, Virtual Computational Chemistry Laboratory - Design and Description. Journal of Computer-Aided Molecular Design, 2005. 19(6): p. 453–463.

88. Chang, C.-C. and C.-J. Lin, LIBSVM: a library for support vector machines. ACM Transactions on Intelligent Systems and Technology (TIST), 2011. 2(3).

89. MOE (Molecular Operating Environment), 2013. Chemical Computing Group, Inc., http://www.chemcomp.com/.

90. Nunes, C.A. and M.P. Freitas, aug-MIA-QSPR on the modeling of sweetness values of disaccharide derivatives. LWT – Food Science and Technology, 2013. 51(2): p. 405–408.

91. ChemSketch, 2013, ACD Labs, Inc., http://www.acdlabs.com/.

92. Kennard, R.W. and L.A. Stone, Computer aided design of experiments. Technometrics, 1969. 11(1): p. 137–148.

93. Nunes, C.A., et al.,, Chemoface: a novel free user-friendly interface for chemometrics. Journal of the Brazilian Chemical Society, 2012. 23(11): p. 2003–2010.

94. Nunes, C.A. and M.P. Freitas, aug-MIA-QSPR study of guanidine derivative sweeteners. European Food Research and Technology, 2013. 237(4): p. 565–570.

95. Mitra, I., A. Saha, and K. Roy, *Exploring quantitative structure-activity relationship studies of antioxidant phenolic compounds obtained from traditional Chinese medicinal plants.* Molecular Simulation, 2010. 36(13): p. 1067–1079.
96. Ghose, A.K., A. Pritchett, and G.M. Crippen, *Atomic physicochemical parameters for three dimensional structure directed quantitative structure-activity relationships III: Modeling hydrophobic interactions.* Journal of Computational Chemistry, 1988. 9(1): p. 80–90.

CHAPTER 11

QSAR STUDIES OF 1,4-BENZODIAZEPINES AS CCK$_A$ ANTAGONIST

SUMITRA NAIN[1], PONNURENGAM M. SIVAKUMAR[2], and SARVESH PALIWAL[1]

[1]Department of Pharmacy, Banasthali University, Banasthali 304022, Rajasthan, India

[2]FPR, Nanomedical Engineering Lab, RIKEN, Wako, Japan

E-mail: nainsumitra@gmail.com; Fax: +91-1438-228365; Tel.: +91-1438-228341 Extn. 348.

CONTENTS

ABSTRACT

Cholecystokinin (cck-33), a 33-amino acid peptide (gastrointestinal hormone), was discovered by isolation from porcine duodenum. [1]CCK exerts its biological effects by binding to specific receptors on its target tissues. In the gastrointestinal tract CCK receptors have been found on the gallbladder, stomach, pancreas, ileum, and colon. The CCK_A receptors are found predominantly in the periphery, whereas CCK_B receptors are found specifically in the interpeduncular nucleus, area postrerna, the nucleus tractus, and hypothalamus. It helps in secretion of digestive enzymes and bile from the pancreas and gallbladder, respectively. It also acts as a hunger suppressant. This chapter includes the quantitative structure–activity relationship study of 1,4 benzodiazepine as CCK_A antagonists.

11.1 INTRODUCTION

11.1.1 CHOLECYSTOKININ

Cholecystokinin (CCK) is a Greek-derived word which means chole, "bile"; cysto, "sac"; kinin, "move"; hence, moves the bile-sac (gallbladder). Cholecystokinin (cck-33), a 33-amino acid peptide (gastrointestinal hormone), was discovered by isolation from porcine duodenum [1, 2]. Mutt and Jorpes in the 1960s culminated the sequencing of the CCK 33 [1]. CCK and gastrin were found to have the same 5 carboxyl-terminal amino acids. Gastrin is a peptide, which was isolated from stomach in 1964[3]. CCK is much more distributed than gastrin. Many similarities between them suggested that they may arise from a common precursor[4] but later on it was found that they are arise from separate prohormones[4]. In this chapter we discuss about the CCK, CCK structure, CCK receptor antagonist, quantitative structure–activity relationship (QSAR) as well as different QSAR studies reported by different scientist regarding CCK.

11.1.2 STRUCTURE OF CCK

The cloning of complementary DNA (cDNA) of rat sequence has enhanced the knowledge for the structure of pre-pro-CCK[5]. It was further followed by the cloning of the human and porcine cDNA. The proposed basic structure for CCK and gastrin is shown in **Figure 1**.

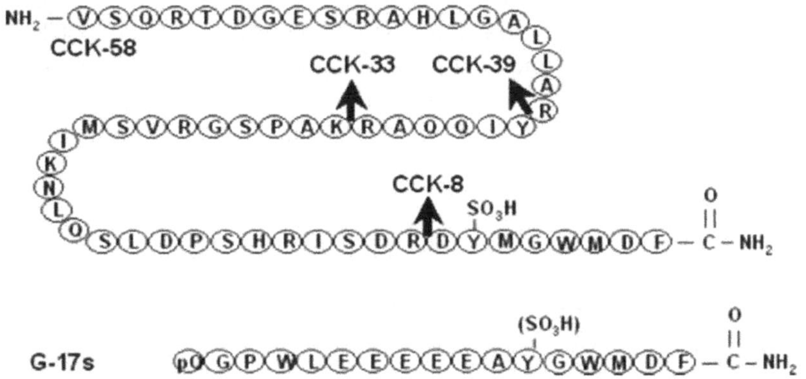

FIGURE 1   CCK and Gastrin[5].

CCK is a peptide hormone, which is responsible for stimulating digestion of fat and proteins in the body. In the rat brain, a gastrin-like immune
reactive peptide was found in 1975[6] which was later known as CCK-8[7–9]. A
large amount of CCK was found in various areas of the central nervous system
(CNS) and also in peripheral nerve endings[10–12]. CCK and gastrin are encoded by two distinct genes which are located on chromosomes 3p22-p21.3 and
17q21, respectively, that is, the human CCK gene is found on the third chromosome, while the gastrin gene is found on the 17th position[13]. They are produced
through multistep processing of large peptidic precursors[14–17].

Addition of sulfur group to the tyrosine at position 7 from the COOH termi-
nus in CCK is found in biologically active peptides and at position 6 in gastrin,
as well as COOH-terminal amidation. Nonsulfated forms of biologically active
gastrins and CCK are also found to exist. In fact, half of the endogenous gastrins
are nonsulfated[14, 15, 18, 19]. CCK and gastrin share some biological and pharmacological effects, because of the sequence similarity in their bioactive region. In
their mature forms, these peptides exert their biological functions by interacting
with CCK receptors (G protein-coupled receptors) located on multiple cellular
targets in the CNS and peripheral organs.

11.1.3   FUNCTIONS OF CCK

It helps in secretion of digestive enzymes and bile from the pancreas and gallbladder, respectively. It also acts as a hunger suppressant. Recent
evidence also suggest that it also plays a major role in inducing drug tolerance to opioids like morphine and heroin, and is partly implicated in experiences
of pain and hypersensitivity during opioid withdrawal[20, 21]. CCKs are found to

be responsible for anxiety[22–24] as well as they are also involved in numerous other mental illnesses such as schizophrenia[25–30] and addictions.[31–36]. CCK concentration in cortex and limbic regions [37, 38] supports its role in the regulation of many behavioral activities, including satiety and appetite, [39] thermoregulation, [40, 41] sexual behavior, [42, 43,] anxiety,[43, 44] memory[45], and response to drugs of abuse.[46]

11.1.4.1   1, 4-BENZODIAZEPINES

CCK antagonists are further classified as follows:
1.   Derivatives of cyclic nucleotides
2.   Benzodiazepine type derivatives
3.   Nonpeptidic fragments extracted from CCK[47]

The nonpeptidic antagonists provided a great hope to find the substitutes of peptidic analogues, with which there is always a problem of achieving good oral bioavailability. Benzodiazepine derivatives were widely investigated [48–55] among variety of nonpeptidic ligands studied. The benzodiazepine series of nonpeptide CCK receptor antagonists were designed from natural product asperlicin as shown in **Figure 2**, which have been well documented.[56]

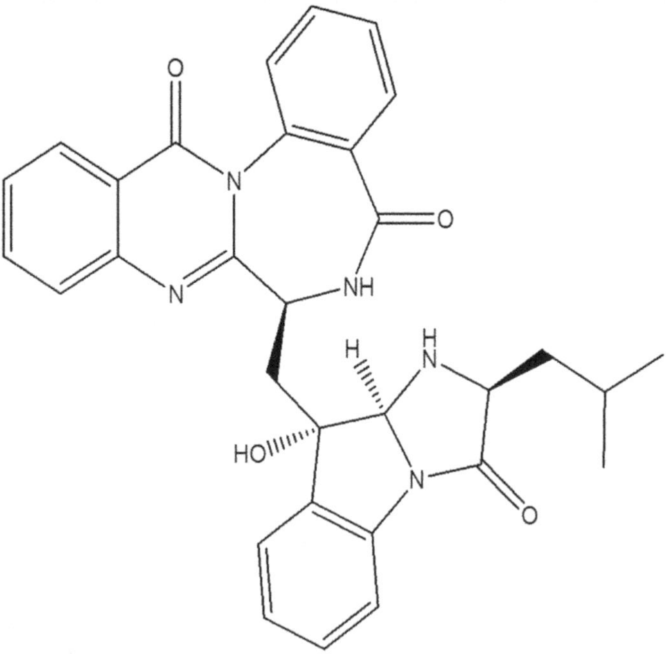

FIGURE 2 Asperlicin[57].

11.2 INTRODUCTION TO QSAR

11.2.1 QUANTITATIVE STRUCTURE–ACTIVITY RELATIONSHIP

QSAR represents a relation between the structure of chemical compounds and their specific empirical properties. QSAR helps to form a quantitative relationship between the chemistry (i.e., the structure) as well as biological effects (i.e., the activity) of each of the chemicals. A QSAR model is comprised of steps as shown in **Figure 3**[58].

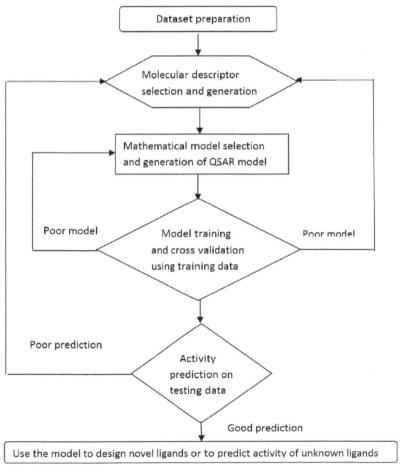

FIGURE 3 General scheme of QSAR model development including systematic training and testing processes[59].

11.2.2   NEED OF QSAR

QSAR is required to gain an insight into structural features of compounds related to different biological activities and at the same time, it also suggests some new substituents which help to enhance the activity. QSAR is used to attain a relationship between molecular structure, their chemistry, and biology. The purpose of these studies includes the following:

- Prediction of biological activities and physico-chemical properties.
- Helps to comprehend and rationalize different mechanisms of action within a series of compounds.
- Other than these aims, several other reasons to develop these models are the following:
- Helps to reduce cost of product development.
- Preprediction of activity may also reduce the requirement for expensive animal tests.
- Prediction of biological activities helps in reducing animal use and the discomfort caused to them.
- Also helps in promoting green chemistry[58].

11.2.3   BASIC REQUIREMENTS IN QSAR STUDIES

- Compounds belonging to a congeneric series
- Compounds having same mechanism of action
- Compounds binding in a comparable manner
- Isosteric replacement effects are predictable
- Binding affinity of compounds should be correlated to interaction energies
- Biological activities must be correlated to binding affinity

TABLE 1   Molecular Properties and Their Parameters[60]

Molecular Property	Corresponding Interaction	Parameters
Lipophilicity	Hydrophobic interactions	log P, π, f, RM, c
Polarizability	van der Waals interactions	MR, parachor, MV
Electron density	Ionic bonds, dipole–dipole interactions, hydrogen bonds, charge transfer interactions	s, R, F, k, quantum chemical indices
Topology	Steric hindrance geometric ft	Es, rv, L, B, distances, volumes

11.2.4 DETERMINATION OF QSAR MODEL

(a) Biological activity: A data set of a series of synthesized compounds which are also tested for its desired biological activity is required for QSAR analysis. Activity of all the chemicals selected must be studied by a common mechanism for a valid and reliable QSAR data. The quality of the model depends upon the quality of the data used for studying the models.

Biological activity can be of two types:

- Continuous response: MEC, IC50, ED50, % inhibition
- Categorical response: Active/inactive

(b) Molecular descriptors: They can be illustrated as a numerical representation of chemical information which is encoded within a molecular structure through a mathematical procedure.

(c) Variable selection methods: For developing a QSAR model, a large number of molecular descriptors are available. Among them an optimal subset of the descriptors are sorted out which plays an important role in determining the activity. The variable selection method is used and they are divided mainly into two categories:

- Systematic variable selection: This method helps to add/delete descriptor in steps one-by-one in a model.
- Stochastic variable selection: This method is based on simulation of various physical or biological processes. These methods aids in creating a model starting from randomly generated model(s) and then modifying these model(s) with the help of different process operator(s) (e.g., perturbation, crossover, etc.) to get an efficient model(s).

(d) Statistical methods: A variable selection method coupled with a suitable statistical method allows the data to be analyzed and establish a QSAR model with the descriptors' subset. They statistically help determining the biological activity of different chemical compounds.

(e) Selection of training and test set: QSAR models help to screen chemical databases and/or virtual chemical libraries to discover a bioactive molecule. These developments helps in emphasizing the importance of many model validations which ensures that the models have both the ability to describe the variance in the biological activity, that is, internal validation and also the acceptable predictive power, that is, external validation. Model validation can be done by dividing the dataset into test set (for examining its predictive ability) and training set (for building the QSAR model). The methods used for the division of the dataset into training and test set are as follows:

- Manual selection: The selection of the variation in the chemical and biological space of the given data set is done by visualizing.
- Random selection: Random distribution is used to create a training and
  test set.
- Sphere exclusion method: It is a rational method which ensures that the
  points in both sets are uniformly distributed with respect to chemical and
  biological space for creation of a training and test set.
- Others: Experimental design, onion design, cluster analysis, principal
  component analysis, self-organizing maps (SOM).

(f) Validate the equation: To evaluate the validity of any model by how well
it will predict data cross-validation technique is used by leave-one-out (LOO)
scheme analysis.

(g) Predict the biological activity: The biological activity of proposed compounds can be calculated by already developed QSAR models[61].

11.3   QSAR STUDIES OF 1,4 BENZODIAZEPINES AS CCKA ANTAGONIST

Here onward QSAR studies of CCK antagonist made by several other scientists
is discussed briefly, which includes the electronic descriptors and substitutions
required for synthesizing new and effective derivatives of CCK receptor antagonist.

Harikumar et al., (2013) proposed the molecular basis of drug action which
can facilitate development of some more potent and selective drugs. They
also explored the molecular basis of action of a small molecule ligand type 1
CCK receptor agonist and type 2 CCK receptor antagonists, GI181771X. They
characterized the binding and utilized the structurally related radio iodinated
ligands selective for CCK receptor subtypes. It was found that CCK utilizes
the same allosteric ligand-binding pocket and by using wild type receptors
and chimeric constructs exchanging the distinct residues lining this pocket.
Biological activity was evaluated using intracellular calcium assays. Molecular
models were developed using a ligand-guided refinement approach for docking
small molecule agonists to the type 1 CCK receptor. The optimal model was
mechanistically consistent with the current mutagenesis data and was distinct
from the previous antagonist model for the same receptor. Leu7.39 was predicted
to interact with the isopropyl group in the N1 position of the benzodiazepine that
acts as a "trigger" for biological activity[62].

Gupta et al., (2012) performed mapping of five chemo types of CCK-BR antagonist from the proposed test set to the selected pharmacophore. In search of
a reliable study for finding some essential structural requirements for CCK-2R

antagonism a quantitative pharmacophore model was developed using benzotri-azepine as CCK-2R antagonists and a training set of 34 substituted anthranilic sulfonamides. The best hypothesis consisted of five features, viz. one aromatic hydrophobic, two aliphatic hydrophobic, one H-bond acceptor, and one ring aromatic feature having excellent correlation for 34 training set (r^2 training = 0.83) and 58 test set compounds (r^2 test = 0.74). Further, 99% significance of this model was found to be in the F-randomization test. The model was also well observed and explained the CCK-2R antagonist activity. Thus, the developed pharmacophore model may not only be useful in finding new anthranilic sulfon-amides having better activity than the benzotriazepine class of CCK-2R antago-nists but may also help in design and develop new chemical entities (NCEs) as potent CCK-2R antagonists before their synthesis[63].

Kirandeep kaur *et al.,* (2008) reported a large number of CCK_2 antagonists playing an important role in nervous system related disorders, controlling gas-tric acid related conditions, and certain types of cancer. To obtain some helpful information for designing potent antagonists with novel structures and to inves-tigate the quantitative structure–activity relationship of a group of 62 different CCK_2 receptor antagonists with varying structures and potencies, comparative molecular field analysis (CoMFA), comparative molecular similarity indices analysis (CoMSIA), and hologram quantitative structure–toxicity relationships (HQSAR) studies were carried out on a series of 1,3,4-benzotriazepine-based CCK_2 receptor antagonists. By applying leave-one-out (LOO) cross-validation study QSAR models were derived from a training set of 49 compounds, cross-validated r^2_{cv} values of 0.673 and 0.608 and noncross-validated r^2_{ncv} values of 0.966 and 0.969 were obtained for the CoMFA and CoMSIA models, respective-ly. The predictive ability of the CoMFA and CoMSIA models were determined using a test set of 13 compounds, indicating a predictive correlation coefficients of 0.793 and 0.786, respectively. HQSAR was also carried out as a complemen-tary study, and the best HQSAR model was generated using atoms, bonds, hy-drogen atoms, and chirality as fragment distinction with fragment size (2–5) and six components showing r^2_{cv} and r^2_{ncv} values of 0.744 and 0.918, respectively. CoMFA steric and electrostatic, CoMSIA hydrophobic and hydrogen bond ac-ceptor fields, and HQSAR atomic contribution maps were used to analyze the structural features of the data sets that govern their antagonistic potency[64].

Irina G. (2007) proposed that computer-aided drug design has become an important part of G-protein-coupled receptors (GPCR) drug discovery process and that it aids in improving the efficiency of derivation and optimization of novel ligands. It also represents the combination of methods using structural information of a receptor-binding site of known ligands to design new ligands. In their report, they provide a brief description of ligand-binding sites in CCK and gastrin receptors (CCK1R and CCK2R) which were also delineated using experimental and computational methods, and they also explained the use of validated ligand binding sites to design and improve novel ligands[65]. The compounds are found in the hierarchy of most potent, least potent, and moderately potent among all.

Chopra and Mishra (2005) had presented a work showing how chemical features of a set of compounds along with their activities ranging over several orders of magnitudes can be used to generate pharmacophore hypotheses that can successfully predict activity. The models were also predictive with six different classes of diverse compounds and also effectively mapped onto most of the features important for activity. The pharmacophores generated from CCK-BR antagonists may be used as a three-dimensional (3D) query in database searches helps to identify compounds with diverse structures. They are potent antagonist of CCK-BR selectively and help to evaluate how well any newly designed compound maps on the pharmacophore before preceding any further study including synthesis.

Both these applications may help in identifying or designing compounds for further biological evaluation and optimization. The pharmacophore developed in this study using antagonists for CCK-BR showed distinct chemical features which are responsible for the activity of the antagonists. They also utilized the information to precede 3D searches on large databases of drug-like molecules to identify a new generation of cholecystokinin-B/gastrin receptors[66].

S. Tairi-Kellow *et al.,* (2001) proposed QSAR models which were obtained by using electronic descriptors, on a set of nonpeptidic antagonists acting on the peripheral and central receptors of CCK such as benzodiazepine in **Figure 4**. Structural elements which govern the antagonist activity are highlighted by these models. The particular important role of the substituent linked to the asymmetric carbon of the molecule was also revealed. To act as antagonist on CCK1 receptor, optimum electronic effect of this substituent must exist. A neutral electronic effect with a value close to zero for LUMO means no important charge transfer interaction in the binding site. On the other hand, in case of CCK2 receptor an attractor effect of this substituent is favorable for the antagonist activity. In other words, attractor electronic effect for the B group to confer good antagonist activity versus the CCK2 receptor was required.

The calculations further showed the importance of CCK2 antagonists like benzodiazepine systems, by suggesting the possible involvement of the van der Waals type of forces in ligands/receptor interactions. These studies revealed new perspectives in the interpretation of the selectivity of the molecule toward each receptor as well as provide a novel approach to synthesize a potent benzodiazepine antagonist against CCK1 and CCK2 receptors, based on the electronic properties of the substituent needed for increasing the antagonist activity. They also proposed a preferential conformation for each compound, as well as the docking calculations to validate their QSAR results and to elucidate the molecular interaction mechanism of ligand/receptor complexes[67].

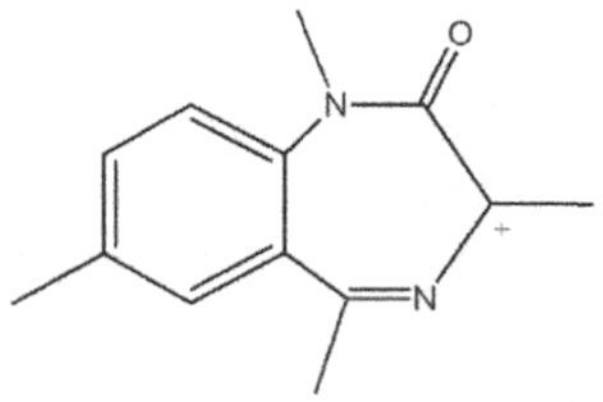

FIGURE 4   Basic moiety for substitution[67].

Ursini *et al.*, (2000) synthesized a series of 5-phenyl-3-ureidobenzodiazepine-2, 4-diones and evaluated it as cholecystokinin-B (CCK-B) receptor antagonists. SAR studies revealed the importance of the N-1 substituent for potent and selective CCK-B affinity. More potent compounds can be synthesized by addition of a urea side chain as substituent. By introduction of bulky substituent such as adamantly methyl at N-1 as well as resolution of racemic ureas may lead to formation of a lead compound GV150013[68].

J. Sinha *et al.*, (1999) suggested a QSAR model obtained from a series of 1,4-benzodiazepine derivatives as shown in **Figure 5**, which act as antagonists for CCK.They act on three different receptor subtypes termed as CCK-A, CCK-B, and gastrin receptor, located in brain, peripheral system, and stomach, respectively. The binding of the compounds found to be significantly dependent upon the lipophilicity of the compounds and their ability to form the hydrogen bonds with the receptor in case of all the three subtypes. However, the binding sites in CCK-A receptor is slightly rigid as compared to those in CCK-B or gastrin receptor and both are found to have similar binding features[51].

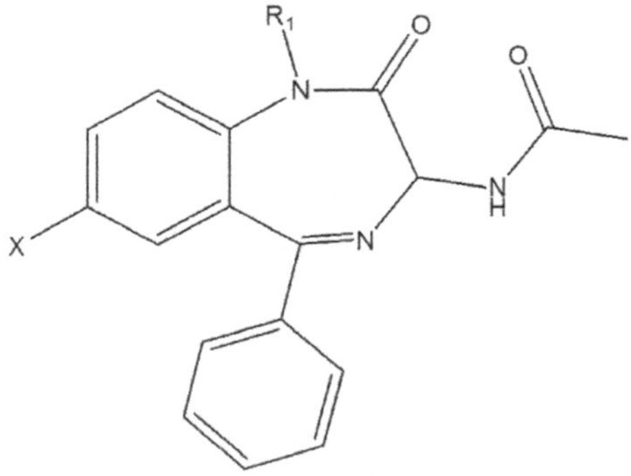

FIGURE 5   Benzodiazepine derivative[51].

Castro *et al.,* (1997) proposed the design, synthesis, and biological activity of a series of high-affinity, basic ligands for the CCK-B receptor. The compounds were found to incorporate a piperidin-2-yl or a homopiperidin-2-yl group, these groups are attached to C5 of a benzodiazepine core structure and are substantially more basic (e.g., 9 d, pKa=9.48) than any antagonists which was already reported based on 5-amino-1,4-benzodiazepines (e.g., 5, pKa=7.1) and have improved aqueous solubility. In respect of their basic nature, it can be suggested that binding of present series of compounds to the CCK-B receptor might be in their protonated form[69].

Cappelli *et al.,* (1996) proposes the synthesis of a series of tifluadom analogues which introduces a methylenic bridge between the 1,4-benzodiazepine nucleus and the (acylamino) methyl group of the parent compound. Close analogues of tifluadom which had the 2-thienyl, 2-fluorophenyl, 4-fluorophenyl, and 2-chlorophenyl substituent had maintained the affinity for the κ1-receptor. Derivatives of these compounds having substitution of chlorine atom at seventh position of the benzodiazepine ring responsible for a marked loss in activity. In this study all the compounds compared to tifluadom had lower affinity for the CCK receptors and so they exhibit a greater CCK-A/κ 1 selectivity ratio. This was particularly evident in compound 7a the 2-[(2-thienylcarbonyl) amino] ethyl derivative, which had a ratio of 60,000 compared to 60 for tifluadom. The newly synthesized ligands allowed us to rationalize quantitatively, with the help of molecular modeling, computational simulations, and correlation analysis, their structure–affinity features. The explained picture of the ligand–receptor interactions emerging from this approach constitutes an important working hypothesis. It will direct the design and synthesis of new congeneric ligands, which will be used to analyze the capability and the limitations of a model[70].

John S. Tokarski and Anton J. Hopfinger (1994) suggested a 3D molecular shape quantitative structure–activity relationship (3D-MSA-QSAR) technique. It has been applied to develop correlations between the calculated physico-chemical properties and the in vitro activities of a series of 3-(Acylamino)-5-phenyl-W-1,4-benzodiazepine shown in **Figure 6**. A varying subsets of 53 analogues were developed by (CCK-A) antagonists. The use of 3D-MSA-QSARs, loss in biological activity and loss in conformational stability principle aids in hypothesizing an active conformation for these compounds. After placing all compounds in the active conformation and performing pairwise molecular shape analysis, it was found that no analog serves as best shape reference compound. Different antagonists are mapped out by nonidentical volumes of allowed receptor space. The accessible receptor space was defined with the help of shape of a reference compound that consists of selected overlapped structures expands. The major factor which contributes to the affinity of this class of compounds, are molecular shape, as represented by common overlap steric volume and non-overlap steric volume. Intramolecular conformational stability, measured by the difference in the global minimum energy conformation, and energy of the active conformation plays an important role. It was concluded from the 3D-MSA-QSAR models that part of the binding pocket for the 3-amido substituent has a preference for lipophilicity. Two indicators variably marking the presence of an N-methyl group and an o-fluoro atom on the 5¢-phenyl substituent of the benzodiazepine ring structure also play a significant role in the 3D-MSAQSAR models. They also proposed a 3D pharmacophore model for the benzodiazepine CCK-A antagonists[71].

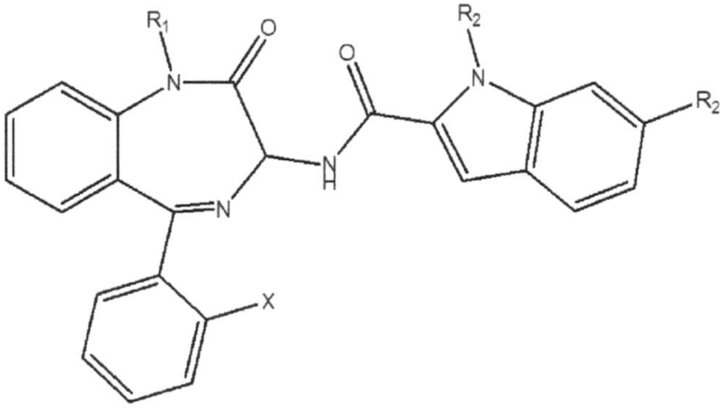

FIGURE 6 Pancreas receptor-binding affinities for 3-(acylamino) benzodiazepines[71].

Arie van der Bent *et al.*, (1992) derived a C_3-substituted benzodiazepines from asperlicin, for example, devazepide (L-364,718, MK-329), which constitute the most potent class of cholecystokinin A-type (CCK_A) receptor antagonists. To gain an insight into the prerequisites for binding, they had examined the conformational properties of both potent and weak moieties of this class with computer assisted molecular modeling (CAMM) techniques. The CAMM results help in determining the binding site for C_3-substituents having planar slot on the CCK_A receptor surface in addition, the proposal of a model also allows to explain the relative binding mode of the less potent R isomers versus S isomers. The latter model illustrates the unique spatial properties of the benzodiazepine moiety, by which they suggest an optimal arrangement of attached substituents[72].

11.4 CONCLUSIONS

This chapter includes a brief introduction about CCK and its antagonists having benzodiazepine moiety. QSAR studies reveal the role of a substituent linked to asymmetric carbon of the 1,4-benzodiazepine nucleus. This substituent shows an optimum electronic configuration, which must be neutral or polar to act as a CCK_A antagonist. This result opens new perspectives in the interaction of the selectivity of molecule toward CCK_A receptor and may provide a novel approach to synthesize potent CCK_A antagonist 1,4-benzodiazepines.

KEYWORDS

- **CCK**
- **Gastrin**
- **QSAR models**
- **Receptor**

REFERENCES

1. Mutt, V.; Jorpes, J.E. *Structure of porcine cholecystokinin-pancreozymin. Cleavage with thrombin and with trypsin. Eur.* J. Biochem. 1968, 6, 156–162.
2. Tsunoda, Y.; Owyang, C. High-affinity CCK receptors are coupled to phospholipase A_2 *pathways to mediate pancreatic amylase secretion. Am J Physiol. Gastrointest. Liver Physiol.* 1995, 269, G435–G444.
3. Gregory, R.A.; Tracy, H.J. The constitution and properties of two gastrins extracted from hog antral mucosa. Gut. 1964, 5, 103–117.
4. McGuigan, J.L. Gastrin mucosal intracellular localization by immunofluorescence. Gastroenterology. 1968, 55, 315–327
5. Deschenes, R.J.; Lorenz, L.J.; Haun, R.S.; Roos, B.A.; Collier, K.J.; Dixon. J.E. Cloning and sequence analysis of a cDNA encoding rat precholecystokinin. Proc. Natl. Acad. Sci. USA. 1984, 81,726–730.
6. Vanderhaeghen, J.J.; Signeau, J.C.; Gepts, W. New peptide in the vertebrate CNS reacting with antigastrin antibodies. Nature.1975, 257, 604–605.
7. Dockray, G.J. *Immunochemical evidence of cholecystokinin-like peptides in brain. Nature. 1976, 264, 568–570.*
8. Rehfeld, J.F. *The new biology of gastrointestinal hormones. Physiol.* Rev. 1998, 78, 1087–1108.
9. Roettger, B.F.; Ghanekar, D.; Rao, R.; Toledo, C.; Yingling, J.; Pinon, D.; and Miller, L.J. *Antagonist-stimulated internalization of the G protein-coupled cholecystokinin receptor. Mol.* Pharmacol. 1997, 51, 357–362.
10. Larsson, L.I; Rehfeld, J.F. *Localization and molecular heterogeneity of cholecystokinin in the central and peripheral nervous system.* Brain Res.1979, 165, 201–218.
11 Rehfeld, J.F. *How to measure cholecystokinin in tissue, plasma and cerebrospinal fluid. Regul.* Pept. 1998, 78, 31–39.
12. Rehfeld, J.F. *The new biology of gastrointestinal hormones. Physiol.* Rev. 1998, 78, 1087–1108.
13. Lund, T.; Geurts van Kessel, A.H.M.; Haun, R.S.; Dixon, J.E. The genes for human gastrin and cholecystokinin are located on different chromosomes. Hum. Genet. 1986, 73, 77–80.

14. Dockray, G.J.; Varro, A.; Dimaline, R.; Wang, T. *The gastrins: their production and biological activities. Annu.* Rev. Physiol. 2001, 63, 119–139.

15. Rehfeld.J.F, Larsson.L.I, Goltermann.N.R, Schwartz.T.W, Holst.J.J, Jensen.S.L, and Morley.J.S. *"Neural regulation of pancreatic hormone secretion by the C-terminal tetrapeptide of CCK". Nature. 1980; 284: 33–38.*

16. Takano, H.; Imaeda, K.; Koshita, M.; Xue, L.; Nakamura, H.; Kawase, Y.; Hori, S.; Ishigami, T.; Kurono, Y.; Suzuki, H. *Alteration of the properties of gastric smooth muscle in the genetically hyperglycemic OLETF rat. J.* Auton. Nerv. Syst. 1998, 70, 180–188.

17. Williams, J.A. *Intracellular signaling mechanisms activated by cholecystokinin-regulating synthesis and secretion of digestive enzymes in pancreatic acinar cells Annu.* Rev. Physiol. 2001, 63, 77–97.

18. Gregory, R.A.; *Tracy, H.J. The constitution and properties of two gastrins extracted from hog antral mucosa Gut. 1964, 46, 103–114.*

19. Gregory, R.A; Tracy, H.J.A note on the nature of the gastrin-like stimulant present in Zollinger-Ellison tumour Gut. 1964, 46, 115–117.

20. Fukazawa, Y.; Maeda, T.; Kiguchi, N.; Tohya, K.; Kimura, M.; Kishioka, S. Activation of spinal cholecystokinin and neurokinin-1 receptors is associated with the attenuation of intrathecal morphine analgesia following electroacupuncture stimulation in rats. J. Pharmacol. Sci. 2007, 104 (2), 159–66.

21. Bradwejn, J. Neurobiological investigations into the role of cholecystokinin in panic disorder. *J. Psych. Neurosci.* 1993, 18,.178–88.

22. Bradwejn, J.; Koszycki, D. The cholecystokinin hypothesis of anxiety and panic disorder. *Ann. N Y Acad. Sci.* 1994, 713, 273–82.

23. Bradwejn, J.; Koszycki, D.; Meterissian, G. Cholecystokinin-tetrapeptide induces panic attacks in patients with panic disorder. *Can. J. Psychiatry.*1990, 35, 835.

24. Bourin, M.; Malinge, M.; Vasar, E.; Bradwejn, J. Two faces of cholecystokinin: anxiety and schizophrenia. *Fundam. Clin. Pharmacol.* 1996,10,116–26.

25. Beinfeld, M.C.; Garver, D.L. Concentration of cholecystokinin in cerebrospinal fluid is decreased in psychosis: relationship to symptoms and drug response. *Prog. Neuro. Psychopharmacol. Biol. Psychiatry.*1991, 15, 601–609.

26. Ferrier, I.N.; Roberts, G.W.; Crow, T.J.; Johnstone, E.C.; Owens, D.G.C.; Lee, Y.C.; *et al.,* Reduced cholecystokinin-like and somatostatin-like immunoreactivity in limbic lobe associated with negative symptoms in schizophrenia. *Life Sci.* 1983,.33, 475–482.

27. Garver, D.L.; Beinfeld, M.C.; Yao, J.K. Cholecystokinin, dopamine and schizophrenia *Psychopharmacol Bull.* 1990, 26, 377–380.

28. Nair, N.P.V.; Lal, S.; Bloom, D.M. Cholecystokinin peptides, dopamine and schizophrenia — a review. *Prog. Neuropsychopharmacol. Biol. Psychiatry.*1985, 9, 515–524.

29. Wang, R.Y. Cholecystokinin, dopamine, and schizophrenia: recent progress and current problems. *Ann. N Y Acad. Sci.*1988, 537, 362–379.

30. Vaccarino, F.J. *Cholecystokinin and anxiety: from neuron to behavior.* Austin. 1995, 127–142.

31. Higgins, G.A.; Sills, T.L.; Tomkins, D.M.; Sellers, E.M.; Vaccarino, F.J. Evidence for the contribution of CCKB receptor mechanisms to individual differences in amphetamine-induced locomotion. *Pharmacol. Biochem. Behav.* 1994, 48, 1019–1024.

32. Crespi, F. The role of cholecystokinin (CCK), CCK-A or CCK-B receptor antagonists in the spontaneous preference for drugs of abuse (alcohol or cocaine) in naive rats. *Methods Find Exp. Clin. Pharmacol.* 1998, 20, 679–697.

33. Crespi, F.; Corsi, M.; Reggiani, A.; Ratti, E.; Gaviraghi, G. Involvement of cholecystokinin within craving for cocaine: role of cholecystokinin receptor ligands. *Expert. Opin. Investig. Drugs.* 2000, 9, 2249–2258.

34. Vaccarino, F.J.; Rankin, J. Nucleus accumbens cholecystokinin (CCK) can either attenuate or potentiate amphetamine-induced locomotor activity: evidence for rostral-caudal differences in accumbens CCK function. *Behav Neurosci.* 1989, 103, 831–836.
35. Wunderlich, G.R.; DeSousa, N.J.; Vaccarino, F.J. Cholecystokinin modulates both the development and the expression of behavioral sensitization to amphetamine in the rat. *Psychopharmacology.* 2000, 151, 283–290.
36. Beinfeld, M.C.; Palkovits, M. Distribution of cholecystokinin (CCK) in the rat lower brain stem nuclei. *Brain Res.* 1982, 238, 260–265.
37. Beinfeld, M.C.; Meyer, D.K.; Eskay, R.L.; Jensen, R.T.; Brownstein, M.J. The distribution of cholecystokinin immunoreactivity in the central nervous system of the rat as determined by radioimmunoassay. *Brain Res.*1981, 212, 517.
38. Fink, H.; Rex, A.; Voits, M.; Voigt, J.P. Major biological actions of CCK — a critical evaluation of research findings. *Exp. Brain Res.* 1998, 123, 77–83.
39. Shian, L.R.; Lin, M.T. Effects of cholecystokinin octapeptide on thermoregulatory responses and hypothalamic neuronal activity in the rat *NaunynSchmiedebergs. Arch. Pharmacol.* 1985, 328, 363–367.
40. Szelenyi, Z. Cholecystokinin and thermoregulation — a mini reviews. *Peptides.* 2001, 22, 1245–1250.
41. Dornan, W.A.; Bloch, G.J.; Priest, C.A.; Micevych, P.E. Microinjection of cholecystokinin into the medial preoptic nucleus facilitates lordosis behavior in the female rat. *Physiol. Behav.*1989, 45, 969–974.
42. Beinfeld, M.C. An introduction to neuronal cholecystokinin. *Peptides.* 2001, 22, 1197–1200.
43. VanMegen, H.J.; Westenberg, H.G.; den Boer, J.A.; Kahn, R.S. Cholecystokinin in anxiety. *Eur. Neuropsychopharmacol.* 1996, 6, 263–280.
44. Huston, J.P.; Schildein, S.; Gerhardt, P.; Privou, C.; Fink, H.; Hasenohrl, R.U. Modulation of memory, reinforcement and anxiety parameters by intra-amygdala injection of cholecystokinin-fragments BOC-CCK-4 and CCK-8S. *Peptides.* 1998, 19, 27–37.
45. Vaccarino, F.J. Nucleus accumbens dopamine–CCK interactions in psychostimulant reward and related behaviors. *Neurosci. Biobehav. Rev.* 1994, 18, 207–214.
46. Harikumar, K.G.; Clain, J.; Pinon, D.I.; Dong, M.; Miller, L.J. Distinct molecular mechanisms for agonist peptide binding to types A and B cholecystokinin receptors demonstrated using fluorescence spectroscopy. J. Biol. Chem. 2005, 280 (2), 1044–1050.
47. Evans, B.E.; Bock, M.G.; Rittle, K.E.; Di Pardo, R.M.; Whitter, W.L.; Veber, D.R.; Anderson, P.S. ; Freidinger, R.M. Design of potent, orally effective, nonpeptidal antagonists of the peptide hormone cholecystokinin. Design of potent, orally effective, nonpeptidal antagonists of the peptide hormone cholecystokinin Design of potent, orally effective, nonpeptidal antagonists of the peptide hormone cholecystokinin. Proc. Natl. Acad. Sci. 1986, 83, 4918.
48. Chang, R.S.L.; Lotti, V.J. Biochemical and pharmacological characterization of an extremely potent and selective nonpeptide antagonist. Proc. Natl. Acad. Sci. USA 1986, 83, 4923.
49. Semple, G.; Ryder, H.; Kendrick, D.A.; Szelke, M.; Ohta, M.; Satoh, M. A.; Muzawa, Nishida, S.; Miyata, K. Bioorg. Med. Chem. 1996, 6, 51.
50. Semple, G.; Ryder, H.; Kendrick, D.A.; Szelke, M.; Ohta, M.; Satoh, M. A.; Muzawa, Nishida, S.; Miyata, K. Bioorg. Med. Chem. 1996, 6, 55.
51. Sinha, J.; Kurup, A.; Paleti, A.; Gupta, S.P. Quantitative structure–activity relationship study on some nonpeptidal cholecystokinin antagonists. Bioorg. Med. Chem. 1999, 7(6), 1127–1130.
52. Huche, M.; Legendre, J.L. Quant. Struct.-Act. Relat. 1997,16,435.
53. Gupta,S.P.; Mulchadani, V.; Das, S.; Subbiah, A.; Reddy,D.N.; Sinha, J. A quantitative structure-activity relationship study on some cholecystokinin antagonists Quant. Struct.-Act. Relat. 1995, 14, 437.

54. Tokarsky, J.S.; Hopfinger, A.J. Three-dimensional molecular shape analysis: quantitative structure activity relationship of a series of cholecystokinin A receptor antagonists. J. Med. chem. 1994, 37, 3639.
55. Chang, R.S.L.; Lotti,V.J.; Monoghan, R.L.; Birnbaum, J.; Stapley, E.O.; Goetz, J M.A..M. Liesch, O.D. Hensens, J.P. A potent nonpeptide cholecystokinin antagonist selective for peripheral tissues isolated from Aspergillus alliaceus Science 1985, 230, 177.
56. Kubota, K.; Sugaya, K.; Matsuda, I.; Matsuoka, Y.; Terawaki, Y. Reversal of antinociceptive effect of cholecystokinin by benzodiazepines and a benzodiazepine antagonist. J. Pharmacol. 1985, 37, 101–105.
57. Stuart W. H.; Xue G.; Yi T.; Christopher T. W. Assembly of asperlicin peptidyl alkaloids from anthranilate and tryptophan: a two-enzyme pathway generates heptacyclic scaffold complexity in asperlicin E. J. Am. Chem. Soc. 2012, 134, 17444–17447.
58. Puzyn T. et al., Challenges and advances in computational chemistry and physics. Recent Advances in QSAR Studies, 2010, 3–11.
59. Myint K.Z.; Xie X. Recent advances in fragment-based QSAR and multi-dimensional QSAR methods Int. J. Mol. Sci. 2010, 11, 3846–3866.
60. Hugo Kubinyi, www.kubinyi.de
http://shodhganga.inflibnet.ac.in/bitstream/10603/6502/11/11_chapter%206.pdf
61. Harikumar et al., Molecular basis for benzodiazepine agonist action at the type 1 cholecystokinin receptor. J. Biol. Chem., 2013, 2–26.
62. Gupta A. K. et al., Toward the identification of a reliable 3D QSAR pharmacophore model for the CCK2 receptor antagonism J. Chem. Inf. Model. 2012, 52 (5), 1376–1390.
63. Kaur Kirandeep et al., 3D QSAR studies of 1,3,4-benzotriazepine derivatives as CCK$_2$ receptor antagonists. J. Mol. Graph. Model. 2008, 27(4), 409–420.
64. Irina, G. et al., Validated ligand binding sites in CCK receptors. Next step: computer-aided design of novel CCK ligands. Curr. Top. Med. Chem. 2007, 7(12), 1243–1247.
65. Chopra, M.; Mishra A.K. Ligand-based molecular modeling study on a chemically diverse series of cholecystokinin-B/gastrin receptor antagonists: generation of predictive model. J. Chem. Inf. Model. 2005, 45 (6), 1934–1942.
66. Kellow, S.T. et al., Electronic descriptors of 1,4 Benzodiazepine derivative related to the antagonist acivity of cholecystokinin receptors. J. Mol. Struct. 2001, 571, 207–223.
67. Ursini, et al., Synthesis/SAR of 5-Phenyl-3-ureido-1,5-benzodiazepines. J. Med. Chem. 2000, 43, 20.
68. Castro, J.L. et al., 5-(Piperidin-2-yl)- and 5-(Homopiperidin-2-yl)-1,4-benzodiazepines: high-affinity, basic ligands for the cholecystokinin-B receptor. J. Med. Chem., 1997, 40 (16), 2491–2501.
69. Cappelli, A.; Anzini, M.; Vomero, S.; Menziani, M.C.; De Benedetti, P.G.; Sbacchi, M.; Clarke, G.D.; Mennuni, L. Synthesis, biological evaluation, and quantitative receptor docking simulations of 2-[(acylamino) ethyl]-1, 4-benzodiazepines as novel tifluadom-like ligands with high affinity and selectivity for kappa-opioid receptors. J. Med. Chem. 1996, 39(4), 860–872.
70. Tokarski, and Hopfinger. 3D-MSA-QSAR of cholecystokinin-A receptor antagonists. J. Med. Chem. 1994, 37, 21.
71. Bent, A.V.; Laak, A.M.T,; Uzerman, A.P.; Soudijin, W. Molecular modelling of asperlicin derived cholecystokinin A receptor antagonists. Eur. J. Pharmacol.: Mol. Pharmacol. 1992, 226(4), 327–334.

CHAPTER 12

DOCKING BASED SCORING PARAMETERS BASED QSAR MODELING ON A DATA SET OF BISPHENYLBENZIMIDAZOLE AS NON-NUCLEOSIDE REVERSE TRANSCRIPTASE INHIBITOR

SURENDRA KUMAR[1] and MEENA TIWARI[1]*

[1]Computer-Aided Drug Design Lab, Department of Pharmacy, Shri Govindram Seksaria Institute of Technology and Science, Indore-452003, India

*Corresponding author: E-mail: mtiwari@sgsits.ac.in; Tel.: +91-9425437039

CONTENTS

ABSTRACT

A newly designed novel approach of docking based scoring parameters based quantitative structure–activity relationship (QSAR) model was developed on a 37 compounds of bisphenylbenzimidazole analogues. The molecular docking simulation was carried out by GLIDE, GOLD, and AutoDock Vina docking programs. All the calculated docking-based scoring parameters were considered in QSAR model development using linear and nonlinear approaches. The linear approach (simulated-annealing) based QSAR model showed better robustness with cross-validated Q^2 of 0.728 and r^2_{pred} of 0.634 over nonlinear approach based QSAR model (Q^2 of 0.697 and r^2_{pred} of 0.603). The developed robust model and approach could be further used as a virtual screening tool to find novel hits for the chosen target. The docking based scoring parameters based QSAR study suggested the importance of hydrophobic substituents, surface area, volume, and flexibility of the ligands. It was also inferred from the present study, that non-nucleoside reverse transcriptase inhibitors should obtain their characteristic butterfly-like orientation for better interaction in the binding pocket of non-nucleoside reverse transcriptase enzyme.

12.1   INTRODUCTION

Acquired immunodeficiency syndrome (AIDS), a degenerative disease of the immune system, caused by the human immunodeficiency virus (HIV) is the fourth leading cause of mortality globally. It is estimated that HIV has infected over 60 million people worldwide. According to the reports of the Joint United Nations Program on HIV/AIDS (UNAIDS), about 2.5 million people became newly infected with HIV in 2011 and an estimate of 34 million peoples were ailing with HIV/AIDS. In 2011, 1.7 million people died from AIDS-related illnesses.[1] There are two species of HIV which infect humans: HIV-1 and HIV-2. HIV-1 is more virulent, easily transmitted, and cause of the majority of HIV infections.[2] HIV-1 displays selective tropism for mature human helper T-lymphocytes, which express the CD4 surface protein.[3]

The investigation of molecular events, critical for HIV-1 replication cycle, identified a number of important biochemical targets for AIDS chemotherapy. HIV-1 entry is mediated by an interaction between CD4 and members of the chemokine receptors.[4, 5] HIV-1 cell entry inhibitors include a chemokine-receptor inhibitor, a CD4-receptor inhibitor, and a membrane-fusion inhibitor. After fusion, HIV-1 releases copies of RNA genome into the cytoplasm and viral reverse transcriptase (RT) enzyme transcribes single-stranded viral RNA into double-stranded DNA that can be integrated into the host genome. The viral integrase enzyme is required for the integration of proviral DNA into the host genome before replication. When the infected cell synthesizes new protein, integrated proviral DNA is also translated into the protein building blocks of new viral progeny. The viral components then assemble on the cell surface and bud out as immature viral particles. The final maturation of newly formed viruses requires the HIV-1 protease to constitute an infectious virion.[6] Thus the inhibition of key enzymes, HIV-1 RT and HIV-1 protease, renders the most attractive targets for the anti-HIV drug development.

RT is a key enzyme, within the HIV-1 virion capsid, which represents an attractive target to inhibit the HIV-1 proliferation for several reasons: (i) it is a crucial enzyme in the viral replication cycle; (ii) its properties are quite different from those of the other cellular DNA polymerases; and (iii) it is active in the cytoplasmic compartment of the infected cell.[7] The inhibitors of RT enzyme are broadly classified into nucleoside and non-nucleoside RT inhibitors. Nucleoside reverse transcriptase inhibitors (NRTIs), act as chain terminators to block the elongation of the HIV-1 viral DNA strand, whereas non-nucleoside reverse transcriptase inhibitors (NNRTIs), a group of structurally diverse compounds, directly inhibit RT enzyme by binding to the allosteric site, that is close to, but distinct from the polymerase active site.[8, 9]

Several studies reported that, in the absence of NNRTI, the non-nucleoside binding pocket does not exist. It is only during the binding of an inhibitor that the aromatic residues Tyr181, Tyr188, and Trp229 reorient to create a hydrophobic pocket of sufficient volume to accommodate the inhibitor. By binding to this allosteric site, the NNRTI increases the distance between the nucleic acid primer grip and dNTP binding site in RT, suggesting this as a possible mechanism for inhibition of polymerase activity.[10] The structural features that seem important for NNRTI binding, include the presence of planar π-electron systems and ability of these systems to adopt a conformation designated as "butterfly-like" orientation.[11] Despite these general features, the structures of different NNRTIs bound to RT vary considerably. This complexity arises from the ability of side chain residues surrounding the pocket to adapt to each bound NNRTI in a highly specific manner, closing down around the surface of the drug to make tight van der Waals contacts. Because of this unique binding, NNRTIs do not inhibit other polymerases (not even HIV-2 RT) and are thus potentially highly effective and nontoxic drugs.[12]

The replication of HIV-1 in infected patients can be reduced considerably by highly active antiretroviral therapy (HAART), a highly active combination of drugs with multiple targets.[13, 14] A multiple-drug treatment approach avoids or delays emergence of resistant viral strains and contributed to declining morbidity and mortality among HIV-infected patients. However, certain factors restrict the selection of agents for combination therapy, including drug compatibilities, adverse effects, and cross-resistance.[15] Therefore, the development of selective, potent, safe, inexpensive NNRTIs that are also effective against mutant HIV strains, remains a worthwhile goal.

In the search of potent non-nucleoside RT inhibitors that are effective against the wild type (WT) viruses, Chimirri et al.,[16, 17] discovered 1-(2,6-difluorophenyl)-1H,3H-thiazolo[3,4-a]benzimidazole (TZB). Later, el Dareer et al.,[18] reported that the therapeutic potential of TZB was hampered by a number of factors, like (1) metabolic oxidation of thiazolo ring leading to the formation of less potent sulfoxides and sulfones metabolites and (2) development of resistance in NNRTI treatment. In order to improve the RT inhibitory activity of TZB, a retrosynthetic analysis of TZB by opening of the thiazole ring, as illustrated in **Figure 1.1**, leads to N-benzyl-2alkylbenzimidazoles. Similar to TZB, N-benzyl-2-alkylbenzimidazoles consisted of two aromatic ring systems that can form a "butterfly-like" conformation critical for binding to the non-nucleoside inhibitor binding pocket (NNIBP).

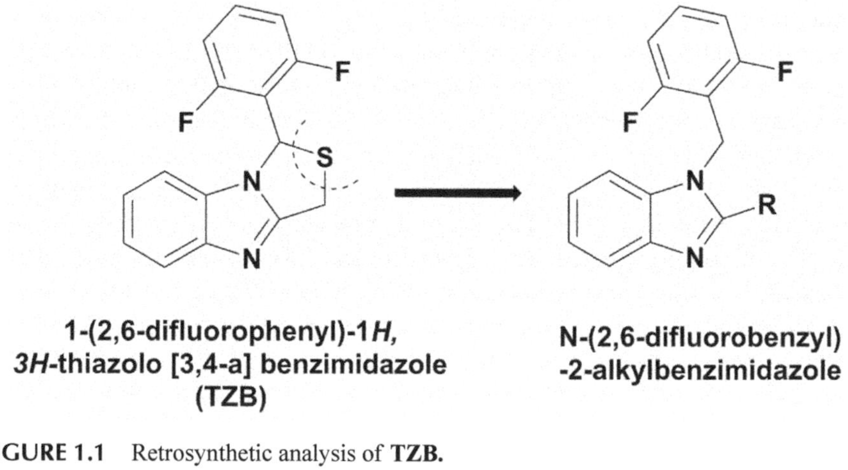

1-(2,6-difluorophenyl)-1H, 3H-thiazolo [3,4-a] benzimidazole (TZB)   **N-(2,6-difluorobenzyl) -2-alkylbenzimidazole**

FIGURE 1.1   Retrosynthetic analysis of **TZB.**

A number of in silico methodologies were developed for the quantitative prediction of the affinity of small molecules to facilitate the process of drug discovery and development and one of them is ligand-based QSAR techniques, which have been applied for many years to rationalize the structure–activity relationships of targets and their inhibitors with an aim to generate models, that can quantitatively predict the activity of new analogues.[19–21] Conversely, structure-based methodologies are based on the prediction of free energy of binding from the receptor–ligand complexes.[22–23] However, these methods for prediction of receptor–ligand affinity are either computationally expensive, for high-throughput virtual screening purposes, or unable to correctly rank the docked compounds according to their experimental activity to yield meaningful affinity rankings. However, these methods have a sufficient level of accuracy to discriminate between binders and nonbinders. Therefore, the combination of methodologies of molecular docking and QSAR might contribute to the construction of robust consensual models and facilitate their application in search of novel and structurally diverse lead compounds by means of virtual screening techniques.

Since a number of computational approaches, viz. QSAR, molecular docking, and free energy perturbations, were applied on the bisphenylbenzimidazole analogues (BPBIs) to rationalize the structural requirement for inhibitory activity or to predict the binding affinity.[19, 24, 25] In this chapter, we have combined both the approaches of drug discovery, viz. QSAR and molecular docking together to find the target inhibitors; originating a novel approach of QSAR, which is based on docking based scoring parameters. The docking based scoring numerical values can be used to estimate the affinity of a compound relative to others. So, if a set of ligands with their experimental activity is available, this can be used as a training set in order to develop a QSAR model, that can correlate docking scores values with the experimental activity through linear or nonlinear regression analysis. Then, the activity of a new ligand can be deduced on the basis of the calculated relationship between docking scores and experimental activity values.

12.2 MATERIALS AND METHODS

12.2.1 DATA SET AND BIOLOGICAL DATA

The data set used in this study was taken from the literature[24–27] comprising of thirty seven 1-(2,6-difluorobenzyl)-2-(2,6-difluorophenyl) benzimidazole (BPBIs) derivatives with RT enzyme inhibition activity (**Table 1**). The EC_{50} value was converted to pEC_{50} by taking the negative logarithm to base 10 of EC_{50} (pEC_{50}). The whole data set has wide distribution of activity (pEC_{50}), which ranged from 4.500 to 7.398 with a mean of 6.135 and a variance of 0.611.

TABLE 1 Structure and activity (pEC$_{50}$) of the BPBI derivatives

S. No	R$_1$	R$_2$	R$_3$	Experimental Activity	
				EC$_{50}$ (μM)	pEC$_{50}$(M)
1	2,6-F$_2$Bn	Ph	H	6.06	5.218
2	2,6-F$_2$Bn	2,6-F$_2$Ph	H	1.70	5.770
3	2,6-F$_2$Bn	2,6-F$_2$Ph	4-CH$_3$	0.44	6.357
4	2,6-F$_2$Bn	4-Py	4-CH$_3$	3.50	5.456
5	2,6-F$_2$Bn	3-Py	4-CH$_3$	31.6	4.500
6	Bn	2,6-F$_2$Ph	4-CH$_3$	0.75	6.125
7	2,6-Cl$_2$Bn	2,6-F$_2$Ph	4-CH$_3$	3.16	5.500
8	2-FBn	2-FPh	H	2.62	5.582
9	2,6-F$_2$Bn	2,6-F$_2$Ph	6-CH$_3$	4.89	5.311
10	2,6-F$_2$Bn	2,6-F$_2$Ph	5-CH$_3$	7.35	5.134
11	2,6-F$_2$Bn	2,6-F$_2$Ph	5-(2,6-F$_2$Bn), 6-OCH$_3$	31.22	4.506
12	2,6-F$_2$Bn	2,6-F$_2$Ph	4-OCH$_3$	0.08	7.097
13	2,6-F$_2$Bn	2,6-F$_2$Ph	4-Cl	0.40	6.398
14	2,6-F$_2$Bn	2,6-F$_2$Ph	4-NHCH$_3$	2.40	5.620
15	2,6-F$_2$Bn	2,6-F$_2$Ph	4-NO$_2$	0.45	6.347
16	2,6-F$_2$Bn	2,6-F$_2$Ph	4-NH$_2$	0.53	6.276
17	2,6-F$_2$Bn	2-OCH$_3$,5-F-Ph	4-NH$_2$	2.71	5.567
18	2,6-F$_2$Bn	2,6-F$_2$Ph	4-CH$_2$OH	0.05	7.301
19	2,6-F$_2$Bn	2,6-F$_2$Ph	4-CH$_2$Cl	0.16	6.796
20	2,6-F$_2$Bn	2,6-F$_2$Ph	4-CH$_2$NH$_2$	1.36	5.867
21	2,6-F$_2$Bn	2,6-F$_2$Ph	4-CH$_2$CH$_3$	0.82	6.086
22	2,6-F$_2$Bn	2,6-F$_2$Ph	4-C(O)NH$_2$	0.37	6.432
23	2,6-F$_2$Bn	2,6-F$_2$Ph	4-CH$_2$OC(O)CH$_3$	0.06	7.222
24	2,6-F$_2$Bn	2,6-F$_2$Ph	4-C(O)H	0.10	7.000
25	2,6-F$_2$Bn	2,6-F$_2$Ph	4-NHC(O)CH$_3$	1.65	5.783
26	2,6-F$_2$Bn	2,6-F$_2$Ph	4-N(CH$_3$)C(O)CH$_3$	0.04	7.398

(*Continued*)

27	2,6-F$_2$Bn	2,6-F$_2$Ph	4-Br	0.37	6.432
28	2,6-F$_2$Bn	2,6-F$_2$Ph	4-OH	0.65	6.187
29	2,6-F$_2$Bn	2,6-F$_2$Ph	4-N(CH$_3$)	2.37	5.625
30	2,6-F$_2$Bn	2,6-F$_2$Ph	4-CN	0.43	6.367
31	2,6-F$_2$Bn	2,6-F$_2$Ph	4-CNH(NHOH)	0.19	6.721
32	2,6-F$_2$Bn	2,6-F$_2$Ph	4-Isopropyl	6.34	5.198
33	2,6-F$_2$Bn	2,6-F$_2$Ph	4-Isoprenyl	1.44	5.842
34	2,6-F$_2$Bn	2,6-F$_2$Ph	4-CH$_2$N$_3$	0.045	7.347
35	2,6-F$_2$Bn	2,6-F$_2$Ph	4-CH$_2$NCH$_3$C(O)CH$_3$	0.58	6.237
36	2,6-F$_2$Bn	2,6-F$_2$Ph	4-CH$_2$OCH$_3$	0.06	7.222
37	2,6-F$_2$Bn	2,6-F$_2$Ph	4-CH$_2$CN	0.06	7.222

†Experimental EC$_{50}$ values (μM) were converted into pEC$_{50}$ (M); *Test Set compounds; Exp. Act.: Experimental Activity

12.2.2 LIGAND PREPARATION

All the structures of data set were built using the builder tool of Maestro v9.3[28] and a multistep minimization protocol was performed using the OPLS_AA force-field, which includes Steepest descent, Polak-Ribiere Conjugate Gradient followed by default settings of LigPrep v2.5[29], to obtain the low energy minimized structure. The LigPrep produces a single low energy 3D structure with correct chiralities for each input structure and can also produce a number of structures from each input structure with various ionization states, tautomers, stereochemistry, and ring conformations. The obtained energy minimized 3D structures were further used for generation of conformers using default parameters of mixed torsional/low-mode sampling function.[30] The conformers were filtered with a maximum relative energy difference of 5 kcal/mol to exclude redundant conformers.

12.2.3 PROTEIN PREPARATION

The HIV-1 RT enzyme in complex with THR-50 (PDB ID: 2B6A) was selected for the molecular docking study.[31] To prepare the protein for docking simulation, the respective protein file with a resolution of 2.65 Å was downloaded and imported into workspace of Maestro v9.3 and the protein preparation wizard was started. The protein structure was prepared by following these steps: (1) All the hydrogens were added; (2) bond orders were corrected; (3) All the water molecules were removed; (4) Missing side chains and loops were added, using the prime module of maestro v9.3; (5) H-bonding network and orientation of Asn, Gln, and His residues were optimized, and (6) finally the entire complex was minimized using *Impref* and the minimization terminated when the root mean square deviation (RMSD) of the heavy atoms in the minimized structure relative to the X-ray structure exceeded 0.3 Å. This helps in maintaining the integrity of the prepared structures relative to the corresponding experimental structures, while eliminating severe bad contacts between heavy atoms.[32]

12.2.4   MOLECULAR DOCKING

The energy minimized low energy conformers of the data set were selected for docking into the binding pocket of the non-nucleoside RT enzyme with three different kinds of docking programs, viz. AutoDock Vina[33], GOLD[34], and GLIDE[35, 36] for comparison and selection of various different docking based scoring parameters.

12.2.4.1   VALIDATION OF THE DOCKING PROGRAM

Before docking of the data set compounds, the selected docking program parameters were validated by following the redocking approach. In this approach, the bound co-crystallized ligand was extracted and docked back into the binding pocket of the enzyme. The docking program should reproduce the orientation and position of inhibitor as observed in the crystal structure. The selection of the target protein was based on considering the fact that the bound co-crystallized ligand (T50_561), was structurally similar to the selected data set compounds. The redocking approach was performed by extracting the bound ligand T50_561, from the protein and docking back into the corresponding binding pocket to determine the ability of all the three docking program parameters to reproduce the orientation and position of the inhibitor as observed in the crystal structure. After the validation of the docking program, all the data set compounds of BPBIs were docked in to the non-nucleoside binding pocket using all the three docking programs.

12.2.4.2   MOLECULAR DOCKING OF BPBI DERIVATIVES INTO THE

NON-NUCLEOSIDE BINDING POCKET USING AUTODOCK VINA

AutoDock Vina, has improved accuracy of binding mode prediction over Autodock 4. Therefore, Autodock Vina was used for the docking of data set compounds. The input ligands and protein were prepared seperatly by, adding hydrogen atoms, assigning Gasteiger Huckel charges on the ligands, and Kollman all united atom charges on protein. The nonpolar hydrogens were merged. A grid box of size $60 \times 60 \times 60$ Å dimension with x, y, and z coordinates of 145.7015, –25.0175, and 74.823, respectively was fixed. Docking was performed using exhaustiveness value of 10 and all other parameters were used as defaults. All rotatable bonds within the ligand were allowed to rotate freely, and the receptor was considered rigid. Finally, AutoDockVina binding affinities were calculated for all the data set ligands.

Furthermore, a force-field based in situ minimization with rescoring protocol was performed on docking poses obtained from AutoDock Vina in order to calculate additional scoring parameters. The best poses of AutoDock Vina, were imported into the Molecular Operating Environment 2009.10[37] and a script named as Dock_Score.svl was used for calculation of various scoring parameters, viz. U_Dock (ASEDock) scoring[38], Affinity_dG scoring[39], and London_ dG scoring[39]. During the force-field based in situ minimization, a constrain was applied on the backbone of the protein and side chains encompassing 4.5Å from the center of the binding site were allowed to move.

12.2.4.3 MOLECULAR DOCKING OF BPBI DERIVATIVES INTO THE

NON-NUCLEOSIDE BINDING POCKET USING GOLD

GOLD uses a genetic algorithm to explore the rotational flexibility of receptor hydrogens and ligand conformational flexibility. For docking simulation of BPBI derivatives into the non-nucleoside binding pocket, prepared ligands and protein files were imported into the SYBYL-X suite[40] and charges were assigned on ligands and protein with Gasteiger Huckel[41] and Kollman all united atom[42], respectively. Binding site was defined on co-crystallized ligand with x, y, and z, coordinates of 145.7015, –25.0175, and 74.823, respectively and a radius of 10 Å. A total number of 10 GA runs were performed and the GOLD_ Fitness_Score function was selected for ranking the compounds. In addition to GOLD_Fitness_Score, some individual contributing parameters to GOLD_ Fitness_Score like S_{hb_ext}, S_{vdw_ext}, S_{int} were also selected.

12.2.4.4 MOLECULAR DOCKING OF BPBI DERIVATIVES INTO THE

NON-NUCLEOSIDE BINDING POCKET USING GLIDE

GLIDE is a Grid-based Ligand Docking with Energetics program. The program was developed to find the favorable interactions between one or more ligand molecules and a receptor molecule. Therefore, in search of ligand poses, which makes some favorable interactions with receptor molecule, a series of hierarchical filters were used, which evaluate the ligands interaction with the receptor. The filtered ligand poses, were then energy minimized on the precomputed OPLS-AA van der Waals and electrostatic grids for the receptor and finally the GlideScore is computed on energy minimized ligand poses. The prepared protein structure was carried forward for the generation of the receptor-grid. A grid box capable of accommodating ligands with up to 10 Å of a geometric length was created at x, y, and z coordinates of 145.7015, −25.0175, and 74.823, respectively, with all other parameters kept at their default settings. The docking calculation was performed using the Glide XP (Xtra precision) mode and Glide Score was computed for each ligand.

GScore = a*vdW + b*Coul + Lipo + Hbond + Metal + BuryP + RotB + Site

where vdW, van der Waal energy; Coul, Coulomb energy; Lipo, lipophilic contact term; HBond, hydrogen-bonding term; Metal, metal-binding term; BuryP, penalty for buried polar groups; RotB, penalty for freezing rotatable bonds; Site, polar interactions at the active site; and the coefficients of vdW and Coul are a = 0.05, b = 0.150.

The data set ligands were ranked in the binding pocket of non-nucleoside RT enzyme with glide GScore, and glide eModel. In addition to GScore and eModel, some individual contributing parameters like glide EvdW (van der Waal energy), glide Ecoul (coulomb energy), and glide Einternal (internal energy) were also selected.

12.2.5 MODEL DEVELOPMENT AND VALIDATION

QSAR modeling of all the calculated docking based scoring parameters were performed using linear and nonlinear regression analysis, considering the scoring/binding affinity values as independent variables and the biological activity of the data set as the dependent variable. Linear regression analysis has been found to be a very useful, interesting, and popular method for model development in QSAR studies because of its simplicity and easy interpretation. This approach requires the selection of relevant descriptors from a large number of descriptors available. However, in some cases, the relationship between the biological activity and physical properties of molecules is not linear. So considering both conditions, in the present work, both approaches for QSAR modeling like simulated annealing[43–45] coupled with linear regression and artificial neural network (ANN)[46] as nonlinear regression tools were used.

In the simulated annealing search the following settings: the Monte Carlo steps: 1,000; initial temperature: 0.5, and final temperature: 0.05; were selected for variable selection. When the variables were picked up, a multiple linear equation with optimum number of steps was generated based on them. The variable selection (simulated annealing approach) based on multiple linear regression was performed using Canvas v1.5[47].

A sigmoidal transfer function and descent gradient with momentum and adaptive learning rate back-propagation in ANN were used to predict the biological activity of the data set used in this study. The back-propagation learning algorithm is the most widely used training algorithms in multilayers feedforward network. All the ANN calculation was performed by Molegro Data Modeller v2.6.[48] Before the training process, the input and output values were normalized between 0.1 and 0.9. After the simulation, the values of the predicted data were transformed to the true values. The parameter values in ANN modeling were max training epochs: 1,000; learning rate: 0.30; output layer learning rate: 0.30; momentum: 0.20; number of neurons in first hidden layer: 3; number of neurons in second hidden layer: 0, and the rest of the parameters were kept default. The robustness, accuracy, reliability, and predictability of the developed model were assessed by internal and external validation processes. The internal validation was done by calculating the cross-validation (Q^2) parameters[49]; normally, a high Q^2 value ($Q^2 > 0.5$) suggests a reasonably robust model. Furthermore, to ensure the high-predictive power of the developed QSAR model, an external test set of compounds that were not included in building of QSAR model was used. The external predictivity of the developed QSAR model was judged by predictive r^2 (r^2_{pred}).[50]

12.3 RESULTS AND DISCUSSIONS

12.3.1 MOLECULAR DOCKING STUDIES AND BINDING MODE ANALYSIS

The molecular docking analysis helps us to understand the interactions between the RT enzyme and its inhibitors. The docking reliability was validated by using the redocking approach and the results showed that all the three docking programs determined the optimal orientation of the docked inhibitor, T50_561 to be close to that of the original orientation found in the co-crystallized bound ligand (**Figure 1.2**). The low RMS deviation (**Table 1.2**) between the docked and crystal ligand coordinates indicates a very good alignment of the experimental and calculated positions, especially considering the resolution of the crystal structure (2.65 Å).

TABLE 1.2   RMSD values from all the three docking programs

Docking Program	Protein	Ligand	RMSD (Å)
AutoDock Vina	2B6A	T50_561	0.2354
GOLD	2B6A	T50_561	0.4488
GLIDE	2B6A	T50_561	0.2055

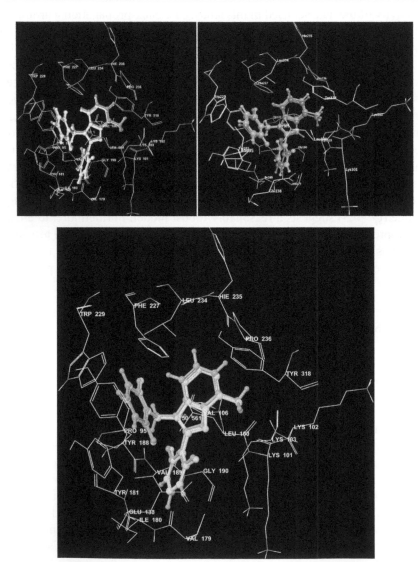

FIGURE 1.2   Conformation of T50_561 crystal structure (red) as compared to the docked conformation of T50_561 (a) AutoDock Vina; (b) GOLD; (c) GLIDE.

After the validation of the docking program parameters, the data set molecules were docked into the non-nucleoside binding pocket. Top ranked docked poses for all the compounds of the data set (**Figure 1.3**) showed similar binding mode as compared to the co-crystallized bound ligand.

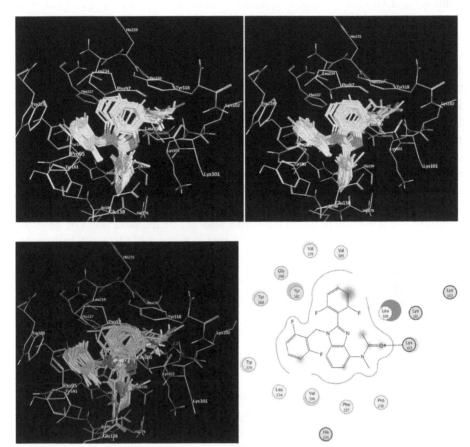

FIGURE 1.3 Conformation of docked poses of bisphenylbenzimidazole derivatives from (a) AutoDock Vina; (b) GOLD; (c) GLIDE docking programs, and (d) schematic ligand interaction diagram for compound 26. A H-bond network with a distance of 2.1 Å was observed between the oxygen atom (compound 26) and backbone atom of Lys103.

A qualitative analysis of the binding mode found in all docked bisphenyl-benzimidazoles and non-nucleoside RT enzyme complexes showed that the BPBI derivatives bind to RT enzyme in a "butterfly-like" binding conformation. The non-nucleoside RT binding pocket comprised of Pro95, Leu100, Lys101, Lys103, Val106, Val109, Val179, Tyr181, Tyr188, Phe227, Trp229, and Tyr318 amino acid residues, which make favorable interactions with inhibitors. Visual analysis of the docked complex of the most potent compound of the data set (compound 26) showed that the 2,6-diflurophenyl group at C-2 position occupy the channel formed between the residues Lys101, Val179 (both from p66 subunit) and Glu138 (fromp51 subunit). The 2,6-difluorobenzyl group at N-1 position makes π–π interactions with hydrophobic amino acid residues Tyr181, Pro95, Tyr188, Trp229, and Leu234. The substituents present at C-4 position on benzimidazole ring system interacts with the backbone atoms, especially with Lys101, Lys103 and side chain residues Val106 and Tyr318. Moreover, one of the important and characteristic features of available non-nucleoside RT inhibitors is that they make a H-bond with backbone residues of Lys101 and Lys103. Most of the compounds of the data set showed a characteristic H-bond network between the nitrogen atoms of the backbone Lys103 and the oxygen atoms of the inhibitors. A mutational modeling study performed by Morningstar et al.,[25] on the same data set, showed that inhibitors with hydrogen bonding groups at C-4 position are unable to effectively block the replication of viruses with mutation at Lys103 position. **Figures 1.4 and 1.5** show the binding interaction of the least potent compounds (05 and 11) of the data set. The binding mode analysis of compound 05 suggests that the favorable interaction formed by group of side chains Lys101, Val179, and Glu138 was lost by the presence of pyridine ring system in place of 2,6-difluorphenyl group due to the loss of hydrophobicity in that area of binding, whereas in compound 11, the presence of bulky 2,6-difluorobenzyl group at C-5 position makes an unfavorable hydrophobic clashing with side chain residue Tyr318 and backbone residues Lys101, Lya103, Pro236, and Val106.

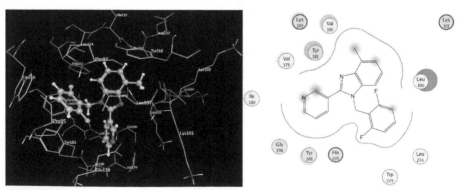

FIGURE 1.4   Binding interaction of compound 05 (a, b).

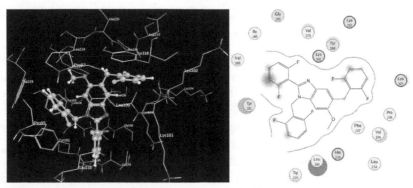

FIGURE 1.5 Binding interaction of compound 11 (a, b).

All the docking programs produce a similar kind of binding orientation for all the data set compounds. It was inferred after observing the binding mode interaction that binding affinities and scoring values were dependent on the substituents present over N-1, C-2, and C-4 positions, which make favorable/unfavorable interactions with the key amino acid residues and are responsible for the variation in scoring values and further activity. Considering the following observation, the docking-based scoring parameters viz. AutoDock Vina binding affinities, U_Dock(ASEDock), Affinity_dG, London_dG, GOLD Fitness score, S(vdw_ext), S(int), S(hb_ext), GlideScore, EvdW, eModel, Ecoul, and Einternal were selected for further analysis. **Table 1.6** shows the list of calculated docking based scoring parameters for data set compounds.

12.3.2 DEVELOPMENT OF DOCKING BASED SCORING PARAMETERS BASED QSAR MODEL

A multiple linear (simulated-annealing) and nonlinear (ANN) regression analysis was performed on the selected data set using a total of 13 docking based scoring functions as independent parameters and experimental activity as the dependent parameter. The data set was randomly divided into training (29) and a test set (8) with the consideration that, both sets consist of high-, medium-, and low-active compounds. Initially a simulated annealing search for variable selection was performed on all the independent parameters and a five parametric SA-MLR based QSAR model was developed. Compound 12 was identified as an outlier (residual of 1.530); so, after removing the outlier, QSAR model was developed on 28 training set compounds. Finally a five parametric simulated annealing based multiple linear (SA-MLR) QSAR model was developed with the following statistics.

$pEC_{50} = 0.463 + (-0.634)*Affinity\_dG + (0.134)*S(int) + (-0.262)*GLIDEScore + (0.028)*EvdW + (-0.042)*GOLD\_Fitness\_Score$

$N_{training}$ = 28; r = 0.853; r^2 = 0.728; Q^2 = 0.728; Q^2_{loo} = 0.586; F = 11.776; SD = 0.411; N_{test} = 8; r^2_{pred} = 0.634; $r^2_{(test)}$ = 0.664; $RMSE_{(test)}$ = 0.411

The regression coefficients of QSAR models were significant at 95% confidence level. $N_{training}$ is the number of compounds in the training set; r^2, the squared correlation coefficient; Q^2, the cross-validated squared correlation coefficient; SD, the standard deviation; F, the Fisher's F-value; r^2_{pred}, the predictive correlation coefficient; $r^2_{(test)}$, the squared correlation coefficient based on test set; $r^2_{m(test)}$, modified correlation coefficient based on test set and $RMSE_{(test)}$ stands for root mean squared error of the test set.

In the above model, Affinity_dG, GLIDEScore, and GOLD_Fitness_Score contribute negatively, whereas, S(int), and EvdW contributes positively toward the RT inhibition activity. A coefficient relevance score was calculated from the multiple linear regression model using descriptors contributing to the model. Each coefficient relevance score was calculated by multiplying the coefficient value with the standard deviation of the corresponding descriptor and dividing the product with the standard deviation of the target variable. The calculated coefficient relevance scores for the used independent parameters are Affinity_dG (0.900), S(int) (0.273), GLIDEScore (0.326), EvdW (0.353), and GOLD_Fitness_Score (0.283).

Furthermore, a (6-4-1) five parametric ANN (nonlinear) based QSAR model was developed and validated on the test set data:

// sigmoid(x) = 1/(1+exp(-x))
IN_0 = Affinity_dG*0.147 + 2.023
IN_1 = AutoDock Vina*0.116 + 1.7
IN_2 = S(int)*0.108 + 1.161
IN_3 = GLIDEScore*0.181 + 2.688
IN_4 = EvdW*0.015 + 0.915
HL_0 = sigmoid(-3.847*IN_0 - 0.744*IN_1 + 1.317*IN_2 - 1.679*IN_3 + 2.062*IN_4 + 1.959)
HL_1 = sigmoid(1.546*IN_0 - 0.099*IN_1 - 0.075*IN_2 + 0.633*IN_3 - 1.606*IN_4 - 0.657)
HL_2 = sigmoid(-1.409*IN_0 - 0.405*IN_1 + 0.356*IN_2 - 0.699*IN_3 + 0.973*IN_4 - 0.431)
OUT = (sigmoid(4.030*HL_0 - 2.089*HL_1 + 1.205*HL_2 - 1.947) + 1.142) / 0.276

$N_{training}$ = 28; r = 0.844; r^2 = 0.712; Q^2 = 0.697; Q^2_{loo} = 0.561; F = 10.878; SD = 0.433; N_{test} = 8; r^2_{pred} = 0.603; $r^2_{(test)}$ = 0.687; $RMSE_{(test)}$ = 0.428

A descriptor relevance score was calculated by following all paths from the input neuron (IN) to the output neuron (including hidden layers [HLs]). For each path, the product of all the connection weights (in absolute values) is added to the score. Afterward, all the relevance scores are normalized in the range between 0 and 100. In the above ANN based QSAR model, the relevance score was calculated and their order was Affinity_dG (100), GLIDEScore (43), EvdW (62), S(int) (28), and AutoDock Vina (16).

The statistical and validation parameters from both QSAR models showed that the linear regression (simulated annealing based QSAR) model yielded the best regression approach to build the QSAR models. The simulated annealing based QSAR model has higher value for square of correlation coefficient (r^2= 0.728), and Fisher value (F=11.776), whereas lower value for standard deviation (SD=0.411), than that of the ANN based QSAR model, suggesting that statistical parameters of simulated-annealing based QSAR model have better robustness. The orthogonality among the descriptors in the model was judged through intercorrelation among the parameters selected for the QSAR model development. All the parameters were fairly independent to each other (**Table 1.3**). It was also observed that the model developed using the linear regression approach is superior to the nonlinear regression approach not only in the statistical parameters of regression, but also in its predictability. The values obtained with simulated annealing based QSAR ($Q^2_{(LOO)}$=0.586) are higher than corresponding ANN-based QSAR ($Q^2_{(LOO)}$ = 0.561).

TABLE 1.3 Correlation Matrix for the significant parameters

	pEC_{50}	A	B	C	D	E	F
pEC_{50}	1.000	0.551	0.162	0.159	0.465	0.123	0.272
A	0.551	1.000	0.400	0.100	0.370	0.443	0.539
B	0.162	0.400	1.000	0.259	0.193	0.799	0.149
C	0.159	0.100	0.259	1.000	0.178	0.241	0.186
D	0.465	0.370	0.193	0.178	1.000	0.128	0.408
E	0.123	0.443	0.799	0.241	0.128	1.000	0.266
F	0.272	0.539	0.149	0.186	0.408	0.266	1.000

Abbreviations: pEC_{50}: Experimental activity; A: Affinity_dG; B: AutoDock_ VINA; C: S(int); D: GLIDEScore; E: EvdW; F: GOLD_Fitness_Score

Comparing the statistical and validation parameters of the developed QSAR models, it was expected for the simulated annealing based QSAR model to be better predictors for HIV-1 RT inhibitors over ANN based QSAR model. For the purpose of prediction of inhibitory activity, that is, r^2_{pred}, a test set consisting of eight bisphenylbenzimidazole derivatives (not considered throughout the model development) was employed. The simulated annealing based QSAR model (r^2_{pred} = 0.634), showed superiority over ANN based QSAR model (r^2_{pred} =

0.603), thus verifying the predictive ability of the proposed model. Furthermore, to confirm the robustness of the derived models, a Y-randomization test was performed by scrambling the experimental activity at 1,000 random numbers of trial considering the same number and definition of descriptors. The results so obtained showed that the original model obtained was not due to a chance correlation (**Table 1.4**). Moreover, to further validate the predictive QSAR models, R^2_p parameter as suggested by Roy *et al.*, was calculated and R^2_p for simulated annealing based QSAR (0.540) and ANN-based QSAR (0.516), a value above 0.5 suggests an acceptable model. A scatter plot between the experimental activity and predicted activity shows all the compounds were well predicted by linear and nonlinear regression model (**Table 1.5**).

TABLE 1.4 Ten random squared correlation coefficients from the pEC_{50} activity (Y) randomization study of developed QSAR models

S. No. †	SA-MLR based QSAR Model		ANN based QSAR Model	
	r^2	$Q^2_{(LOO)}$	r^2	$Q^2_{(LOO)}$
1.	0.589	0.304	0.633	0.470
2.	0.565	0.198	0.626	0.166
3.	0.525	0.148	0.606	0.370
4.	0.522	0.255	0.553	0.213
5.	0.521	0.202	0.550	0.000
6.	0.509	0.000	0.547	0.293
7.	0.465	0.200	0.530	0.336
8.	0.464	0.223	0.506	0.241
9.	0.456	0.000	0.488	0.000
10.	0.448	0.000	0.467	0.080

†values of 10 high y-randomization recorded from 1,000 random shuffles

TABLE 1.5 Experimental and predicted activity of bisphenylbenzimidazole derivatives

CMPD No.	SA-MLR					ANN			
	Exp. Act. (pEC_{50})	Pred. Act. (pEC_{50})	Res.	Pred. Act. (LOO) (pEC_{50})	Res.	Pred. Act. (pEC_{50})	Res.	Pred. Act. (LOO) (pEC_{50})	Res.
COMP01^t	5.218	5.278	-0.060	-	-	5.083	0.135	-	-
COMP02	5.770	6.046	-0.276	6.086	-0.317	6.010	-0.240	6.006	-0.237
COMP03	6.357	6.145	0.211	6.134	0.222	6.319	0.038	6.208	0.148
COMP04	5.456	5.383	0.073	5.372	0.084	5.470	-0.014	5.451	0.005

(*Continued*)

COMP05	4.500	4.816	-0.316	4.962	-0.462	4.973	-0.473	5.263	-0.762
COMP06[t]	6.125	6.248	-0.123	-	-	6.396	-0.271	-	-
COMP07	5.500	5.458	0.042	5.357	0.143	5.493	0.007	5.192	0.308
COMP08	5.582	5.656	-0.075	5.669	-0.087	5.570	0.012	5.506	0.075
COMP09[t]	5.311	6.151	-0.840	-	-	6.074	-0.763	-	-
COMP10	5.134	5.514	-0.380	5.693	-0.559	5.152	-0.018	5.153	-0.019
COMP11	4.506	4.426	0.080	3.797	0.708	4.584	-0.078	4.685	-0.179
COMP12*	7.097	5.567	1.530	-	-	5.749	1.348	-	-
COMP13	6.398	6.186	0.212	6.163	0.235	6.227	0.171	6.156	0.242
COMP14[t]	5.620	5.769	-0.149	-	-	6.081	-0.461	-	-
COMP15	6.347	6.552	-0.205	6.601	-0.254	6.485	-0.138	6.473	-0.126
COMP16	6.276	5.917	0.359	5.878	0.398	6.096	0.180	6.039	0.237
COMP17	5.567	5.614	-0.047	5.622	-0.055	5.850	-0.283	5.913	-0.346
COMP18	7.301	7.276	0.025	7.270	0.031	7.113	0.188	7.100	0.201
COMP19[t]	6.796	6.216	0.580	-	-	6.452	0.344	-	-
COMP20	5.867	6.177	-0.310	6.235	-0.369	6.571	-0.704	6.667	-0.801
COMP21[t]	6.086	6.214	-0.128	-	-	6.429	-0.342	-	-
COMP22	6.432	6.082	0.350	6.034	0.398	6.410	0.022	6.402	0.030
COMP23	7.222	7.484	-0.263	7.682	-0.460	7.185	0.037	7.150	0.072
COMP24	7.000	6.720	0.280	6.664	0.336	6.821	0.179	6.795	0.205
COMP25	5.783	5.676	0.107	5.624	0.158	5.625	0.157	5.522	0.260
COMP26	7.398	6.601	0.797	6.543	0.855	6.689	0.709	6.534	0.864
COMP27	6.432	6.221	0.210	6.198	0.234	6.409	0.023	6.362	0.070
COMP28	6.187	6.318	-0.131	6.336	-0.149	6.353	-0.166	6.342	-0.155
COMP29	5.625	6.170	-0.545	6.271	-0.645	6.476	-0.850	6.557	-0.931
COMP30	6.367	6.473	-0.107	6.481	-0.114	6.625	-0.258	6.650	-0.284
COMP31	6.721	7.322	-0.601	7.541	-0.820	7.154	-0.433	7.243	-0.522
COMP32	5.198	6.152	-0.954	6.300	-1.102	6.485	-1.287	6.560	-1.362
COMP33	5.842	5.971	-0.130	6.006	-0.164	6.364	-0.523	6.483	-0.642
COMP34[t]	7.347	7.026	0.321	-	-	7.051	0.296	-	-
COMP35[t]	6.237	6.626	-0.389	-	-	6.744	-0.508	-	-
COMP36	7.222	6.119	1.103	5.966	1.255	6.401	0.821	6.048	1.173
COMP37	7.222	6.730	0.492	6.651	0.570	6.896	0.326	6.829	0.393

Exp. Act.: Experimental Activity; Pred. Act.: Predicted Activity; Res.: Residual between Experimental Activity and Predicted Activity; [t]Test Set Compounds;

TABLE 1.6   Docking based scoring parameters for data set of bisphenylbenzimidazole derivatives

CMPD No.	Exp. Act.	A	B	C	D	E	F	G	H	I	J	K	L	M
COMP01	5.218	-12.387	-10.066	-11.012	-10.600	61.310	47.550	-4.080	0.000	-10.895	-46.312	-0.863	-71.687	1.279
COMP02	5.770	-34.432	-11.203	-11.990	-12.800	62.250	47.920	-3.640	0.000	-11.186	-48.050	-1.079	-78.930	0.535
COMP03	6.357	-34.843	-11.728	-12.714	-13.500	66.690	51.580	-4.240	0.000	-11.616	-50.874	-1.037	-83.722	0.133
COMP04	5.456	-38.359	-10.582	-12.040	-12.300	66.750	51.090	-3.490	0.000	-10.980	-49.715	-0.891	-79.564	0.984
COMP05	4.500	-33.924	-9.526	-11.913	-12.400	65.760	50.400	-3.540	0.000	-11.207	-49.414	0.005	-78.200	1.176
COMP06	6.125	-30.764	-11.801	-12.149	-13.100	68.240	51.410	-2.450	0.000	-11.062	-49.954	-0.816	-79.021	0.235
COMP07	5.500	-21.040	-11.675	-13.211	-13.000	63.540	53.370	-9.850	0.000	-11.527	-51.178	-0.852	-86.742	0.240
COMP08	5.582	-34.346	-10.472	-11.356	-12.100	62.140	47.450	-3.110	0.000	-11.039	-46.746	-0.962	-73.855	0.496
COMP09	5.311	-31.479	-11.476	-12.658	-12.900	60.810	47.810	-4.920	0.000	-11.402	-48.538	-1.092	-73.023	0.767
COMP10	5.134	-26.558	-10.168	-12.850	-11.900	54.930	43.710	-5.160	0.000	-11.109	-46.554	-1.843	-63.835	0.620
COMP11	4.506	-11.429	-7.624	-11.917	-6.900	54.210	45.720	-8.650	0.000	-9.894	-1.022	-1.070	39.466	23.426
COMP12	7.097	-31.887	-10.870	-13.051	-12.600	68.290	52.200	-3.480	0.000	-11.557	-52.781	-0.901	-87.906	0.523
COMP13	6.398	-38.023	-11.723	-12.697	-13.200	63.720	49.790	-4.740	0.000	-11.508	-50.351	-0.732	-86.193	0.463
COMP14	5.620	-32.304	-11.447	-13.139	-12.800	70.080	54.810	-5.280	0.000	-12.165	-53.006	-2.089	-93.203	0.118
COMP15	6.347	-36.207	-12.442	-13.809	-12.900	65.060	49.450	-3.650	0.710	-11.440	-56.119	-0.637	-92.781	2.757
COMP16	6.276	-41.843	-10.888	-12.982	-12.800	66.600	50.600	-2.970	0.000	-12.071	-50.511	-3.042	-85.227	0.095
COMP17	5.567	-37.565	-10.824	-13.792	-11.500	70.330	53.570	-3.340	0.010	-11.635	-48.420	-1.980	-86.526	0.666
COMP18	7.301	-41.961	-12.506	-14.584	-13.000	71.440	54.060	-2.890	0.000	-13.817	-48.073	-5.113	-94.652	0.655
COMP19	6.796	-33.567	-12.108	-13.444	-12.800	70.070	54.400	-4.740	0.000	-11.986	-52.949	-1.897	-90.330	1.241

(Continued)

Compound	Exp. Act.	A	B	C	D	E	F	G	H	I	J	K	L	M
COMP20	5.867	-47.490	-11.315	-13.999	-13.000	71.770	54.250	-3.490	0.650	-13.012	-49.461	-5.221	-88.615	0.781
COMP21	6.086	-28.566	-12.103	-13.389	-13.100	68.970	53.760	-4.940	0.000	-11.921	-53.001	-1.186	-89.579	0.797
COMP22	6.432	-30.070	-11.410	-14.474	-13.500	71.030	52.840	-2.420	0.790	-12.344	-54.960	-3.239	-92.962	0.512
COMP23	7.222	-8.633	-12.999	-15.714	-11.600	71.800	55.130	-4.010	0.000	-12.781	-36.274	-2.447	-73.110	1.104
COMP24	7.000	-38.198	-11.798	-13.352	-13.200	68.710	51.600	-2.880	0.640	-13.376	-51.877	-2.357	-94.369	0.191
COMP25	5.783	-11.349	-11.889	-14.617	-12.800	65.690	51.190	-4.840	0.140	-9.896	-53.833	-3.718	-7.190	7.757
COMP26	7.398	-4.190	-12.436	-15.006	-12.000	69.650	53.790	-4.320	0.000	-12.218	-51.466	-2.818	-73.382	2.087
COMP27	6.432	-36.038	-11.819	-13.067	-13.300	68.540	52.070	-3.070	0.000	-11.427	-51.312	-0.721	-88.078	0.145
COMP28	6.187	-45.244	-11.379	-13.200	-12.800	62.970	48.840	-4.180	0.000	-12.212	-48.258	-4.843	-84.785	0.607
COMP29	5.625	-21.877	-12.382	-13.896	-12.200	73.730	56.880	-4.480	0.000	-11.593	-52.893	-1.903	-86.223	3.851
COMP30	6.367	-40.983	-11.937	-14.311	-13.800	67.830	51.640	-3.250	0.070	-12.313	-53.437	-1.617	-89.267	1.355
COMP31	6.721	-27.825	-13.057	-15.790	-13.300	75.290	55.730	-3.370	2.040	-14.321	-55.530	-5.974	-106.388	3.233
COMP32	5.198	-20.828	-12.333	-14.306	-12.800	72.680	56.690	-5.270	0.000	-11.842	-52.537	-0.977	-84.990	3.521
COMP33	5.842	1.323	-12.049	-14.878	-11.500	75.770	58.270	-4.350	0.000	-11.839	-52.330	-2.273	-85.273	5.241
COMP34	7.347	-29.668	-13.073	-14.130	-12.600	73.320	56.190	-3.940	0.000	-10.769	-33.574	0.518	-17.598	3.117
COMP35	6.237	40.446	-13.035	-15.742	-9.800	77.470	58.230	-2.750	0.160	-11.577	-53.970	-1.865	-88.427	1.806
COMP36	7.222	-33.220	-11.967	-14.656	-12.000	71.230	55.590	-5.380	0.180	-12.390	-52.206	-3.420	-91.322	2.414
COMP37	7.222	-29.385	-12.658	-15.289	-12.300	74.610	56.750	-3.510	0.090	-12.361	-49.685	-1.770	-79.379	3.970

Exp. Act.: Experimental activity; A: U_Dock(ASEDock); B: Affinity_dG; C: London_dG; D: AutoDock_VINA; E: GOLD_Fitness_Score; F: S(vdw_ext); G: S(int); H: S(hb_ext); I: GLIDEScore; J: EvdW; K: Ecoul; L: eModel; M: Einternal

In both, linear and nonlinear regression models, coefficient/descriptor relevance score suggested that a significant contribution was observed from Affinity_dG, GLIDEScore, EvdW, S(int), and GOLD_Fitness_Score for modulating the inhibitory activity. The Affinity_dG parameters represent the enthalpic contribution from free binding energy and its sign of the regression coefficient in SA-MLR model is negative, which suggest that, for a compound to show better inhibition, the free binding energy should be in more negative values. Therefore, the reason for moderate to high potent compounds (compounds no. 18, 19, 23, 26, 31, and 37) to show good binding affinity as compared to least potent compounds (compounds 01, 05, 10, and 11) can be explained by observing the descriptor data table. Another negatively contributing parameter is GLIDEScore, which estimates the binding affinities between the inhibitor and their target. The GLIDEScore values calculated for least potent compounds showed a similar pattern as compared to Affinity_dG values. However, for moderate to highly active compounds not much differentiation in GLIDEScore was observed. GOLD_Fitness_Score contributes negatively toward the biological activity, suggesting that decreasing the value of GOLD_Fitness_Score will enhance the biological activity. As can be seen from the descriptor data table (Table 1.6), some of the low-active compounds (compounds no. 20, 29, 32, and 33) show higher value for GOLD_Fitness_Score values, as compared to moderate to high active compounds (compounds no. 03, 13, 24, 26, and 30). EvdW is an individual contribution from GLIDE docking and represents the energy of van der Waals interaction between the substituents and key amino acid residues. The contribution of EvdW toward the biological activity is positive, which suggests that van der Waals interactions play an important role in governing the biological activity. As it was observed, the binding pocket of the non-nucleoside RT enzyme is hydrophobic in nature, so the substitution of appropriate sized hydrophobic groups on bisphenylbenzimidazole nucleus, modulate the inhibitory activity. It was also observed that excessively abundant bulky groups will cause a detrimental effect on the activity. As can be seen in data set compounds (**Table 1**) and descriptor data **Table 1.6**, presence of bulky groups on compound no. 05 creates a steric hindrance to accommodate well into the hydrophobic pocket of enzyme, whereas small bulky groups make better interaction and accommodate well in the binding pocket. Most of the data set molecules contain the -F, -Cl, -Br, and -CH$_3$ substituents present over the bisphenylbenzimidazole nucleus and their steric size is small enough to be accommodated in the binding pocket to cause better inhibitory effects. Another positively contributing parameter is the S(int), which is based on intermolecular strain resulted from vdW and torsional energy. S(int) parameter suggests the importance of hydrophobic substituents and the flexibility of the ligand. It was inferred that non-nucleoside RT inhibitors should obtain their characteristic butterfly-like orientation for better interaction in the binding pocket of non-nucleoside RT enzyme. The butterfly-like orientation is only obtained by substitution of less bulky substituents over the bisphenylbenzimidazole nucleus, which provides unrestricted flexibility of the molecules into the binding pocket.

12.4 CONCLUSIONS

Ligand based QSAR techniques have been applied for many years to rationalize the structure–activity relationships of targets and their inhibitors with an aim to generate robust models that can quantitatively predict the activity of new analogues. In this chapter, we have developed and applied a novel approach of docking based scoring parameter based QSAR modeling on a data set of thirty-seven BPBIs active against RT enzyme. The data set compounds were docked into the binding pocket of RT enzyme (PDB ID: 2B6A) using three molecular docking programs (AutoDock Vina, GOLD, and GLIDE). The docking based scoring parameters calculated for data set compounds were selected and used as independent parameters for robust QSAR model development by linear (simulated annealing based QSAR) and nonlinear (ANN-based QSAR) regression approaches, considering experimental activity as dependent parameters. Based on statistical and validation parameters, simulated annealing based QSAR (linear approach) (r^2=0.728; Q^2=0.728; and r^2_{pred}=0.634) model showed better result as compared to ANN-based QSAR (nonlinear approach) (r^2 = 0.712; Q^2 = 0.697; and r^2_{pred} = 0.603) model. The docking based scoring parameters based QSAR study suggested that the hydrophobicity, volume, and shape of molecules influence the inhibitory activity of molecules. Therefore, it can be concluded from the above result analysis, that the docking based scoring parameters based QSAR model can be considered as a virtually screening model to search novel hits, with similar structural analogy from available databases and their activity can be further predicted based on selected QSAR model.

KEYWORDS

- **Artifical neural network**
- **Docking based scoring parameters**
- **QSAR**
- **Simulated annealing search**

REFERENCES

1. UNAIDS Global Fact Sheet. http://www.unaids.org/en/media/unaids/contentassets/documents/epidemiology/2012/gr2012/20121120_FactSheet_Global_en.pdf (accessed 20 November 2012).
2. Reeves, J. D.; Doms, R. W. Human Immunodeficiency virus type 2. *J. Gen. Virol.***2002**, 83, 1253-1265.
3. Klatzmann, D.; Champagne, E.; Chamaret, S.; Gruest, J.; Guetard, D.; Hercend, T.; Gluckman, J. C.; Montagnier, L. T-lymphocyte T4 molecule behaves as the receptor for human retrovirus LAV. *Nature***1984**, 312, 767–768.
4. Clapham, P. R.; McKnight, A. Cell surface receptors, virus entry and tropism of primate lentiviruses. *J. Gen. Virol.***2002**, 83, 1809–1829.
5. Hoxie, J. A.; LaBranche, C. C.; Endres, M. J.; Turner, J. D.; Berson, J. F.; Doms, R. W.; Matthews, T. J. CD4-independent utilization of the CXCR4 chemokine receptor by HIV-1 and HIV-2. *J. Reprod. Immunol.***1998**, 41, 197–211.
6. Kilby, J. M.; Eron, J. J. Novel therapies based on mechanisms of HIV-1 cell entry. *N. Eng. J. Med.***2003**, 348, 2228–2238.
7. Tarrago-Litvak, L.; Andreola, M. L.; Nevinsky, G. A.; Sarih-Cottin, L.; Litvak, S. The reverse transcriptase of HIV-1: from enzymology to therapeutic intervention. *FASEB J.* **1994**, 8, 497–503.
8. De Clercq, E. Non-nucleoside reverse transcriptase inhibitors (NNRTIs): past, present, and future. *Chem. Biodivers.* **2004**, 1, 44–64.
9. Guillemont, J.; Pasquier, E.; Palandjian, P.; Vernier, D.; Gaurrand, S.; Lewi, P. J.; Heeres, J.; de Jonge, M. R.; Koymans, L. M.; Daeyaert, F. F.; Vinkers, M. H.; Arnold, E.; Das, K.; Pauwels, R.; Andries, K.; de Bethune, M. P.; Bettens, E.; Hertogs, K.; Wigerinck, P.; Timmerman, P.; Janssen, P. A. Synthesis of novel diarylpyrimidine analogues and their antiviral activity against human immunodeficiency virus type 1. *J. Med. Chem.***2005**, 48, 2072–2079.
10. Kroeger Smith, M. B.; Rouzer, C. A.; Taneyhill, L. A.; Smith, N. A.; Hughes, S. H.; Boyer, P. L.; Janssen, P. A.; Moereels, H.; Koymans, L.; Arnold, E.; Ding, J.; Das, K.; Zhang, W. Molecular modeling studies of HIV-1 reverse transcriptase nonnucleoside inhibitors: total energy of complexation as a predictor of drug placement and activity. *Protein Sci.* **1995**, 4, 2203–2222.
11. Ding, J.; Das, K.; Moereels, H.; Koymans, L.; Andries, K.; Janssen, P. A.; Hughes, S. H.; Arnold, E. Structure of HIV-1 RT/TIBO R 86183 complex reveals similarity in the binding of diverse nonnucleoside inhibitors. *Nat. Struct. Biol.***1995**, 2, 407–415.
12. Tantillo, C.; Ding, J.; Jacobo-Molina, A.; Nanni, R. G.; Boyer, P. L.; Hughes, S. H.; Pauwels, R.; Andries, K.; Janssen, P. A.; Arnold, E. Locations of anti-AIDS drug binding sites and resistance mutations in the three-dimensional structure of HIV-1 reverse transcriptase. Implications for mechanisms of drug inhibition and resistance. *J. Mol. Biol.***1994**, 243, 369–387.
13. Dubey, S.; Satyanarayana, Y. D.; Lavania, H. Development of integrase inhibitors for treatment of AIDS: an overview. *Eur. J. Med. Chem.***2007**, 42, 1159–1168.
14. Alterman, M.; Sjöbom, H.; Säfsten, P.; Markgren, P. O.; Danielson, U. H.; Hämäläinen, M.; Löfås, S.; Hultén, J.; Classon, B.; Samuelsson, B.; Hallberg, A. P1/P1' modified HIV protease inhibitors as tools in two new sensitive surface plasmon resonance biosensor screening assays. *Eur. J. Pharm. Sci.***2001**, 13, 203–212.
15. Barreca, M. L.; Balzarini, J.; Chimirri, A.; De Clercq, E.; De Luca, L.; Hltje, H. D.; Hltje, M.; Monforte, A. M.; Monforte, P.; Pannecouque, C.; Rao, A.; Zappal, M. Design, synthesis, structure-activity relationships, and molecular modeling studies of 2,3-diaryl-1,3-thiazolidin-4-ones as potent anti-HIV gents. *J. Med. Chem.***2002**, 45, 5410–5413.

16. Chimirri, A.; Grasso, S.; Monforte, A. M.; Monforte, P.; Zappala, M. Anti-HIV agents. I: synthesis and in vitro anti-HIV evaluation of novel 1H,3H-thiazolo[3,4-a] benzimidazoles. *Farmaco* **1991**, 46, 817–823.

17. Chimirri, A.; Grasso, S.; Monforte, A. M.; Monforte, P.; Zappala, M. Anti-HIV agents II. Synthesis and in vitro anti-HIV activity of novel 1H,3H-thiazolo[3,4-a]benzimidazoles. *Farmaco* **1991**, 46, 925–933.

18. el Dareer, S. M.; Tillery, K. F.; Rose, L. M.; Posey, C. F.; Struck, R. F.; Stiller, S. W.; Hill, D. L. Metabolism and disposition of a thiazolobenzimidazole active against human immunodeficiency virus-1. *Drug Metab. Dispos.* **1993**, 21, 231–235.

19. Kumar, S.; Tiwari, M. Variable selection based QSAR modeling on bisphenylbenzimidazole as inhibitor of HIV-1 reverse transcriptase. *Med. Chem.* **2013**, 9, 955–967.

20. Kumar, S.; Singh, V.; Tiwari, M. QSAR modeling of the inhibition of reverse transcriptase enzyme with benzimidazolone analogs. *Med. Chem. Res.* **2011**,20, 1530–1541.

21. Kumar, S.; Tiwari, M. Grid potential analysis, virtual screening studies and ADME/T profiling on N-arylsulfonylindoles as anti-HIV-1 agents. *J. Chemometr.* **2013**, 27, 143–154.

22. Chipot, C.; Rozanska, X.; Dixit, S. B. Can free energy calculations be fast and accurate at the same time? Binding of low-affinity, non-peptide inhibitors to the SH2 domain of the src protein. *J. Comput. Aided Mol. Des.* **2005**, 19, 765–770.

23. Foloppe, N.; Hubbard, R. Towards predictive ligand design with free-energy based computational methods? *Curr. Med. Chem.* **2006**, 13, 3583–3608.

24. Kroeger Smith, M. B.; Hose, B. M.; Hawkins, A.; Lipchock, J.; Farnsworth, D. W.; Rizzo, R. C.; Tirado-Rives, J.; Arnold, E.; Zhang, W.; Hughes, S. H.; Jorgensen, W. L.; Michejda, C. J.; Smith, R. H. Molecular modeling calculations of HIV-1 reverse transcriptase non-nucleoside inhibitors: correlation of binding energy with biological activity for novel 2-aryl-substituted benzimidazole analogues. *J. Med. Chem.* **2003**, 46, 1940–1947.

25. Morningstar, M. L.; Roth, T.; Farnsworth, D. W.; Smith, M. K.; Watson, K.; Buckheit, R. W., Jr.; Das, K.; Zhang, W.; Arnold, E.; Julias, J. G.; Hughes, S. H.; Michejda, C. J. Synthesis, biological activity, and crystal structure of potent non-nucleoside inhibitors of HIV-1 reverse transcriptase that retain activity against mutant forms of the enzyme. *J. Med. Chem.* **2007**, 50, 4003–4015.

26. Roth, T.; Morningstar, M. L.; Boyer, P. L.; Hughes, S. H.; Buckheit, R. W., Jr.; Michejda, C. J. Synthesis and biological activity of novel nonnucleoside inhibitors of HIV-1 reverse transcriptase. 2-Aryl-substituted benzimidazoles. *J. Med. Chem.* **1997**, 40, 4199–4207.

27. Rao, A.; Chimirri, A.; De Clercq, E.; Monforte, A. M.; Monforte, P.; Pannecouque, C.; Zappala, M. Synthesis and anti-HIV activity of 1-(2,6-difluorophenyl)-1H,3H-thiazolo[3,4-a]benzimidazole structurally-related 1,2-substituted benzimidazoles. *Farmaco* **2002**, 57, 819–823.

28. Schrodinger Suite 2012: Maestro, version 9.3, Schrödinger, LLC, New York, NY, **2012**.

29. Schrodinger Suite 2012: QikProp, version 3.5, Schrödinger, LLC, New York, NY, **2012**.

30. Watts, K. S.; Dalal, P.; Murphy, R. B.; Sherman, W.; Friesner, R. A.; Shelley, J. C. ConfGen: a conformational search method for efficient generation of bioactive conformers. *J. Chem. Inf. Model.* **2010**, 50, 534–546.

31. http://www.rcsb.org/pdb/explore.do?structureId=2b6a.

32. Schrödinger Suite 2012 Protein Preparation Wizard; Epik version 2.3, Schrödinger, LLC, New York, NY, **2012**; Impact version 5.8, Schrödinger, LLC, New York, NY, 2012; Prime version 3.1, Schrödinger, LLC, New York, NY, **2012**.

33. Trott, O.; Olson, A. J. AutoDock Vina: improving the speed and accuracy of docking with a new scoring function, efficient optimization, and multithreading. *J. Comput. Chem.* **2010**, 31, 455–461.

34. Jones, G.; Willett, P.; Glen, R. C.; Leach, A. R.; Taylor, R. Development and validation of a genetic algorithm for flexible docking. *J. Mol. Biol.* **1997**, 267, 727–748.

35. Schrodinger Suite 2012: Glide, version 5.8, Schrödinger, LLC, New York, NY, 2012.

36. Friesner, R. A.; Banks, J. L.; Murphy, R. B.; Halgren, T. A.; Klicic, J. J.; Mainz, D. T.; Repasky, M. P.; Knoll, E. H.; Shelley, M.; Perry, J. K. Glide: a new approach for rapid, accurate docking and scoring. 1. Method and assessment of docking accuracy. *J. Med. Chem.***2004**, 47, 1739–1749.

37. Molecular Operating Environment (MOE), 2009.10; Chemical Computing Group Inc., 1010, Sherbooke St. West, Suite #910, Montreal, QC, Canada, H3A 2R7, **2009.**

38. Goto, J.; Kataoka, R.; Muta, H.; Hirayama, N. ASEDock-docking based on alpha spheres and excluded volumes. *J. Chem. Inf. Model.***2008**, 48, 583–590.

39. Weber, J.; Rupp, M.; Proschak, E. Impact of X-ray structure on predictivity of scoring functions: PPARγ case study. *Mol. Inf.***2012**, 31, 631–633.

40. SYBYL-X 2.0, Tripos International, 1699 South Hanley Rd., St. Louis, Missouri, 63144, USA.

41. Gasteiger, J.; Marsili, M. Iterative partial equalization of orbital electronegativity – A rapid access to atomic charges. *Tetrahedron***1980**, 36, 3219–3228.

42. Weiner, S. J.; Kollman, P. A.; Nguyen, D. T.; Case, D. A. An all atom force field for simulations of proteins and nucleic acids. *J. Comput. Chem.***1986,** 7, 230–252.

43. Kirkpatrick, S.; Gelatt, C. D., Jr.; Vecchi, M. P. Optimization by simulated annealing. *Science***1983,** 220, 671–680.

44. Itskowitz, P.; Tropsha, A. kappa nearest neighbors QSAR modeling as a variational problem: theory and applications. *J. Chem. Inf. Model.***2005,** 45, 777–785.

45. Sutter, J. M.; Dixon, S. L.; Jurs, P. C. Automated descriptor selection for quantitative structure-activity relationships using generalized simulated annealing. *J. Chem. Inf. Comp. Sci.***1995,** 35, 77–84.

46. Devillers, J. Strengths and Weaknesses of the backpropagation neural network in QSAR and QSPR studies. In *Neural Networks in QSAR and Drug Design*; Academic Press: London, 1996; pp 1–46.

47. Schrodinger Suite 2012: canvas, version 1.5, Schrödinger, LLC, New York, NY, 2012.

48. Molegro Data Modeller, Version 2.6, CCL Bio, Denmark.

49. Picard, R. R.; Cook, R. D. Cross-validation of regression models. *J. Am. Statist. Assoc.***1984,** 79, 575–583.

50. Golbraikh, A.; Tropsha, A. Beware of q2! *J. Mol. Graph. Model.***2002**, 20, 269–276.

CHAPTER 13

POTENTIAL ANTI-INFLAMMATORY AND ANTIPROLIFERATIVE AGENTS AND 1H-ISOCHROMEN-1-ONES AND THEIR THIO ANALOGUES AND THEIR QSAR STUDIES

F. NAWAZ KHAN[1, 3]* PONNURENGAM M. SIVAKUMAR[2], MUKESH DOBLE[2], P. MANIVEL[1], and EUH D. JEONG[3]

[1]Organic & Medicinal Chemistry Research Laboratory, School of Advanced Sciences, VIT University, Vellore;Tel.: 91-416 220 2334, Fax: 91-416 224 3092, Cell: 094442 34609, Email: nawaz_f@yahoo.co.in.

[2]Department of Biotechnology, Indian Institute of Technology Madras, Adyar, Chennai - 600036, India

[3]Division of High Technology Materials Research, Busan Center, Korea Basic Science Institute (KBSI), Busan 618-230, Republic of Korea
E-mail: edjeong@kbsi.re.kr

CONTENTS

ABSTRACT

A series of 1H-isochromen-1-ones and their thio analogues (1H-isochromen-1-thione) has been considered for evaluation of their cytotoxic effect on the H460 cancer cells by a propidium iodide assay. A quantitative structure–activity relationship has been developed between the cytotoxicity against H460 (at 0.1 μM) and the structural features of the compounds. Statistical measures such as r^2 (0.86), q^2 (0.58), pred-r^2 (0.94), and F-ratio (15.22) were found to be in an acceptable range.

13.1 INTRODUCTION

The 1H-isochromen-1-ones and their analogues possess a broad spectrum of pharmacological properties and contain b-unsaturated carbonyl group as a Michael acceptor, and an active moiety often employed in the design of anticancer drugs [1–10]. Based on the above facts and in continuation of our research interest [11–17], some 1H-isochromen-1-ones, their thio analogues were obtained and their anti-inflammatory activity has been evaluated by the production of lipopolysaccharide (LPS)-induced tumor necrosis factor-a (TNF-a) and interleukin-6 (IL-6). Similarly, the antiproliferative activity of such compounds has been assessed on the H460 (human large-cell lung carcinoma line). A quantitative structure–activity relationship (QSAR) model was developed between the structural properties of the 1H-isochromen-1-ones and their thio analogues and their cytotoxicity against H460 cell lines. The synthesized 1H-isochromen-1-ones, 1a-f and 1H-isochromen-1-thiones, 2a-f have been tested for their ability to inhibit tumor-promoting activity.

In overall, the present results on antiproliferation studies have suggested that 1H-isochromen-1-ones and 1H-isochromen-1-thiones could be effective anti-inflammatory and antiproliferative agents for lung cancer treatemt. This chemopreventive effect, may involve multiple mechanisms including induction of apoptosis and decrease in cell proliferation. Pretreatment with 1H-isochromen-1-oness and thio analogue decreased tumor development at a very low concentration (nmoles per application). However, it is possible that it may provide complete protection at relatively higher concentrations.

QSAR studies have also suggested that the growth inhibitory activity of 1H-isochromen-1-ones and their thio analogues (GI$_{50}$ at 0.1 μM concentration) is dependent on the size (molecular weight [MW]) and the topology (shape). The statistical measures for the QSAR model developed were found to be satisfactory for both the training (r^2, q^2, r^2adj, and F-ratio) and test set (pred-r^2) data. MW showed a negative contribution toward the activity which was also observed by other researchers too. MW is related to the diffusion of the compounds through the cell membrane. Thus, the QSAR study provides valuable input to design newer 1H-isochromen-1-ones and their thio analogues as growth inhibitory agents.

13.2 PHARMACOLOGY

The 1H-isochromen-1-ones, 1a-f and 1H-isochromen-1-thiones, 2a-f have been tested for their ability to inhibit tumor-promoting activity. Cell viability was monitored by propidium iodide assay. The IC_{50} values were calculated from curves by plotting suppression ratio (%) against the sample concentration. Each assay, as well as the whole experiment, was carried out in triplicates. The test samples 1a-f and 2a-f were also evaluated for their cytotoxicity in vitro against H460 (human large-cell lung carcinoma line). The 50% growth inhibition concentrations (GI_{50}) of these compounds were summarized. Showing that compounds 1a-f and 2a-f exhibited significant antitumor activity with moderate GI_{50} values. The GI_{50} values of the test samples were determined using the propidium iodide assay as described in the methods; values are mean ± standard deviations (SD) of the triplicate determination. The anti-inflammatory activity of the compounds was evaluated by the production of LPS-induced TNF-a and IL-6.

Growth inhibitory activity of the 1H-isochromen-1-ones and their thio analogues against the H460 cell line was measured at various concentrations namely, 0.1, 1, 10, and 30 µM. The QSAR model was developed for the cytotoxicity measured at the lowest concentration (0.1 µM). The growth inhibitory or cytotoxicty of the compounds (GI_{50}) was converted to $-\log (GI_{50})$ in order to facilitate the development of the regression model. The structure of the 1H-isochromen-1-ones and their thio analogues were built and their energy was minimized using consistent valence force field (CVFF) using Cerius^2 software (Accelrys Inc., USA). Further, 249 physico-chemical properties or descriptors, which consist of electronic, quantum mechanical, topological, spatial, structural, and thermodynamic for these 12 structures were considered and evaluated using the software. Several reports about these descriptors were published earlier [18–20]. Genetic function approximation (GFA) statistical technique was used to select the appropriate descriptors from this large pool of 249 descriptors for developing the regression model.

The quality of the regression models were tested using various statistical parameters such as r^2, r^2 adj, cross-validated r^2 (q^2), pred-r^2 (for test set), F-ratio, predicted residual sum of squares (PRESS), and standard error of estimate. The best QSAR equation was selected from this set of regression models [21, 22].

The total of 12 compounds was divided into training and test sets. The former had eight and later consisted four of compounds (1b, 1f, 2a, and 2b). The former was used to build the QSAR model and the later was used to test the predictive ability of the equation; this approach is known as external validation method.

13.3   RESULTS AND DISCUSSION

All the tested 1H-isochromen-1-ones, 1a-f showed dose-dependent cytotoxicity toward H460 cell line (**Figure. 1**). The activities were found to be significant, inhibiting the growth at even low concentration. Compound 1c was found to be most potent as its IC_{50} is 0.12 μM. At the concentration of 10 μM, the cell death was 77%; however, at higher concentration (30 μM) the cell death remained the same. The IC_{50} for 1e was 1.18 μM and at the concentration of 30 μM the cell death was determined as 92% when compared with the control. The compound, 1e has high potency in the growth inhibition even though the IC_{50} was comparatively less than 1c. The compound 1f also showed a significant cytotoxicity with an IC_{50} value of 17.2 μM and 75% cell death at a concentration of 30 μM. Compounds 1b and 1d showed 23 and 26.3 μM as IC_{50}, respectively. The cell death was 55% for 1b and 53% for 1d at 30 μM. Among the tested compounds, the 1a was less toxic and the maximum toxicity observed was 54% at 10 μM as well as at 30 μM.

		R
	a	CH_3
	b	C_6H_5
	c	$pCH_3C_6H_4$
	d	$pClC_6H_4$
	e	$pNO_2C_6H_4$
1a-f **2a-f**	f	$pOCH_3C_6H_4$

Of all the tested 1H-isochromen-1-thiones, strongest cytotoxicity was observed in 2b (**Figure. 2**). The cytotoxicity was evaluated as concentration and time dependent inhibitory effect on the growth of H460 cells. The concentration of 2b inhibiting 50% of the H460 cells was 5.7 μM. However, 40% cell death was observed when the concentration was increased to 30 μM. Morphological examination of the 2b treated cells showed a typical apoptotic characteristics such as cell shrinkage and membrane blabbing. The second most potent compound was 2d that showed a significant cytotoxicity toward H460 cells. The IC_{50} was found to be 12.5 μM and there was 75% cell death with 30 μM of 2d. Compounds 2c and 2a showed growth inhibition with an IC_{50} of 18.6 and 28.1 µM, respectively. However, compound 2c showed a strong cytotoxicity (72% cell death) with increased concentration (30 µM).

The anti-inflammatory activity of the compounds was evaluated by the production of LPS-induced TNF-a and IL-6 and the results indicate that the compounds inhibited the cytokine expression to various degrees (**Figures 3, 4**). The compound 1f is highly active in the inhibition of the cytokine production. The inhibition of TNF-a and IL-6 by 1f at 30 µM was found to be 92 and 97%, respectively. At 10 µM, the compound showed 90% inhibition of IL-6 which is significant. The compound 1b was also more potent in inhibiting the LPS-induced TNF-a and IL-6 expression. However, no IL-6 expression was observed in the enzyme-linked immunosorbent assay (ELISA) assay when the cells were treated with compound 1b at 30 µM, whereas the TNF-a production inhibition was found to be 81%. The compound showed similar activity as 1f and selectively inhibited the IL-6, but not TNF-a at a dose of 10 µM. Among other compounds, 1c and 1d are more potent in inhibiting LPS-induced IL-6 expression. The tested samples selectively inhibited the IL-6 at lower concentrations. At 30 µM the compounds showed better activity toward both TNF-a and IL-6. Compound 1d showed less inhibitory effects on TNF-a and there was no activity on IL-6 at all the concentrations tested. This compound showed activity at a concentration of 0.1 µM, but no activity was observed at 30 µM. The compound 1a had no activity at any of the concentrations tested.

Compounds 1f and 1b showed stronger inhibitory effect on IL-6 and moderate activity on TNF-a. Compound 1b showed the best inhibitory activity on IL-6. Compounds 1c and 1d also exhibited better inhibitory activity on LPS-induced IL-6 expression. The stronger inhibitory activity by the compounds indicates that these compounds could be favorable for the anti-inflammatory activity.

Among the 1H-isochromen-1-thiones, 2f showed strong inhibition toward TNF-a. At the concentration of 30 µM, the total inhibition was found to be 96%. However, no inhibition was observed at 0.1 µM. However, when the concentration increased to 1 µM the inhibition was found to be 15% and the same was 77% with 10 µM 2f. It also showed significant inhibition against IL-6 (61%). The 2b also showed a strong inhibitory activity against TNF-a and exhibited 91% inhibition with 30 µM 2b, whereas the inhibition was 81% with 10 µM 2b. However, it did not show any significant activity toward IL-6. Further, 30% inhibition was recorded with 30 µM 2b. The 2d showed inhibitory activity on both TNF-a and IL-6. At 30 µM concentration 2d inhibited respectively 66% and 90% against TNF-a and IL-6. The inhibitory effect of 2c against IL-6 was 85%, but no activity was observed for TNF-a round 30% inhibition was observed for 2a for both TNF-a and IL-6. No activity was found with the compound 2e.

The cytotoxicity of the synthesized compounds was evaluated by growth in-hibition of H460 cells. **Figures 1 and 2** show the cytotoxicity of the compounds with IC_{50} value. The sensitivity of the H460 cell lines to the tested compounds is relatively stronger. Prominent higher cytotoxicity was found in compound 2c; however, the toxicity was not increased at higher concentration. The compound 1e also showed excellent cytotoxicity toward H460 and dose dependently in-hibits the cell growth. The 1H-isochromen-1-ones series have shown strong cy-totoxicity and anti-inflammatory activity when compared with thio analogues. In general, all the tested compounds are toxic to the cells at any concentration tested, indicating the higher cytotoxicity of the compounds.

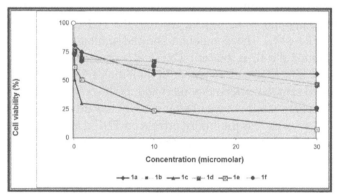

FIGURE 1   The in vitro cytotoxicity of 1H-isochromen-1-ones against H460 (human large-cell lung carcinoma line) cell viability versus the concentration of the compounds in hours, at increasing concentrations of secondary metabolite.

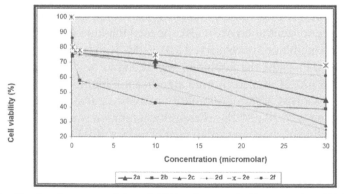

FIGURE 2   The in vitro cytotoxicity of 1H-isochromen-1-thiones against H460 (human large-cell lung carcinoma line) cell viability versus the concentration of the compounds in hours, at increasing concentrations of secondary metabolite.

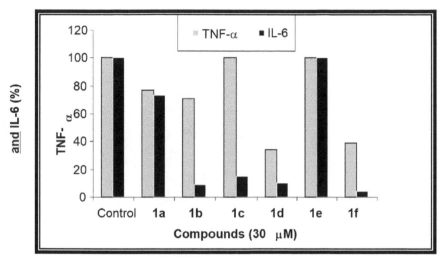

FIGURE 3 Anti-inflammatory activities of 1H-isochromen-1-ones were examined by measuring the inhibitory effect on LPS-induced TNF-a and IL-6 expression in TH1 cell lines using ELISA-based assay.

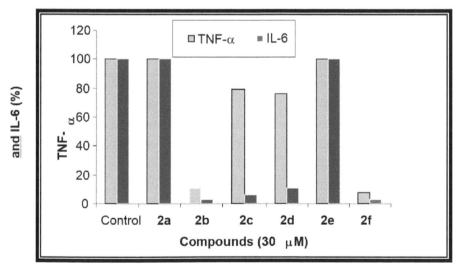

FIGURE 4 Anti-inflammatory activities of 1H-isochromen-1-thiones were examined by measuring the inhibitory effect on LPS-induced TNF-a and IL-6 expression.

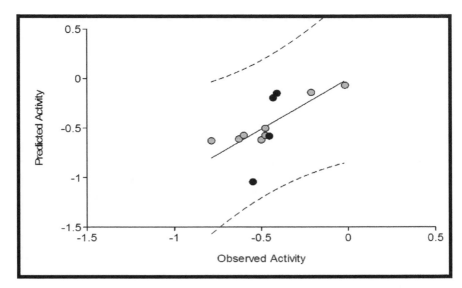

FIGURE 5 Pairty plot between observed H460 growth inhibition and model prediction (⊄-training set, ⊄-test set) (dotted lines indicate 99% confidence limits).

TABLE 1 Observed and predicted activities and descriptor values in QSAR for H460 cell line

Com- pound No.	Observed Activity ($-\log(GI_{50})$)	MW	Zagreb	Predicted Activity
1a	−0.62973	160.172	62	−0.60883
1b	−0.41017	222.2428	90	−0.14773
1c	−0.01737	236.2696	96	−0.06845
1d	−0.5006	256.6879	96	−0.6177
1e	−0.21261	267.2404	106	−0.14057
1f	−0.43196	252.269	100	−0.19444
2a	−0.54967	176.2326	62	−1.04086
2b	−0.45426	238.3034	90	−0.57976
2c	−0.47712	252.3302	96	−0.50048
2d	−0.47712	283.301	106	−0.5726
2e	−0.60206	283.301	106	−0.5726
2f	−0.78837	268.3296	100	−0.62647

In brief, in this report the cytotoxicity of the compounds was determined by PI assay on H460 cell lines and the anti-inflammatory activities were examined by measuring the inhibitory effect on LPS-induced TNF-a and IL-6 expression in TH1 cell lines using ELISA-based assay. The tested compounds have shown strong cytotoxic activity as well as an even better effect on TNF-a and IL-6 inhibition. However, the selective cytotoxicity of the compounds for cancer cell lines and the underlying mechanisms needs to be studied. In addition, the mechanism for the inhibition of LPS-induced TNF-a and IL-6 expression remains unknown. Nevertheless, the above findings suggest that the synthesized compounds have potential therapeutic effect as anticancer and anti-inflammatory activity, which requires further investigations in future. QSAR between growth inhibitory activity of 1H-isochromen-1-ones (GI_{50} at 0.1 µM concentration) and their thio analogues and their physico-chemical descriptors is given as follows:

$$H460 = -1.0184 - 0.0269*MW + 0.0761*Zagreb$$

$$n = 8, r^2 = 0.86, r^2adj = 0.80, q^2 = 0.58, \text{pred-}r^2_{\text{test set}} = 0.94, F\text{-ratio} = 15.22$$

The biparametric equation has two descriptors, the MW and Zagreb index (topology parameter) respectively, showing a negative and positive contribution toward the growth inhibitory activity. The cytotoxicty of these molecules is dependent on their permeability through the cell wall membrane. Researchers have proved that permeation through the stratum corneum depends on certain physico-chemical parameters including water solubility, octanol/water partition coefficient, and MW [23]. European Technical Guidance Documents (ETGD) also suggests that 100% dermal absorbance is obtained if the MW is less than 500 kDa. Hence, MW plays an important role in the absorption and penetration of drugs in cell lines.

Lipinski's rule of 5—a useful tool to find the drug likeliness property of active compounds—also suggested that the MW of the test samples should not exceed 500 kDa, and if it exceeds this limit, will lack permeability and solubility [24]. The current analysis also indicates that increasing MW decreases the activity, which may due to reduced permeability of high MW compounds. Further Camenisch et al., also stated that compounds with MW of 200 and 350 ± 150 kDa are able to diffuse without any restriction and MW approximately more than 500 kDa decreases membrane diffusion [25].

Zagreb is a topological descriptor. In general, topological indices are calculated based on graph theory concepts. These indices are used to differentiate and classify the molecule based on size, degree of branching, flexibility, and their overall shape [26].

Zagreb index is calculated using the following formula and is defined as the sum of the squares of vertex valencies [27].

$$\mathrm{Zagr} = \sum_i \delta_i^2$$

Other researchers also reported the contribution of topological descriptors toward anticancer activity of acridines [28–30]. **Table 1** lists the observed and predicted activities and descriptors involved in the QSAR for the training and test set compounds. **Figure 5** shows the comparison of observed and predicted growth inhibitory activity data (GI_{50} at 0.1 µM concentration).

13.4 EXPERIMENTAL

13.4.1 INSTRUMENTS AND CHEMICALS

The chemicals were purchased from Sigma–Aldrich and Merck, India and were used without any additional purification. All reactions were monitored by thin layer chromatography (TLC) on gel F254 plates. The silica gel (230–400 meshes) for column chromatography was purchased from Spectrochem Pvt. Ltd., India. Infrared (IR) spectra were recorded on Nucon Infrared spectrophotometer using KBr pellets. ^{1}H-NMR (400 MHz) and ^{13}C-NMR (100 MHz) spectra were recorded on a Bruker 400 MHz spectrometer in $CDCl_3$ or DMSO (with TMS for ^{1}H and DMSO for ^{13}C-NMR as internal references).

13.4.2 GENERAL PROCEDURE FOR THE PREPARATION OF 3-SUBSTITUTED 1H-ISOCHROMEN-1-ONES 1A-F

A mixture of homophthalic acid, (20 mmol) and acid chlorides (80 mmol) was heated under reflux at 200°C in an oil bath for 4 to 5 h. The completion of the reaction was monitored by TLC and then purified by column chromatography on silica gel using hexane and ethyl acetate as eluant. The product 3-substituted 1H-isochromen-1-ones were obtained in good yield and purity. The products were characterized by LC-MS, ^{1}H-NMR, and ^{13}C-NMR techniques and compared with our earlier report [14-17].

13.4.3 GENERAL PROCEDURE FOR THE PREPARATION OF 3-SUBSTITUTED 1H-ISOCHROMEN-1-THIONES 2A-F

Reaction of the 1H-isochromen-1-ones, 1a-f with the Lawesson reagent in a 1:1.2 molar ratio in toluene at reflux temperature results in an O/S-exchange at the carbonyl carbon atom with formation of the 1H-isochromen-1-thiones, 2a-f in good yield. The reaction proceeds smoothly and is complete within a maximum of 5 to 6 h. The product has been isolated by chromatography using hexane/EtOAc mixture (9:1). The solid obtained was characterized by LC-MS, ^{1}H-NMR, and ^{13}C-NMR techniques and compared with our earlier report [14–17].

13.4.4 ANTIPROLIFERATIVE ASSAY

PREPARATION OF STOCK SOLUTION

The lyophilized compound was used to prepare stock using distilled water (1 mg/mL) and filtered through 0.2 μm filter (Sartorius, India) to avoid contamination. The appropriate concentrations of the compounds were made by serial dilutions.

CELL CULTURE

H460 (human large-*cell* lung carcinoma *line)* was obtained from ATCC and maintained in RPMI 1640 (Invitrogen, India) medium supplemented with 10% FBS (v/v) and 100 mg/L streptomycin and 100 μg/mL penicillin (Himedia, India) at 37°C in a CO_2 incubator with 5% carbon dioxide.

13.4.5 CYTOTOXICITY BY PROPIDIUM IODIDE ASSAY

The cytotoxicity of the test samples in H460 cells were tested by propidium iodide assay as described earlier [31]. The compounds were diluted in 0.5% DMSO and the desired concentrations (0, 0.1, 1, 10, and 30 μg/mL) were made by diluting the stock solution with medium. The cells were seeded in 96-well plate (1×10^5 cells/well); the test samples were added and incubated for 48 h. After incubation, the medium was removed and 25 μL of propidium iodide (50 μg/mL in medium) was added into each well. The plates were frozen at –80°C for 24 h and were thawed at room temperature. Then readings were taken at 520 nm (excitation) and 620 nm (emission) using Magellan plate reader (Tecan). The cellular activity is proportional to the number of living cells. The wells with only culture medium or cells treated with 0.5% of DMSO served as control. The percentage of cytotoxicity was calculated using the formula

% cytotoxicity = OD control – OD treated/OD control × 100

A graph was plotted with cell viability against the concentration of the compounds, in hours at increasing concentrations of secondary metabolite. The mean and the IC_{50} values were calculated by nonlinear regression analysis using the data analysis software (Prism) from three independent experiments.

13.4.6   QUANTIFICATION OF CYTOKINES PRODUCTION

The cytokines were measured in THP-1 (human monocytic leukemia) cell line. The cells were cultured in 24 flat bottom plates at a concentration of 5×10^5 per ml of RPMI 1640 medium supplemented with 5% FBS. The cytokine release was induced by LPS (1 μg/ml). After incubation for 24 h (for TNF-α) or 48 h (for IL-6) the supernatants were collected and the cytokine concentrations were measured by ELISA-based assay in 96-well plates. The cytokine release was measured using TNF-OptEIA set and IL-6-OptEIA set (both from BD Pharmingen, San Diego, CA, USA). The user manual was followed for the assays, and the percentage inhibition was calculated using the formula

$$\text{OD induced} - \text{OD test/OD induced} \times 100$$

A standard curve was run on each assay plate using recombinant TNF-α and IL-6 in serial dilutions and the results were expressed in picogram per milliliter. The kits were specific to TNF-α and IL-6 and do not measure other.

13.5   CONCLUSION

QSAR studies have also suggested that the growth inhibitory activity of 1H-isochromen-1-ones and their thio analogues (GI_{50} at 0.1 μM concentration) is dependent on the size (MW) and the topology (shape). The statistical measures for the QSAR model developed were found to be satisfactory for both the training (r^2, q^2, r^2adj, and F-ratio) and test set (pred-r^2) data.

ACKNOWLEDGMENTS

The authors thank the VIT University for their support and facilities.

KEYWORDS

- 1H-isochromen-1-one
- 1H-isochromen-1-thione
- Anti-proliferative agents
- Cell growth, QSAR.

REFERENCES

1. Indian Council of Medical Research, Annual Report, 2003, www.icmr.nic.in.
2. L.W. Wattenberg, Chemoprevention of cancer by naturally occurring and synthetic compounds, in: L.W. Wattenberg, M. Lipkin, C. Boone and G.Kelloff, (Eds.), Cancer Prevention, CRC Press, Boca Raton, New york, 1992, pp. 19–39.
3. B. Haefner, *Drug Discov. Today* 8, (2003) 536.
4. H. Fahmy, S.I. Khalifa, T. Konoshima, and J.K. Zjawiony. Mar. Drugs 2, (2004) 1–7.
5. H. Fahmy, J.K. Zjawiony, T. Konoshima, H. Tokuda, S. Khan and S.Khalifa. Mar. Drugs 4, (2006) 28–36.
6. V. Kundoor, X. Zhang, S. Khalifa, H. Fahmy and C. Dwivedi. Mar. Drugs 4, (2006) 274.
7. P. Traxler and P. Furet. Pharmacol. Ther. 82, (1999) 195–206.
8. A.J. Bridges. Chem. Rev. 101, (2001) 2541–2550.
9. R.M. Myers, N.N. Setzer, A.P. Spada, P.E. Persons, C.Q. Ly, M.P. Maguire, A.L. Zulli, D.L. Cheney, A. Zilberstein, S.E.Johnson, C.F. Franks anf K.J. Mitchell. Bioorg. Med. Chem. Lett. 7, (1997) 421–424.
10. Y. D.Wang, K. Miller, D.H. Boschelli, F. Ye, B. Wu, M.B. Floyd, D.W. Powell, A. Wissner, J.M. Weber and F. Boschelli. Bioorg. Med. Chem. Lett. 10, (2000) 2477–2480.
11. Nitin T. Patil, F. Nawaz Khan and Y.Yamamoto. Tetrahedron Lett. 45, (2004) 8497–8499.
12. F. Nawaz Khan, R.Jayakumar and C. N. Pillai. J. Mol. Cat. A, Chemical, 195, (2003)139–145.
13. F. Nawaz Khan, R. Jayakumar and C. N. Pillai. Tetrahedron Lett. 43, (2002) 6807–6809.
14. S. Syed Tajudeen and F. Nawaz Khan. Synth. Commun. 37, (2007) 3649–3656.
15. Venkatesha R. Hathwar, P. Manivel, F. Nawaz Khan and T. N. Guru Row. Acta Cryst. E, 63, (2007) 03707.
16. Venkatesha R. Hathwar, P. Manivel, F. Nawaz Khan and T. N.Guru Row. Acta Cryst. E, 63, (2007) 03708.
17. Venkatesha R Hathwar, P. Manivel, F. Nawaz Khan and T. N. Guru Row. Crysteng. Comm. **11, (2009) 284–291.**
18. R.Todeschini, M.Lasagni and E. Marengo. J. Chemom. 8, (1994)263–273.
19. R.Todeschini and V. Consonni, (2000) Handbook of Molecular Descriptors. Wiley-VCH, Weinheim.
20. M. Karelson (2000) Molecular Descriptors in QSAR/QSPR. Wiley Interscience, New York.
21. P. M. Sivakumar, G. Sheshayan and M. Doble. Chem. Biol. Drug. Des. 72, (2008) 303–313.
22. P.M. Sivakumar, S. Prabu Seenivasan, Vanaja Kumar and Mukesh Doble. Bioorg. Med. Chem. Lett., 17, **(2007)** 1695–1700.
23. http://home.planet.nl/~wtberge/qsarperm.html (11.04.2011).
24. C. A. Lipinski, F. Lombardo, B. W. Dominy and P.J. Feeney. Adv. Drug Deliv. Rev. 46, (2001) 3–26.
25. G. Camenisch, J Alsenz, H van de WaterbeemdandG Folkers. Eur. J. Pharm. Sci. 6, **(1998)** 313–319.
26. B. Debnath, S. Gayen, S. Bhattacharya, S. Samanta and T. Jha. Bioorg. Med. Chem. 11, **(2003)** 5493–5499.
27. L.B. Kier, and L.H.Hall. Molecular connectivity indices in chemistry and drug research, in: G. deStevens (Eds.), Medicinal Chemistry, Vol 14, Academic Press, New York, (1976).
28. D.Bonchev. Information Theoretic Indices for Characterization of Chemical Structures, in: D.D. Bawden (Eds.), Chemometrics Series, Vol 5, Research Studies Press Ltd, New York, (1983).
29. A. Thakur, M. Thakur, N. Kakani, A. Joshi, S. Thakur and A. Gupta. ARKIVOC 14, (2004) 36–43.
30. N.S.H.N. Moorthy, C. Karthikeyan and P. Trivedi. Indian J. Chem. 46B, (2007) 177–184.
31. K. Wrobel, E. Claudio, F. Segade, S. Ramos and P.S. Lazo. J. Immun. Methods, 189, (1996) 243–249.

CHAPTER 14

QSAR STUDIES ON DIHYDROFOLATE REDUCTASE ENZYME: FROM MODEL TO BIOLOGICAL ACTIVITY

RAJESH RENGARAJAN[1], GARIMA MATHUR [2], ANU SHARMA[2], PONNURENGAM M.SIVAKUMAR[3], and SUMITRA NAIN[2]

[1]Chemistry Department, Faculty of Science, North Jeddah, King Abdulaziz University P. O. Box 80205, Jeddah 21589, Saudi Arabia

[2]Department of Pharmacy, Banasthali University, Banasthali 304022, Rajasthan, India

[3]FPR, Nanomedical Engineering Lab, RIKEN, Wako, Japan

E-mail: nainsumitra@gmail.com; Fax: +91-1438-228365; Tel.: +91-1438-228341 Extn. 348

CONTENTS

ABSTRACT

Dihydrofolate reductase (DHFR) is an enzyme that has a role in the synthesis of tetrahydrofolate and is used as a target for antineoplastic, antiprotozoal, antifungal, and antimicrobial action. The nicotinamide adenine dinucleotide phosphate-dependent reduction of dihydrofolate to tetrahydrofolate by catalysis of DHFR inhibitors plays an essential role in the synthesis of numerous amino acids. In this chapter, a quantitative structure–activity relationship study on dihydroreductase inhibitors is included.

14.1   INTRODUCTION

Chemotherapy is an essential way of controlling infectious diseases and cancer. Cancer chemotherapy is a novel molecularly intended therapeutics, which is vastly selective and not associated with the severe toxicities of predominant cytotoxic drugs [1]. Methotrexate is an antimetabolite and antifolate drug developed by Yellapragada Subbarao. Methotrexate originated to swap the more toxic antifolate aminopterin in the 1950s. Methotrexate competitively inhibits dihydrofolate reductase (DHFR) enzyme. Methotrexate binding on DHFR enzyme was significantly used to develop drugs for the cancer treatment and is also constructive in the treatment of acute lymphocytic leukemia [2]. Methotrexate, a folate analogue is used in the prevention of acute lymphoblastic leukemia, ovarian cancer, osteosarcoma, rheumatoid arthritis, psoriasis, inflammatory bowel disease, and for prevention of graft-versus-host disease after transplantation [3]. DHFR enzyme converts dihydrofolate to tetrahydrofolate and is used as a target by antineoplastic, antiprotozoal, antifungal, and antimicrobial drugs [4]. The nicotinamide adenine dinucleotide phosphate (NADPH)-dependent reduction of dihydrofolate to tetrahydrofolate by catalysis of DHFR enzyme has role in synthesis of numerous amino acids, thymidylate, and purine. The DHFR enzyme inhibitors namely pyrimethamine, trimethoprim, and diaveridine have only effect on parasite growth inhibition and sometimes produce side effects in acquired immune deficiency syndrome (AIDS) patients. DHFR enzyme inhibitors used in combination with macrolide are effective against the inhibition of *Plasmodium carinii* and the in vitro activity of alone lytic peptides [5]. Some combinations like pyrimethamine and sulfonamide, now effectual against toxoplasmosis especially in case of immunosuppressed patients and also effective against *P. falciparum* in Haiti due to enlargement of resistance to chloroquine [6]. The valuation of dihydrofolate synthetase or its combination with DHFR enzyme resulted in redundancy against the treatment of malaria parasite in Haiti [7]. This is because methotrexate resistant DHFR enzymes are different from the normal human cell DHFR enzyme [8].

14.2   STRUCTURE

Molecular weight of DHFR is 18,000–20,000 Da and it is relatively a water soluble protein synthesized on the activation of human DHFR located on q22 region of chromosome no. 5 as shown in **Figure 1**.

In general DHFR enzyme as shown in **Figure 2** is about 1000-fold of folate in the central eight-stranded b-pleated sheet that is responsible for the polypeptide backbone folding of DHFR [9]. The structure consists of seven strands in parallel positions and eight run in antiparallel positions. Four a-helices are connected with b-strands [10]. Residues 9–24 are termed "Met20" or "loop 1" and, along with other loops, form part of the major subdomain that surrounds the active site [11]. The active site was situated in the N-terminal half of the sequence, which includes a conserved Pro Trp dipeptide; however, the tryptophan has been shown to be involved in the binding of substrate by the enzyme [12].

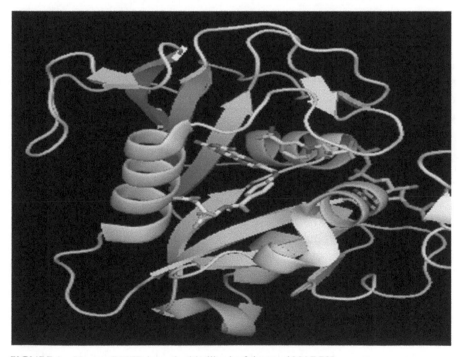

FIGURE 1   Human DHFR bound with dihydrofolate and NADPH.

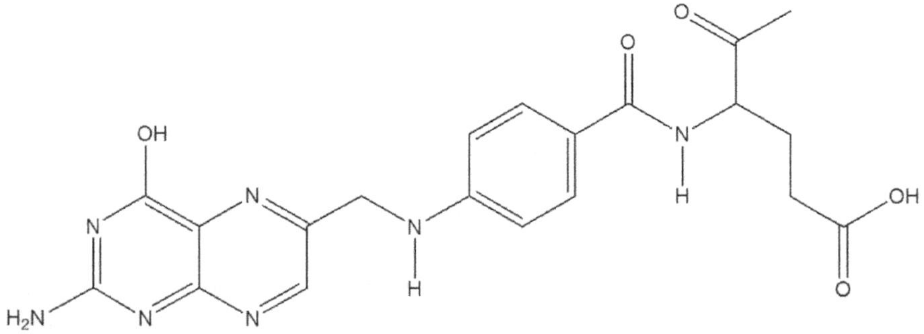

FIGURE 2   Dihydrofolatereductase.

14.2.1   CLASSIFICATION OF DHFR INHIBITORS

DHFR inhibitors are further classified into two groups as classical and nonclassical antifolate. The classical antifolate bear p-aminobenzoyl glutamic acid side chain, example is methotrexate, the nonclassical antifolate has a lipophilic side chain.

14.2.1.1   CLASSICAL DHFR INHIBITORS

The structural activity of classical dihydrofolate inhibitors is similar to folic acid. These groups are based on aspteridines, aryl, and a glutamic group. These types of substances have intracellular enzyme folylpolyglutamyl synthetase that is well known as polyglutamated form and responsible for DHFR inhibition. For example, methotrexate is N-{4-[[(2, 4-diamino-6-pteridyl) methyl]-N10-methylamino]} benzoyl glutamic acid as shown in **Figure 3**.

14.2.1.2   NONCLASSICAL DHFR INHIBITORS

The nonclassical DHFR inhibitors are more potent analogues that have lipophilic side chains, and are developed to overcome side effects of classical antifolate. They generally consist of diaminopyrimidine moiety, an aryl moiety, and a pteridine moiety.

14.2.2 STRUCTURE OF DHFR INHIBITORS

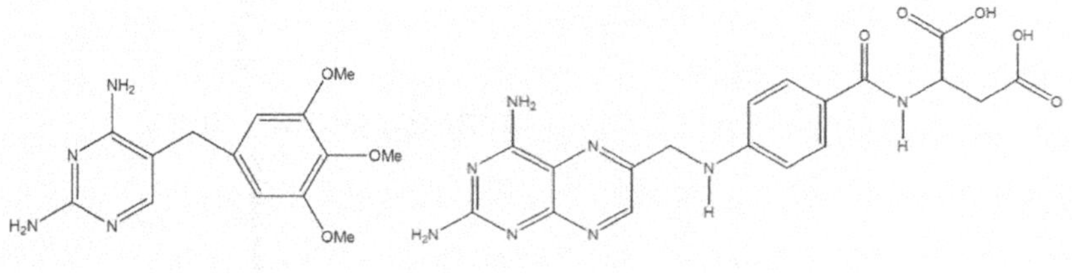

Trimethoprim methotrexate

FIGURE 3 Structure of DHFR inhibitors.

14.2.3 FUNCTIONS OF DHFR

DHFR inhibitor converts the dihydrofolate to the active tetrahydrofolate. The NADPH-dependent reduction of dihydrofolate to tetrahydrofolate by the catalysis of DHFR inhibitor has a role in the synthesis of several amino acids, thymidylate and purine as shown in **Figures 4 and 5**. DHFR is about 1000-fold compared to folate and folic acid and is essential for the de novo synthesis of the nucleoside thymidine, required for the DNA synthesis. Due to these types of folate coenzyme in the biosynthesis of nucleic acids, the biosynthetic pathways and folate have been recognized as targets in cancer chemotherapy. Tetrahydrofolate plays a key role in cell development and also can be used in the synthesis of nucleic acid precursor. DHFR-like genes have been identified on separate chromosomes and functional DHFR gene has been mapped to chromosome 5, multiple introns less processed pseudogenes [13].

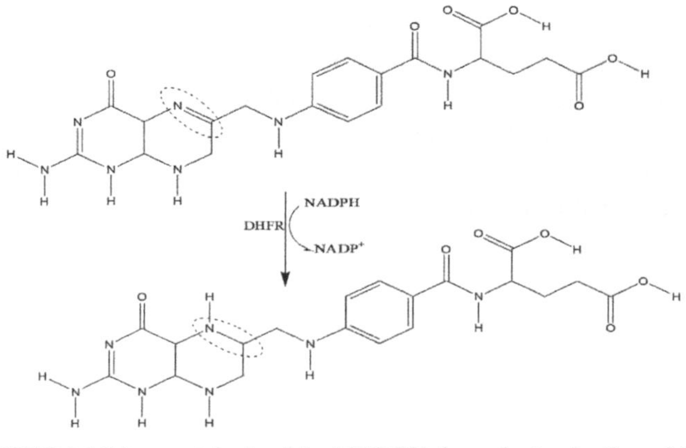

FIGURE 4 DHFR inhibitors catalysis of the NADPH-dependent reduction of dihydrofolate to tetrahydrofolate [13].

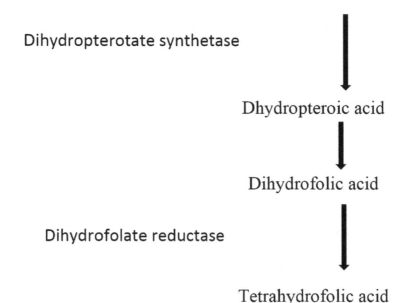

Dihydropterotate synthetase

Dhydropteroic acid

Dihydrofolic acid

Dihydrofolate reductase

Tetrahydrofolic acid

FIGURE 5   The pathway of formation of tetrahydrofolic acid[14].

14.2.4 MECHANISM OF ACTION OF DHFR

DHFR has a role in the reduction of 7,8-dihydrofolate (DHF) to 5,6,7,8-tetra-hydrofolate (THF) by the transfer of NADPH cofactor to the C_6 atom of protein ring with protonation of N_5 atom as shown in **Figure 6.**

7,8-Dihydrofolate + NADPH + H $\longrightarrow$ 5, 6, 7, 8-tetrahydrofolate + NADP

DHFR converts the dihydrofolate that produce tetrahydrofolate [15] as shown in **Figure 6** and at the end NADPH is oxidized to $NADP^+$ and dihydrofolate is reduced to tetrahydrofolate. The active site is essential for promoting the release of the product, tetrahydrofolate. The Met20 loop helps to stabilize the nicotinamide ring of the NADPH to promote the transfer of hydride from NADPH to dihydrofolate [16].

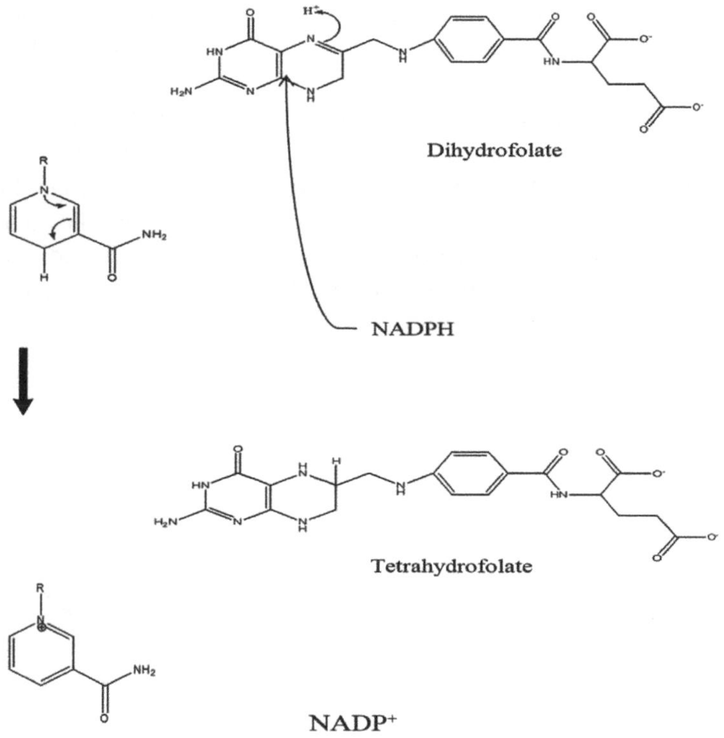

FIGURE 6   The reaction mechanism of dihydrofolate that reduced to tetrahydrofolate and NADPH is oxidized to NADP+ [16].

14.2.5 THERAPEUTIC APPLICATION AND DISEASE APPLICABILITY

DHFR can be targeted in the treatment of cancer which is responsible for the levels of tetrahydrofolate in a cell, and the inhibition of DHFR can result in inhibition of growth and proliferation of cells that are characteristics of cancer. Methotrexate is a competitive inhibitor of DHFR, and is only one among many other anticancer drugs that inhibits DHFR [17]. Some other drugs trimethoprim and pyrimethamine can be used as antitumor and antimicrobial agents [18].

Trimethoprim is effective againsta number of varieties of Gram-positive bacterial pathogens [19]. However, resistance of trimethoprim and some other DHFR inhibitors, may arise due to variety of mechanisms, limiting the success of their therapeutically uses [20, 21]. Resistance due to mutations in DHFR enzyme decreases in the uptake of the drugs, DHFR enzyme gene amplification, among others. Trimethoprim and sulfamethoxazole combination has been used as an antibacterial agent [22].

For cell growth folic acid is required and the metabolic pathway for synthesis of folic acid can be used for the development new anticancer drugs [23]. DHFR enzyme was effectively used for targeted-anticancer drugs. Fluorouracil, doxorubicin, and methotrexate as shown in **Figure 7** were shown to prolong survival in patients with advanced gastric cancer [24]. Further studies on DHFR enzyme inhibitors can help to develop new drugs for the treatment of cancer.

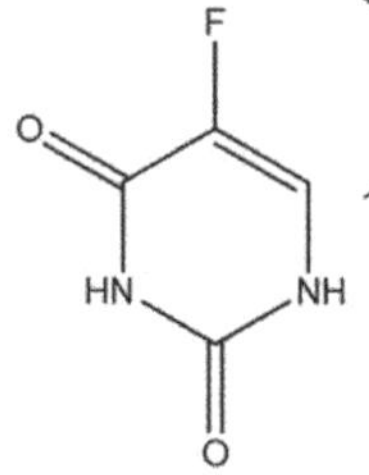

Fluorouracil

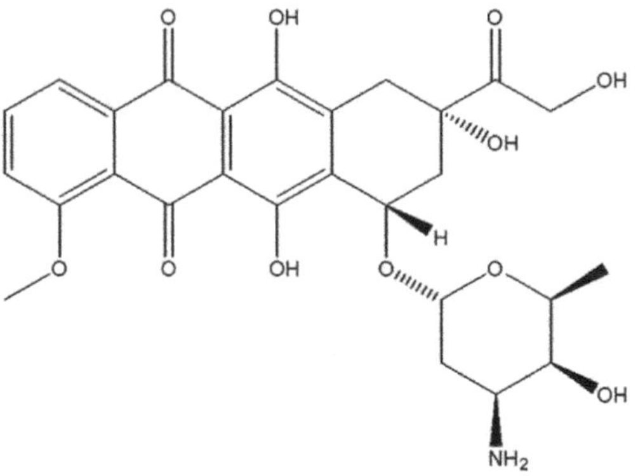

Doxorubicin

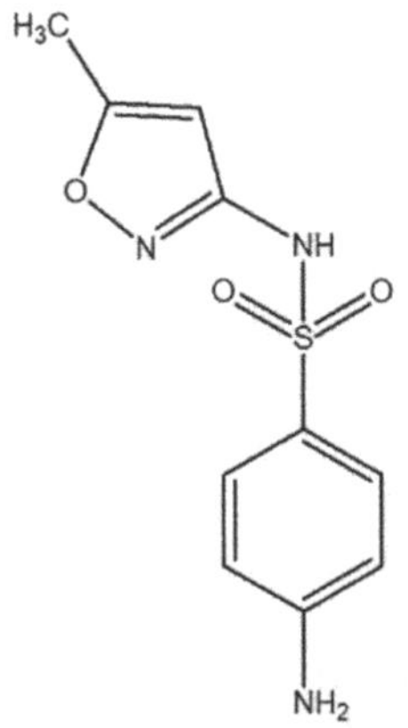

Sulfamethoxazole

FIGURE 7   Some drugs that are inhibitor of DHFR.

A large number of molecules have been formulated by clinical importance of DHFR, which stimulated a great deal of work in several fields.

Quantitative structure–activity relationship (QSAR) and quantitative structure–property relationships (QSPRs) are mathematical models that relate the structure derived from a compound to its biological or physico-chemical activity. These physico-chemical descriptors include parameters for hydrophobicity, topology, electronic properties, and steric effects. These descriptors are determined empirically or, more recently, by computational methods. Other techniques included quantitative structure–toxicity relationship (QSTR) and quantitative structure–pharmacokinetic relationship (QSPkR). QSAR works on structurally similar compounds with similar activity, to predict the biological activity (e.g., IC50) as shown in **Figure 8.** QSAR models starts with the collection of data and necessary to exclude low-quality data, as they will lower the quality of the model.

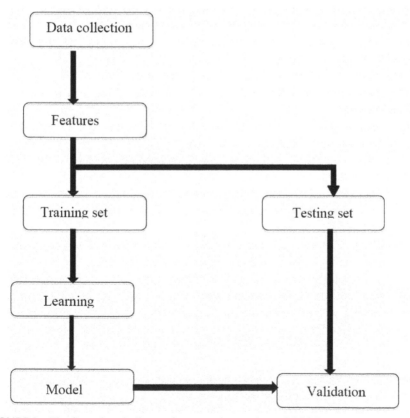

FIGURE 8   The flow chart indicates the general procedure of QSAR.

14.3   QSAR

(a) Biological activity

In QSAR analysis, a data set of a series of synthesized molecules is tested for its desired biological activity which is valid and reliable for QSAR. The quality of the model is totally dependent on the quality of the experimental data that are used for building the model.

Biological activity can be of two types:

1. Continuous response: MEC, IC50, ED50, and % inhibition
2. Categorical response: Active/inactive

(b) Molecular descriptors

Molecular descriptors are numerical representations of chemical information encoded within a molecular structure via mathematical procedure.

(c) Selection of training and test set

QSAR models are used to determine the chemical databases or virtual chemical libraries for potentially bioactive molecules. These developments emphasize the importance of rigorous model validation to ensure that the models have both the ability to explain the variance in the biological activity and also the acceptable predictive power.

For model validation, the data set is required to be divided into training and test sets. The following methods are used for division of the data set into training and test sets:

1.   Manual selection: These can be achieved by visualizing the variation in the chemical and biological space of the given data set.
2.   Random selection: The method creates training and test set by random distribution.
3.   Sphere exclusion method: It is a rational method for the creation of training and test sets. It ensures uniform distribution with respect to chemical and biological space.
4.   Others: Experimental design, onion design, cluster analysis, principal component analysis, andself-organizing maps (SOM).
5.   Variable selection methods: There many types of molecular descriptors, but not all the descriptors are useful in determining biological activity. Hence, a variable selection method is required to find the optimal subset of the descriptors having important role in determining biological activity. These variables are divided into two categories as explained in the following:
6.   Systematic variable selection: These methods add and/or delete a descriptor in steps one-by-one in a model.
7.   Stochastic variable selection: This method is based on physical or biological processes. It's a created model starting from randomly generated

model(s) and later modifying these model(s) by using different process operator(s) (e.g., perturbation, crossover, etc.).

Statistical methods

This type of method allows analyses of data in order to establish a QSAR model with the subset of descriptors that is statistically significant in determining biological activity.

(f) Validate the equation

Cross-validation technique is used to evaluate validity of a model which predicts data rather than how well it will fit data.

(g) Predict the biological activity

From the developed QSAR model, the biological activity of proposed compounds can be calculated.

In this review, study is focused on structure-based drug design of DHFR inhibitors.

14.4   QSAR STUDY ON DHFR INHIBITORS

QSAR models are highly effective to calculate structural basis of biological activity. A lot of research work has been carried out by different research groups on QSAR studies of DHFR inhibition by different compounds.

T. Timothy. Myoda et al., (1984) performed an assignment on human DHFR gene to the qll >q22 region of chromosome 5 and done the cytogenetic and biochemical analyses of these clones which have shown that the human DHFR gene is located on chromosome 5. Three of these hybrid cell lines contained different terminal deletions of chromosome 5. An analysis of the breakpoints of these deletions has demonstrated that the DHFR gene resides in the qll-q22 region [25].

Selassie et al., (1986) studied QSAR activity on a series of benzylpyrimidines and performed QSAR study on inhibition of chicken liver DHFR [26].

Booth and his co-workers (1987) worked with QSAR study on the cell growth and inhibition of *Leishmania* DHFR by triazines [27].

Selassie et al., (1989) reported QSAR result on inhibition of DHFR from *Lactobacillus casei* and chicken liver by diaminopyrimidines [28] and that of *E. coli* by benzyl pyrimidine [29]. Selassie and co-workers also reported QSAR study on inhibition of leukemia 1210 (L1210) DHFR by triazines [30].

Pineda et al., (2003) performed a study on exceptional resistance to methotrexate but not to trimetrexate of mutant DHFR. They found that mutant DHFR was catalytically active and resistant to methotrexate, bis-methotrexate, and PT 523 but not trimetrexate [31].

Senkovich *et al.,* (2005) studied that the lipophilic antifolate of trimetrexate is potent against trypanosomacruziin in chagas disease. It is an Food and Drug Administration (FDA)-approved drug used in the treatment of *Pneumocystis carinii* infection in AIDS patients [32].

Kashkedikar *et al.,* (2005) performed QSAR analysis of pyrimidine derivatives as DHFR inhibitors and suggest that molecules are able to interact with electron-rich area at the receptor site. DPL_3 is related to the molecular charge distribution in Z-component. These electronic parameters can be altered through the incorporation of electronegative groups [33].

Hikaru Saito and co-workers (2006) studied QSAR analysis on a new strategy of high-speed screening to evaluate human ATP (adenosine triphosphate)-binding cassette transporter ABCG2–drug interactions. Basically this strategy was considered effective and can be used for the molecular designing of new ABCG2 modulators [34].

Hachet *et al.,* (2008) identified the best QSAR model using MOE descriptors and nonlinear models optimized by evolutionary computation. These models were used to identify key descriptors for DHFR inhibition and are useful for the high-throughput screening of novel drug leads [35].

Patel *et al.,* (2011) studied *in silico* 2-D QSAR based on the certain topological and constitutional descriptors. Methotrexate is a DHFR inhibitor that can be used for the treatment of rheumatoid arthritis. But due to potential neurotoxicity, patients had to terminate their chemotherapy. In this survey, DHFR inhibitors were structurally similar to methotrexate with biological activity in *Toxoplasma gondii* and *L. casei* [36].

Goodey *et al.,* (2011) worked on conformational changes associated with inhibitor binding in the development of a fluorescently labeled thermo stable DHFR. DHFR is used to determine the kinetic and protein conformational changes with the methotrexate binding and provides a new tool for flurophore with sensitive *Bacillus starothermophillus* [37].

NutanPrakash *et al.,* performed QSAR analysis on antimalarial drugs as shown in **Figure 9**. They recognized a proguanil using Argus lab and Hex software and found that some of the modified analogues are better than the commercially marketed drugs [38].

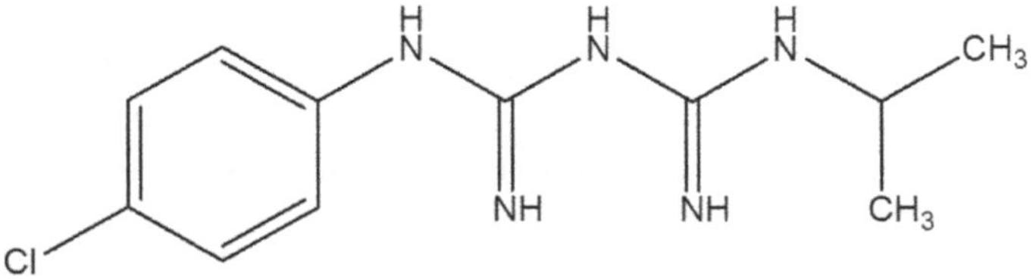

FIGURE 9   Proguanil.

Srivastava *et al.,* optimized a molecular docking approach, resulting in a reliable and good correlation coefficient model and IC_{50} values by a new shape-based method [39].

Adane and Bharatam (2011) performed *in silico* study using computer-aided molecular design approach that involved molecular orbital and density functional theory calculations, along with molecular electrostatic potential analysis, and molecular docking studies to design 1H-imidazole-2,4- diamine derivatives as potential inhibitors of Pf-DHFR (Pf-*P. falciparum*) enzyme. Visual inspection of the compounds demonstrated that all interact via H-bond interactions, with key amino acid residues (Asp54, Asn/Ser108, Ileu/Leu164, and Ile14) similar to WR99210 as shown in **Figure 10** in the active site of the enzymes used in the study. These interactions are known to be essential for enzyme inhibition. Using TOPKAT software *in silico* toxicity study was performed that showed that the compounds are nontoxic [40].

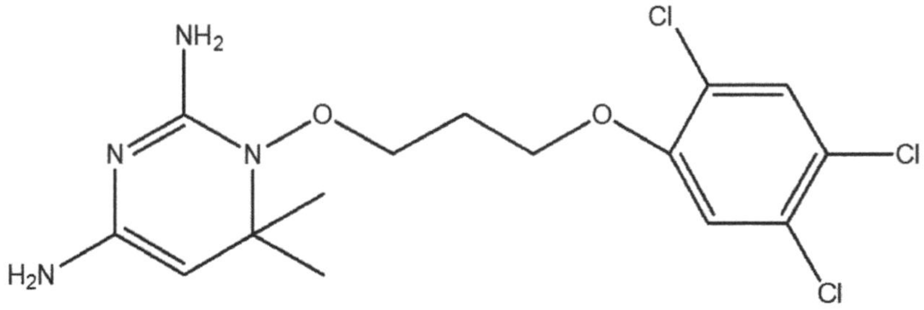

FIGURE 10   WR99210.

A newly potent and small-peptide inhibitors, as shown in **Figure 11**, against *Mycobacterium tuberculosis* DHFR can be used *in silico* structure-based approach for antituberculosis drugs discovery because of small difference between the human DHFR and *Mycobacterium* DHFR active site. The difference was effective for designing of new class of antitubercular drugs. Docking study on the designed tripeptide inhibitors indicated that compounds have high potency and selectivity. Due to recent advances in the drug delivery technique, the opportunities for peptide drug development are significantly enhanced. Thus the designing of small peptides can be done using structure-based approach with the help of crystal structure of *M. tuberculosis* DHFR complex with NADPH and methotrexate and human DHFR complexes NADPH with PT523 [41].

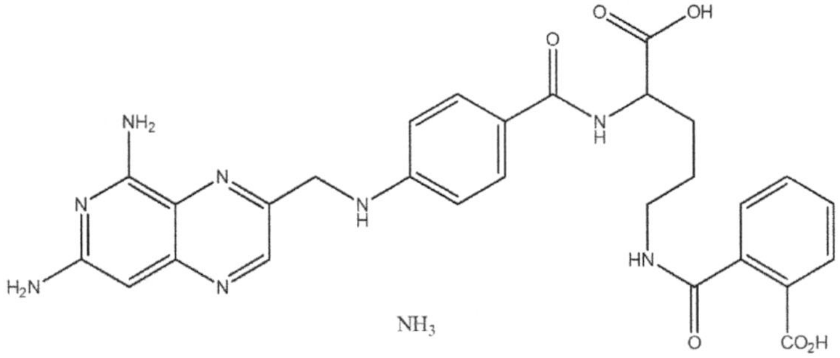

PT 523

FIGURE 11   PT523.

3D QSAR analysis of ligand–receptor binding models using free energy for the 18 structurally different compounds like pyrimethamine, cycloguanil, methotrexate, aminopterin, and trimethoprim shown in **Figures 12 and 13** pyrrolo [2,3-d] pyrimidine's were done. 3D QSAR analysis enabled calculation of important descriptors and structural features that are relevant to resistance of current antimalarial drugs [42].

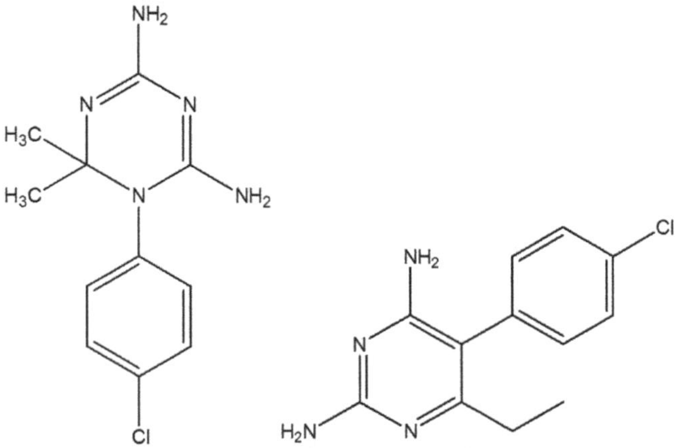

CycloguanilPyrimethamine

FIGURE 12   Structure of some current antimalarial drugs.

The computational approach used to check the affinity and selectivity of 2,4-diaminopteridine and 2,4-diaminoquinazoline as inhibitors of DHFR. By molecular dynamic simulation, the binding energy was calculated by a force field evaluation and thermal sampling. The huge difference between pteridine and quinazoline binding strength was useful in new drug discovery for determination of binding energy of new inhibitors before synthesis [43].

Vijjulatha *et al.,* (2011) performed a study on a building bridge between the docking studies of homology modeled bovine DHFR proteinase as well as ligand- and target-based 3D-QSAR techniques of comparative molecular field analysis (CoMFA) and comparative similarity indices analysis (CoMSIA) [44].

Xiang Maa *et al.,* (2012) studied 3D-QSAR on dihydro-1,3,5-triazines and their spiro derivatives as DHFR inhibitors by CoMFA. Computational analyses resulted in a reliable model with the parameters that the steric and electrostatic properties predicted by CoMFA contours can be related to the DHFR inhibitory activity [45].

Gacchea *et al.,* (2013) studied *in silico* screening of chalcone derivatives as potential inhibitors of DHFR. Assessments using molecular docking of chalcone derivatives with human as well as Mycobacterial DHFR, followed by paired potential and hydrophobic potential analysis were carried out to understand the novel chalcone DHFR interactions [46].

El-Subbagh *et al.,* (2013) performed a molecular modeling study on non-classical antifolates of some new 2-heteroarylthio-quinazolin-4-ones for their in vitro DHFR inhibition, antimicrobial, and antitumor activities. This research group recognized that the two key amino acids, namely Arg38 and Lys31 are essential for the binding and biological activities. The obtained model could be useful for the development of new DHFR inhibitors revealed by the flexible alignment, that is, electrostatic and hydrophobic mappings [47].

Konda *et al.,* (2013) performed 3D-QSAR analysis of non-classical DHFR inhibitors by CoMFA and CoMSIA. 3D-QSAR relationship studies involve CoMFA and CoMSIA, performed using *P. carinii* pyridopyrimidine DHFR inhibitors to find out the structural relationship with the predicted activities. Designed compounds resulted nearly equal to that of potent series of compounds [48].

14.5   CONCLUSION

DHFR inhibitor catalyzes the NADPH-dependent reduction of dihydrofolate to tetrahydrofolate and is essential for the synthesis of several amino acids, thymidylate, and purine. DHFR plays an important role in various pathologic conditions like cancer and tuberculosis. DHFR has been used as target for antineoplastic, antiprotozoal, antifungal, and antimicrobial mechanisms. DHFR is considered as a potential target for the development of novel inhibitors analogues. The crystal structures of various DHFR strains are available and can be used in designing of rational inhibitors. Different approaches and designs of novel compound can achieve potent and selective inhibitors of DHFR. QSAR studies provide an important structural insight for designing of novel and potent DHFR inhibitors.

KEYWORDS

- **Chemotherapy**
- **DHFR**
- **NAPDH**
- **QSAR**

REFERENCES

1. Seymour, L. Novel anti-cancer agents in development: exciting prospects and new challenges. Cancer Treat Rev. 1999, 25, 301–312.
2. Meyer, Leo M.; Miller, Franklin R.; Rowen, Manuel J.; Bock, George; Rutzky, Julius. Treatment of Acute Leukemia with Amethopterin (4-amino, 10-methyl pteroyl glutamic acid). Acta Haematol. 1950, 4 (3), 157–167.
3. Ulrich, C.M.; Yasui, Y.; Storb, R.; *et al.,* Pharmacogenetics of methotrexate: toxicity among marrow transplantation patients varies with the methylenetetrahydrofolatereductase C677T polymorphism. Blood. 2001, 98(1), 231–234.
4. Abali, E.E.; Skacel, N.E.; HilalCelikkaya; Yi-Ching Hsieh. Regulation of human dihydrofolate reductase activity and expression vitamins and hormones. 79, 267–287.
5. Klepser, M.E.; Klepser, T.B. Drugs. 1997, 53, 40–73
6. Genestier, L.; Paillot, R.; Fournel, S.; Ferraro, C.; Miossec, P.; Revillard, J.P. Immunosuppressive properties of methotrexate: apoptosis and clonal deletion of activated peripheral T cells. J. Clin. Invest. 2014
7. Carter T.E.; Warner, M.; Mulligan1,C.J.; Existe, A.; Victor, Y.S.; Memnon, G.; Boncy, J.; Oscar, R.; Fukuda, M.M.; Okech, M.A. Evaluation of dihydrofolatereductase and dihydropteroatesynthetase genotypes that confer resistance to sulphadoxine-pyrimethamine in Plasmodium falciparum. Malaria J. 2012, 11, 275.
8. Chen, M.; Shimada, T.; Msoulton, A.; Cline, R.; Humphries, K. The functional human dihydrofolate reductase. Gene 1983, 259(6), 25.
9. Matthews, D.A.; Alden, R.A.; Bolin, J.T.; Freer, S.T.; Hamlin, R.; Xuong, N.; Kraut, J.; Poe, M.; Williams, M.; Hoogsteen, K. Dihydrofolatereductase: x-ray structure of the binary complex with methotrexate. Science. 1997, 197 (4302), 452–455.
10. Filman, D.J.; Bolin, J.T.; Matthews, D.A.; Kraut, J. Crystal structure of Escherichia coli and Lactobacillus caseidihydrofolatereductase refined at 1.7 A resolution. II. Environment of bound NADPH and implications for catalysis. J. Biol. Chem. 1982, 257 (22), 13650–13662.
11. Osborne, M.J.; Schnell, J.; Benkovic, S.J.; Dyson, H.J.; Wright, P.E. Backbone dynamics in dihydrofolate reductase complexes: role of loop flexibility in the catalytic mechanism. Biochemistry. 2001, 40 (33);9846–9859.
12. Bolin, J.T.; Filman, D.J.; Matthews, D.A.; Hamlin, R.C.; Kraut, J. Crystal structures of Escherichia coli and Lactobacillus caseidihydrofolatereductase refined at 1.7 A resolution. I. General features and binding of methotrexate. J. Biol. Chem. 1952, 257 (22); 13650–13662.

13. "Entrez Gene: DHFR dihydrofolatereductase".
14 Shinde, G.H, Pekamwar, S.S, Wadher, S.J. An overview on dihydrofolate reductase inhibitors. Int. J. Chem. Pharm. Sci. 2013, 4 (2).
15. Schnell, J.R.; Dyson, H.J.; Wright, P.E. Structure, dynamics, and catalytic function of dihydrofolatereductase. Ann. Rev. Biophys. Bio. Mol. Struct. 2004, 33 (1), 119–140.
16. Osborne, M.J.; Schnell, J.; Benkovic, S.J.; Dyson, H.J.; Wright, P.E. Backbone dynamics in dihydrofolate reductase complexes: role of loop flexibility in the catalytic mechanism. Biochemistry. 2001, 40 (33), 9846–9859.
17. Li, R.; Sirawaraporn, R.; Chitnumsub, P.; *et al.,* Three-dimensional structure of M. tuberculosis dihydrofolate reductase reveals opportunities for the design of novel tuberculosis drugs. J. Mol. Biol. 2000, 295 (2), 307–323.
18. Benkovic, S.J.; Fierke, C.A.; Naylor, A.M. Insights into enzyme function from studies on mutants of dihydrofolate reductase. Science. 1988, 239 (4844), 1105–1110.
19. Hawser, S.; Lociuro, S.; Islam, K.; Dihydrofolate reductase inhibitors as antibacterial agents. Biochem. Pharmacol. 2006, 71(7), 941–948.
20. Huennekens, F.M. In search of dihydrofolate reductase. Protein Sci. 1996, 5 (6), 1201–1208.
21. Banerjee, D.; Mayer-Kuckuk, P.; Capiaux, G.; Budak-Alpdogan, T.; Gorlick, R.; Bertino, J.R. Novel aspects of resistance to drugs targeted to dihydrofolate reductase and thymidylate synthase. Biochim. Biophys. Acta. 2002, 1587 (2–3), 164–173.
22. Hawser, S.; Lociuro, S.; Islam, K. Dihydrofolate reductase inhibitors as antibacterial agents. Biochem. Pharmacol. 2001, 71(7), 941–948.
23 http://www.ncbi.nlm.nih.gov/pmc/articles/PMC2730961/
24. Murad, A.M.; Santiago, F.F.; Petroianu, A.; Rocha, P.R.; Rodrigues, M.A.; Rausch, M. Modified therapy with 5-fluorouracil, doxorubicin, and methotrexate in advanced gastric cancer. 1993, 72 (1), 37–41.
25. Vicky, L; Funanage, T; Timothy Myoda, Priscilla, A; Moses, Henry, R; Cowell. Assignment of the human dihydrofolate reductase gene to the qll >q22 region of chromosome 5. Mol. Cell. Biol. 1984, 2010–2016.
26. Selassie, C.D.; Fang, Z.X.; Li, R.L.; Hansch, C.; Klein, D.; Langridge, R.; Kaufman, B.T. Inhibition of chicken liver dihydrofolate reductase by 5–(substituted benzyl)–2,4–diaminopyrimidines. A quantitative structure–activity relationship and graphics analysis J. Med. Chem. 1986, 29, 621–626.
27. Booth, R.G.; Selassie, C.D.; Hansch, C.; Santi, D.V. Quantitative structure–activity relationship of triazine– antifolate inhibition of Leishmania dihydrofolate reductase and cell growth. J. Med. Chem. 1987, 30, 1218–1224.
28. Selassie, C.D.; Fang, Z.X.; Li, R.L.; Hansch, C.; Klein, D.; Langridge, R.; Kaufman, B.T. On the structure selectivity problem in drug design. A comparative study of benzyl pyrimidine inhibition of vertebrate and bacterial dihydrofolate reductase via molecular graphics and quantitative structure–activity relationships. J. Med. Chem. 1989, 32, 1895–1905.
29. Selassie, C.D.; Li, R.L.; Poe, M.; Hansch, C. On the optimization of hydrophobic and hydrophilic substituent interactions of 2,4–diamino–5–(substituted–benzyl) pyrimidine's with dihydrofolatereductase. J. Med. Chem. 1991, 34, 46–54.
30. Selassie, C. D.; Strong, C.D.; Hansch, C.; Delcamp, T.J.; Freisheim, J.M.; Khwaja, T.M. Comparison of triazines as inhibitors of L1210 dihydrofolate reductase and of L1210 cells sensitive and resistant to methotrexate. Cancer Res. 1986, 46, 744–756.
31. Pineda, P.; Kanter, A.; Scott McIvor, R.; Benkovic, S.J.; Rosowsky, A.; Wagner, C.R. Dihydrofolate reductase mutant with exceptional resistance to methotrexate but not to trimetrexate. J. Med. Chem. 2003, 46, 2816–2818.
32. Senkovich, O.; Bhatia, V.; Garg, N.; Chattopadhyay, D. Lipophilic antifolate trimetrexate is a potent inhibitor of trypanosomacruzi: prospect for chemotherapy of Chagas disease. Antimicrob. Agents Chemother. 2005, 3234–3238.

33. Jain, P.; Soni, L.K.; Gupta, A.K. Kashkedikar, S.G. QSAR analysis of 2,4-diaminopyrido[2,3-d]pyrimidine's and 2,4-diaminopyrrolo[2,3-d]pyrimidine's as dihydrofolatereductase inhibitors. Indian J. Biochem. Biophys. 2005, 42, 315–320

34. Saito, H.; Hirano, H.; Nakagawa, H.; Fukami, T.; Oosumi, K.; Murakami, K.; Kimura, H.; Kouchi, T.; Konomi, M.; Tao, E.; Tsujikawa, N.; Tarui, S.; Nagakura, M.; Osumi, M.; Ishikawa, T. A new strategy of high-speed screening and quantitative structure-activity relationship analysis to evaluate human ATP-binding cassette transporter ABCG2-drug interactions. JPET 2006, 317(3), 1114–1124.

35. Hecht, D.; Cheung, M.; Fogel, G.B. QSAR using evolved neural networks for the inhibition of mutant PfDHFR by pyrimethamine derivatives. Bio Syst. 2008, 92, 10–15.

36. Patel, S.K.; Prasanth Kumar S.; Pandya H.A.; Jasrai, T.Y.; Patni, M.I.2D-QSAR analysis of dihydrofolate reductase (DHFR) inhibitors with activity in toxoplasma gondiiand lactobacillus casei. J. Adv. Bioinforma. Appl. Res. 2011, 2, 161–166.

37. Goodey, N.M.; Alapa, M.T.; Hagmann, D.F.; Korunow, S.G.; Mauro, A.K.; Kwon, K.S.; Hall, S.M. Development of a fluorescently labeled thermo stable DHFR for studying conformational changes associated with inhibitor binding. Biochem. Biophys. Res. Commun. 2011, 413, 442–447.

38. Prakash, N.; Patel, S.; Faldu, N.J.; Ranjan,R.; Sudheer, D.V.N. Molecular docking studies of antimalarial drugs for malaria. J. Comput. Sci. Syst. Biol. Available onwww.omicsonline.com.

39. Srivastava, V.; Kumar, A.; B.N. Mishra, M.I. Siddiqi. Molecular docking studies on DMDP derivatives as human DHFR inhibitors. Available on www.bioinformation.net.

40. Adane, L.; Bharatam, P.V. Computer-aided molecular design of 1Himidazole- 2,4diamine derivatives as potential inhibitors of plasmodium falciparum DHFR enzyme. J. Mol. Model. 2011, 17, 657–667.

41. Kumar, M.; Vijayakrishnan, R.; SubbaRao, G.; In silico structure-based design of a novel class of potent and selective small peptide inhibitor of Mycobacterium tuberculosis Dihydrofolate reductase, a potential target for anti-TB drug discovery. Mol. Divers. 2010, 14, 595–604.

42. Santos-Filho, O.A.; Mishra, R.K.; Hopfinger, A.J. Free energy force field (FEFF) 3D-QSAR analysis of a set of Plasmodium falciparum dihydrofolate reductase inhibitors. J. Comput.-Aided Mol. Des. 2001, 15, 787–810.

43. Mareliusa, J.; Graffner-Nordbergb, M.; Hanssona, T.; Hallbergb, A.; Åqvist, J. Computation of affinity and selectivity: binding of 2, 4-diaminopteridine and 2, 4- diaminoquinazoline inhibitors to dihydrofolate reductases. J. Comput.-Aided Mol. Des. 1998, 12, 119–131

44. Yamini, L.; MeenaKumari, K.; Vijjulatha, M. Molecular docking, 3D QSAR and designing of new quinazolinone analogues as DHFR inhibitors. Korean Chem. Soc. 2011, 32(7), 2433.

45. Xiang Maa, Guangya Xiang, Chun-Wei Yap, Wai-Keung Chui. 3D-QSAR study on dihydro-1, 3, 5-triazines and their Spiro derivatives as DHFR inhibitors by comparative molecular field analysis (CoMFA). Bioorg. Med. Chem. Lett. 2012, 22, 3194–3197.

46. Dhanaji, S.; Gonda, Rohan J.; Meshrama, Sharad G.; Jadhava, Gulshan.;Wadhwab, Rajesh N.; Gacchea. Insilico screening of chalcone derivatives as potential inhibitors of dihydrofolatereductase: assessment using molecular docking paired potential and molecular hydrophobic potential studies.

47. Fatmah A; M. Al; Omary, Ghada S; Hassan, Shahenda; M, El;Messery, Mahmoud; N, Nagi, El;Sayed, E; Habib, Hussein; I, El;Subbagh. Nonclassical antifolates, synthesis, biological evaluation and molecular modeling study of some new 2-heteroarylthio-quinazolin- 4-ones. Eur. J. Med. Chem. 63, 2013, 33–45.

48. Kulkarni, R.; S. Konda; A. Garlapati. Design of nonclassical DHFR inhibitors by CoMFA and CoMSIA 3D QSAR studies RGUHS. J. Pharm. Sci. 2013.

INDEX

Milton Keynes UK
Ingram Content Group UK Ltd.
UKHW031138141024
449569UK00024B/1232